A TEXTBOOK OF ECONOMICS

BY THE SAME AUTHOR:

A DICTIONARY OF ECONOMICS AND COMMERCE
AN INTRODUCTION TO APPLIED ECONOMICS
ECONOMICS FOR STUDENTS
MONETARY THEORY AND PRACTICE
AN OUTLINE OF MONETARY THEORY
ECONOMIC ASPECTS OF INDUSTRY AND COMMERCE
THE STRUCTURE OF MODERN COMMERCE
THE WORLD OF INDUSTRY AND COMMERCE
LIFE AND WORK (with illustrations by T. D. Kilburn)

A TEXTBOOK OF ECONOMICS

by

J. L. HANSON

M.A., M.Ed. (Leeds), Ph.D., B.Sc.(Econ.) (London)

Formerly Senior Lecturer in Economics
Huddersfield College of Technology

FOURTH EDITION

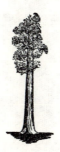

MACDONALD & EVANS, LTD.

8 John Street, London, W.C.1

1966

First published 1953
Reprinted 1954
Second edition June 1956
Reprinted May 1957
Reprinted August 1958
Reprinted July 1959
Reprinted August 1960
Third edition August 1961
Reprinted June 1962
Reprinted January 1963
Reprinted August 1963
Reprinted August 1964
Reprinted August 1965
Fourth edition May 1966
Reprinted August 1967
Reprinted May 1968
Reprinted May 1969

MACDONALD AND EVANS LTD.

1961; 1966

Library edition: S.B.N. 7121 2004 1
Paperback edition: S.B.N. 7121 2008 4

Printed in Great Britain by Richard Clay (The Chaucer Press), Ltd.,
Bungay, Suffolk

PREFACE TO THE FIRST EDITION

THE tendency of professional economists at the present day—as of scientists in other fields—is to specialise in particular aspects of their subject. Students in Technical and University Colleges, however, must cover the whole subject, and if a textbook writer is to be of service to them, he must endeavour to satisfy their wide, non-specialist needs.

The present work attempts to provide a systematic course which will meet the requirements, at all levels, of the numerous professional bodies which set papers in economics, and also the needs, short of what is necessary for the final examinations, of students studying for university degrees. No university student reading for a final degree in economics, or indeed in any subject, would expect to find all his work treated within the covers of a single volume. Nevertheless, it is hoped that even they may find a textbook which ranges over the whole field of service to them by providing a foundation on which wider study can be based. The detailed recommendations for further reading at the end of each chapter will be helpful in this respect, and should be regarded as an integral part of the course.

Appended to each chapter is a representative selection of questions on its subject matter, taken by permission from recent examination papers. These will serve both as tests of the student's mastery of the chapter and as an indication of the type of question he is likely to meet with in the examination room. It would be well if all students attempted at least some of them.

It may be said, generally, that the main purpose in studying economics is to acquire knowledge of the techniques of economic analysis, and the ability to apply that knowledge to the solution of economic problems. In the words of the late Lord Keynes, economics "is a method rather than a doctrine, an apparatus of the mind, a technique of thinking which helps its possessor to draw correct conclusions." Nevertheless, the present volume is not restricted to economic theory; it discusses also some of the outstanding problems of applied economics in relation to the theory upon which their solution depends. It cannot be forgotten that economics is a social science dealing with a particular aspect of human existence: if theory is completely divorced from reality we are left only with the dry bones of the subject. Certainly, the student must learn to use the tools of economic analysis, but he can do so only if he has factual material upon which to work. For this reason descriptions of economic institutions have been included, and more attention than is usual in a general textbook has been given to consideration of such matters as the population problem, the location of industry, the capital market, transport, nationalised industries and public finance.

PREFACE TO THE FOURTH EDITION

For its fourth edition this book has been thoroughly revised to take account of the many economic developments that have taken place since the publication of the previous edition. This has involved the complete rewriting of some sections of the work. The statistics have been brought up to date, and many improvements have been made in the text.

Once again I take the opportunity to thank the many correspondents, both teachers and students, who have written to me since the book was first published. More particularly, I wish to thank my former colleague at the Huddersfield College of Technology, Dr H. Robinson, B.A., M.Ed., Ph.D., Principal Lecturer in charge of Geography, who has given me useful advice on the chapter dealing with the population problem. I also wish to thank Mr P. Haigh, B.A., Senior Lecturer in Applied Economics at the North Staffordshire College of Technology and Mr R. G. D. Evans, B.A.(Com.), A.Inst.M.S.M., Lecturer in Marketing at the Derby and District College of Technology, for their many helpful suggestions. My thanks are also again due to Mr A. Taylor, B.A.(Admin.). B.Sc.(Econ), A.C.I.S., Principal Lecturer in Business Studies at the Huddersfield College of Education (Technical), for his assistance with the chapters dealing with the nationalised industries and the co-operative movement.

Grateful acknowledgment is made to the Controller of Her Majesty's Stationery Office for allowing the use of copyright material taken from White Papers and other Government publications, and also to the Senate of the University of London, and to the Councils of the various professional bodies, listed on pp. xxvii and xxviii for permission to reproduce questions from examination papers set by them.

1966.   J.L.H.

CONTENTS

PART FOUR. THE TOOLS OF ECONOMIC ANALYSIS
(continued)

(ii) The Concept of the Margin

CHAPTER XII

THE BASIS OF DEMAND 199

CHAPTER XIII

THE BASIS OF SUPPLY: (1) UNDER PERFECT
COMPETITION 218

CHAPTER XIX

INTEREST AND PROFIT 325

PART SIX. BANKING AND FINANCE

CHAPTER XX

THE ORIGIN AND FUNCTIONS OF MONEY . . 345

CHAPTER XXIV

THE ENGLISH BANKING SYSTEM: THE BANK OF ENGLAND

CHAPTER XXV

THE CAPITAL MARKET

LIST OF ILLUSTRATIONS

LIST OF TABLES

EXAMINATION QUESTIONS

The following abbreviations are employed to indicate the sources of the examination questions:

R.S.A. Inter. R.S.A. Adv.	Intermediate and Advanced Examinations in Economics of the Royal Society of Arts.
R.S.A. Adv. Com.	Advanced Examination in Commerce of the Royal Society of Arts.
L.C. Com. Econ. L.C. Com. B. & C. L.C. Com. C. & F.	Examinations in Economics, Banking and Currency, and Commerce and Finance of the London Chambers of Commerce.
I.T.	Institute of Transport Graduateship Examination.
Exp.	Examination of the Institute of Export.
B.S. Inter. B.S. Final	Examinations of the Building Societies Institute.
C.I.S. Inter. C.I.S. Final	Examinations of the Chartered Institute of Secretaries
C.C.S. Inter. C.C.S. Final	Examinations of the Corporation of Certified Secretaries
S.I.A.A.	Examination of the Society of Incorporated Accountants and Auditors.
A.I.A.	Intermediate Examination of the Association of International Accountants
A.C.C.A. Inter. A.C.C.A. Final	Examinations of the Association of Certified and Corporate Accountants

I.M.T.A.   Examinations of the Institute of Municipal Treasurers and Accountants

I.B.   Examination in Economics of the Institute of Bankers.

I.H.A.   Intermediate Examination of the Institute of Hospital Administrators

L.G.B.   Intermediate Examination (Administrative Grade) of the Local Government Examinations Board.

University of London Examinations:

D.P.A.   Diploma in Public Administration

G.C.E. Adv.   General Certificate in Education (Advanced Level).

Final Degree   Final B.Sc.(Econ.)

PART ONE

INTRODUCTORY

CHAPTER I

SOME PRELIMINARY IDEAS

I. THE SCOPE OF ECONOMICS

(1) THE SUBJECT-MATTER OF ECONOMICS

Most books on economics open with a discussion of the difficulties of giving in a concise form an adequate definition of the subject. The inadequacy of concise definition is, however, not peculiar to economics, as a glance at the definitions of physics, philosophy, geology and other subjects of study given in any good dictionary will quickly confirm. On account of these difficulties there seem to be almost as many definitions of the subject as there are economists, for few writers on economics appear to be satisfied with the definitions of their predecessors, and almost invariably seem to find it necessary to frame new ones of their own.

Though it may be difficult to agree upon a satisfactory, concise definition of economics, its subject-matter is generally beyond dispute. Almost any business transaction involves the many branches of the subject, for under modern economic conditions most people earn their living by specialising in comparatively narrow fields of activity. A solicitor, for example, spends his time giving legal advice in return for money payments, and because other people have been specialising in the production of food and clothing he is able to obtain these things in exchange for some of the money received from his clients. Specialisation, however, makes the business of production and exchange more complex. If people specialise in different kinds of work it becomes necessary for them to exchange goods and services with one another. The solicitor, for example, prefers to be paid for his services in money because money is a medium of exchange, and the use of money facilitates exchange.

Only a miser desires money for its own sake, and there are probably few misers nowadays—perhaps because paper money is less attractive than bright gold coins. Payment in money is preferred merely because money can be exchanged for food, clothing and many other things, or, if one so wished, deposited in a bank and its spending deferred until a later date. The money the solicitor spends enables him to obtain goods produced in all parts of the world. The fact that he has paid

3

money for these things, however, hides what has really taken place—namely, that he has exchanged his own services for these various commodities. Economists used to refer to this as the "money veil."

Suppose, for example, a man visits his tailor for the purpose of buying a new suit. This simple transaction involves almost the entire complex economic system. He is probably shown bunches of patterns, and, in itself, the very act of choosing involves an economic decision, for choice, as will be shown shortly, is fundamental to economics. Maybe he selects a worsted cloth, woven in the West Riding of Yorkshire. Consider, then, the long chain of events that took place before the cloth reached the tailor's shop: there was the Australian sheep-farmer who sold the wool to a merchant, who arranged for its sale at the wool auctions in Melbourne or London; there was the transport of the wool from Australia to the West Riding, numerous merchants again being involved; then there were the firms that handled the commodity after it had reached Yorkshire—the scourer, the wool-comber, the spinner, the weaver, each employing many people doing different kinds of work; finally there was the merchant who sold the cloth to the retailer.

This by no means exhausts the list of people who in one way or another have had a share in the production of this piece of worsted cloth. Next it might be asked: how were all the various stages of production financed? The banks probably assisted the Australian sheep-farmer, the different manufacturers and possibly the merchants, too; while the risks of loss or damage to the materials in stock or in transit were covered by insurance companies, the transport itself being provided by railways, steamship companies and perhaps airlines. The risks of production were borne by the shareholders in the case of companies, or by the traders themselves if they were working on their own account. The power to drive the machinery in the mills may have been supplied by coal hewn from the earth by the miners of the South Yorkshire coalfield, or electricity, or maybe oil brought four thousand miles across the sea served this purpose. The manufacture of spinning-frames, looms and other machinery may have employed workers in the iron mines of Sweden or Cleveland, and steel-workers in many parts of Great Britain.

If the story be continued to cover the making of the suit it will be necessary to include the people engaged in the Lancashire cotton industry, who made the linings from cotton grown in the United States of America; the workers at Paisley who spun and reeled the thread with which it was sewn together; the button-makers of Birmingham, and many others. One need not stop even here, for while all these people were going about their own individual tasks they had to be fed by the efforts of others who were employed on food production.

Every one of the people mentioned is engaged on some kind of economic activity that is of interest to the economist. He is not interested, however—at least, not in his professional capacity—in the technical aspect of production: how to work this or that machine, how to judge the quality of the wool, or things of that kind. These are problems for the technician. The economist is, however, interested in such questions as: Was the production at various stages of manufacture on a large or small scale? Was one firm responsible for several processes or only for a single process? Was the work done by hand or by machine? The economist then endeavours to discover why one form of production was preferred to another, and what determined the size of the various firms; how much of the different commodities was produced; and why more of one was made than of another. He also wants to know how the different stages of production were financed, and if the banks were responsible for this, how they obtained the money for the purpose. Pursuing his inquiries further, he asks how the prices of the different raw materials and the final finished products were determined; what wages were paid to the different workers, and why some workers received more than others, and how the imports of wool, cotton, iron, etc., were paid for. All these are economic problems. It also falls within the province of economics to describe the working of the basic economic institutions, such as the banking system, and the money and capital markets.

(2) SOME DEFINITIONS OF ECONOMICS

Keeping in mind the sort of questions with which economics attempts to deal, it will be of interest to note some definitions of the subject put forward by different economists.

The earliest definitions were in terms of wealth, by which was meant not only gold and silver but also all kinds of other goods— houses and public buildings, furniture, works of art and other private possessions, as well as ships, workshops, tools and the machines in use at the time for the production of goods. Adam Smith, for example, considered his work to be "an inquiry into the nature and causes of the wealth of nations," while J. S. Mill looked on economics as "the practical science of the production and distribution of wealth"—the definition adopted by the *Concise Oxford Dictionary*. Adam Smith, then, was concerned with the broader aspects of wealth, the means by which the total volume of production could be increased—an important aim of economic policy today. J. S. Mill's definition went a stage further

B

and included problems of both distribution and production, thus covering the two main influences on the standard of living. The greater part of economics, however, is now given up to a study of problems of exchange, and Davenport emphasised this aspect of the subject when he declared economics to be "the science that treats phenomena from the standpoint of price."[1] Important as is the price mechanism, this definition gives little indication of the subject-matter of economics. A. C. Pigou defined economics in terms of welfare, thereby stressing the human as well as the material aspect of the subject,[2] regarding economics as a means of studying how total production could be increased so that the standard of living of a people might be improved. Alfred Marshall's definition appears to form a link between those centred on wealth and those that stress welfare and the standard of living. First he declares somewhat vaguely that economics is "a study of mankind in the ordinary business of life," but then goes on to amplify this statement by saying that economics "examines that part of individual and social action connected with the attainment of the material requisites of well-being," so that the subject becomes "on the one side, a study of wealth; on the more important, a part of the study of man." [3] Like Pigou later, he regarded the accumulation of wealth only as a means towards raising a people's standard of living. Modern economics, however, is based on a theory of *scarcity* and *choice*, and this approach to the subject makes possible the framing of a definition in yet another form. Before this definition can be given, however, it is necessary to find out exactly what the economist means by the two terms, scarcity and choice.

II. SCARCITY AND CHOICE

(3) SCARCITY

To the economist all things are said to be scarce, since by "scarce" he means simply "limited in supply." In ordinary speech, however, the word "scarce" has a more restricted meaning. In the past there was always a danger of a "scarcity" of food as a result of bad harvests. To countries like Great Britain this danger may now seem very remote, but it is still present even today to people in many parts of the world. Nowadays the shops of this country are generally well stocked with all kinds of goods, and there seem to be ample supplies of everything for everybody—for everybody, that is, who has the money with which to

[1] H. J. Davenport: *Economics of Enterprise*, Chapter 2.
[2] A. C. Pigou: *Economics of Welfare*, Part I, Chapters 1 and 2.
[3] A. Marshall: *Principles of Economics*, Book I, Chapter 1.

buy them. However, it is just in conditions such as these that economists say that all goods are scarce. What is meant is that all goods are scarce relative to people's desire for them. Most people would probably like to have more or better things than they possess at present: larger houses, perhaps, in which to live, better furnished with the latest labour-saving devices, such as electric washers, cookers, refrigerators; more visits to the theatre or the concert-hall; more travel, the latest models in motor cars, radio and television sets; and most women exhibit an apparently insatiable desire for more clothes.

People's wants are many, but the resources for making all the things they want—labour, raw materials, factory buildings, machinery—are themselves limited in supply. There are not sufficient productive resources in the world to produce so much of everything to make it possible, therefore, to satisfy the wants of everybody. Consequently, to the economist all things are at all times said to be "scarce," even though improvements in methods of production—that is, in using resources more economically—may appear to make them less scarce.

(4) SCARCITY IS RELATIVE

It is frequently asserted today that we are living in an age of plenty, larger quantities than ever before of all kinds of goods being produced each week. Can this statement be reconciled with a theory of scarcity? Indeed, it can, since by scarcity we mean merely a limited supply relative to demand.

Although the output of all kinds of things has increased enormously during the past fifty years, goods are still scarce relative to the demand for them. It is extremely unlikely that we shall ever be able to produce unlimited quantities of anything, however rapid our rate of economic progress, and so it seems goods will always remain scarce in the sense in which economists use the term, namely, limited in supply.

(5) ECONOMICS AS A STUDY OF THE DISPOSAL OF SCARCE GOODS

Since wants are many and the means for satisfying them are limited, a way has to be found of distributing these scarce goods among those who want them, and the problems associated with this distribution form the subject-matter of economics. In fact, economics has been defined as "the science which studies human behaviour as a relationship between ends and scarce means which have alternative uses."[1] Thus economics justifies its name by becoming a study of a particular kind of

---

[1] L. Robbins: *Nature and Significance of Economic Science*, p. 16.

economising—the economising of resources and their apportionment among all the industries competing for their use. The advantage of this definition is that it covers all kinds of economic activity, in the home as well as in the outside world. Unfortunately, such a definition gives little indication of the scope or subject-matter of economics. It is, in fact, a definition of economics for economists.

(6) CHOICE

If, then, all things are scarce relative to the *desire* for them, and if people have many unsatisfied wants and the means exist for satisfying only some of them, obviously they cannot satisfy all of them, and therefore they must make a choice. In order to be able to enjoy some things it is necessary to do without others. If every human action was perfectly rational everyone would naturally satisfy his more pressing wants first, choosing the things he desired most, and going without those he considered less desirable. By and large, this may be so, though there are few people who have not at some time or other given way to impulse, and made a purchase they have afterwards regretted. Strictly, the economist is not concerned—that is, not concerned as an economist, though he may be vitally interested for other reasons—with the merits or demerits of the choice. The drunkard prefers to go without all sorts of things in order to satisfy his craving for drink; the scholar may stint himself of food so that he may have more books; the traveller may deprive himself of a home in order to allow full play to his urge to see the world. All these people are making choices, enjoying one thing at the expense of another, but whether they are making good or bad choices is a matter not for economics, but for ethics.

A few moments' thought are sufficient to reveal how fundamental to economic problems is this question of choice. How frequently one hears the complaint that a person has not the time to do this or that. It will generally be found, however, that this is merely an excuse for his not doing something that he dislikes, and what he really means is that he prefers to do something else. "I can't find the time to attend a course of lectures on economics," says the young man who spends most evenings at a youth club, and the rest at a dance-hall or viewing television. Time is "scarce," and therefore one has to choose between competing ways of spending it. Most people have little control over the amount of time required of them by their employers, but many others can choose between working overtime or not: if they choose to work overtime they forgo so much leisure. A man may be able to choose between a well-paid, but uncongenial occupation, and a more congenial one at a lower salary.

The greatest amount of choice occurs, however, in the expenditure of one's income. First, one has to decide how much to spend and how much to save, and then how much to spend on such things as rent, food, clothing, holidays, etc. People often say they cannot afford to buy something when they really mean they prefer to spend their money on something else. A man says he cannot afford to go abroad for holidays, but he may run an expensive car, and be a member of an exclusive golf club. Another wishes he could afford to run a car, but spends heavily on drink, tobacco and visits to the theatre. Business men, too, are constantly being confronted with choices. They have to decide what method of production to adopt, whether to employ more or less labour, less or more capital. Cigarettes and motor cars are scarce to consumers, because the available productive resources of land, labour and capital are also scarce to the entrepreneurs—that is, to those responsible for deciding what shall be produced.

Choice in a free economy. Whatever be the method by which choice is decided, choice between alternatives is the fundamental principle underlying all economic activity. In a free economy consumers have a free choice as to what they buy, limited only by the amount of money they have to spend. The relative strength of consumers' demands for various commodities determines the amount of each that entrepreneurs will try to produce. Thus, for example, a big demand for furniture will lead to an expansion of the manufacture of furniture, the industry attracting to itself the required amount of labour and other resources. Industries producing commodities for which there is a small demand will require less productive resources. In this way scarce or limited resources, which have alternative uses, are distributed among the various producers.

Choice in a planned economy. By a planned economy is meant one where the State decides what shall be produced. In such an economy some choice is taken away from consumers. How much choice they retain will depend on the extent of the planning. In a completely planned economy the State will accept entire responsibility for making all the choices—deciding what shall be produced, how much shall be produced and allocating productive resources among the various producers in accordance with these decisions. How much of each commodity is each consumer permitted to enjoy may also be decided by the State, and some scheme of rationing will then be required for the distribution of the limited quantities of goods so produced. In a free economy the consumer himself makes the choice; in the planned economy the choice rests with the State, acting through its planning committee. Nevertheless, whatever form the economic system may take, the fact that all goods and services are scarce relative to the demand for them makes choice necessary.

(7) OPPORTUNITY-COST

It is possible now to answer an important question. What is the real cost of a good? It has just been seen that an individual cannot satisfy all his wants, but must choose between one thing and another. The satisfaction of one want involves going without something else. The real cost of satisfying any want is the alternative that has to be forgone in order to do so. If a man is confronted by a choice between living in a larger house and running a motor car, the real cost of running the motor car, if he chooses that alternative, would be the larger house he has had to do without. The real cost of his books to the poor scholar is the food he has to forgo in order to buy them. In the expenditure of time, this idea of real cost is even more readily understood. If a student misses one of his lectures on economics because he wants to see a particular football match, the cost of this to him is the lecture on economics that he has missed. The real cost of anything in the sense of the alternative that has to be forgone, is known as it "opportunity-cost."

(8) SCALES OF PREFERENCE

In economics it is assumed that when an individual is faced by a particular situation he will always act rationally. Thus, if he has to make a choice between one thing and another, he will always choose the alternative that will yield him the greater satisfaction. This implies too that each individual has a scale of preferences, a sort of list of all his unsatisfied wants arranged in order of preference. Near the top of his scale will be what he regards as his most pressing wants, and he will satisfy these before he pays any attention to wants near the bottom of his scale. Faced, then, with the alternative of satisfying either want No. 2 or want No. 5, he would therefore satisfy No. 2. Few people have such a definite scale of unsatisfied wants, though many may be able to distinguish between their most pressing and their least pressing wants; but for the purpose of economic theory it is necessary to make the assumption that people behave rationally, and it is therefore assumed that each person has his or her own scale of preference, on which his wants are arranged in the order of relative importance. The ethical or moral aspect of the order of preference is not the direct concern of economics. On one person's scale alcoholic drink may occupy a high place, while good food may be quite low; another person may place a "thriller" before a volume of Shakespeare's plays; other people may think both these preferences ill-chosen. Economically, however, the wisdom of the choice is not important.

III. THE SOCIAL SCIENCES

(9) ECONOMICS AS A SOCIAL SCIENCE

The social sciences concern themselves with the study of different aspects of human behaviour, whereas the province of the physical sciences is the study of various aspects of Man's environment, while the concern of the natural sciences may be said to lie with the physical side of animal (including human) life. The early philosophers such as Plato and Aristotle allowed their thoughts to roam over any aspect of the universe that aroused their curiosity. All subjects of study were to them merely different aspects of one great comprehensive subject—philosophy. Increasing knowledge, however, made the study of Man and his environment too vast for a single subject, and in course of time it has split up into an increasing number of separate sciences. The physical and natural sciences were the first to become independent disciplines, but until quite recent times philosophy still embraced all the social sciences. Writers recognised no clear line of demarcation between ethics, politics, economics, etc., and questions concerning one or all of them were indiscriminately discussed.

One by one, however, the social sciences have broken away from philosophy. By dividing up knowledge into ever smaller compartments, the number of subjects has increased, so that the variety of studies offered to students by modern universities forms a formidable list, many of these subjects being unknown not so many years ago.

(10) ECONOMICS, ETHICS, THEOLOGY AND POLITICS

Economic questions were touched upon by the Greek philosophers Plato and Aristotle, but only when incidental to ethical or political problems; for example, it was on ethical grounds that Plato objected to the payment of interest on borrowed money. Similarly, Aristotle for ethical reasons condemned exchange when money was employed instead of barter. Medieval philosophers inherited the Greek and Roman objection to usury, but in their case economics was regarded as subsidiary to theology, the influence of Christian teaching leading to the throwing over of Aristotle's defence of slavery, and the proclaiming instead of the dignity of labour. Though it was taught that all men were equal before God, inequality of station was accepted, as present existence was regarded as merely preparatory for the after-life. When Plato propounded his theory of communism it was because he thought this to be a prerequisite of the good life, and it was for similar reasons that Aristotle favoured private property, the medieval thinkers accepting the Aristotelian argument. The question of value was approached also from the point of view of ethics, and discussion centred round the idea of a "just price."

The Renaissance, the progress of science and the discovery of the New World brought the Middle Ages to an end, to be followed by the Age of Mercantilism, the growth of nationalism and a great expansion of trade. A secular outlook replaced the "other-worldliness" of the medieval period, and economics became the handmaid of politics to point the way towards the creation of strong, prosperous, national states. Increased supplies of silver, following the discovery of new sources of supply in the New World, led to a greater use of money, and made taxation administratively easier, while the accumulation of wealth, previously frowned upon, acquired a degree of respectability. Gold and silver were regarded as *real* wealth, and it was thought that a country's wealth was increased if in its trade with the rest of the world it could achieve an excess of exports over imports, the excess being paid for in gold or silver. The State intervened to regulate trade and industry in order to promote the prosperity of the nation, and so economic matters became political questions.

(ii) ECONOMICS AS AN INDEPENDENT SUBJECT OF STUDY

It remained for the Industrial Revolution completely to free economics from the other social sciences. In the simple economies of the Ancient World economics was a branch of ethics or politics; in the economy of the Middle Ages it had been an adjunct of theology; in the Age of Mercantilism it became a tool of politics of the nation-State. The Industrial Revolution resulted in a vast increase in production and increasing specialisation, with its corollary of increased exchange, so that the economic system became ever more complex. Economics shook itself free from ethics, theology and politics. The development of the doctrine of *laissez-faire*, which favoured a policy of non-interference by the State, assisted its emancipation.

Adam Smith can be considered as the first writer to produce a work devoted purely to economics. Though published in 1776, before the Industrial Revolution had got fully under way, his *Wealth of Nations* is a landmark in the development of economics as an independent subject of study. Since that time the number of writers on economics has gradually increased, until now there is a flood of new work published each year. In fact, economics has now expanded to such an extent that economists themselves have begun to specialise in small branches of the subject—Value, Labour, Money, Banking, Foreign Trade, Taxation, etc.

(12) THE BARRIERS BETWEEN ECONOMICS AND OTHER SOCIAL SCIENCES AGAIN BREAKING DOWN

There is, however, at the present time a tendency to break down the barriers that had been built up between economics and the other social sciences—ethics, theology, politics, sociology and psychology. Not so long ago it used to be emphatically stressed that ethical or political aspects of economic problems were not the concern of the economist. Some modern economists still hold this view, but others are not so sure.

A practical problem may be considered purely from the economic point of view, but if the economist looks upon its solution simply as an intellectual exercise it is likely to bring the study of economics into disrepute. It is well for the inquirer to isolate economic considerations to secure clarity of thinking; but, having done so, it is important then to discover whether his solution conflicts with the findings of workers in other fields. Economic questions are often inextricably entangled with ethical or political implications. As soon as one asks the question, "Is it right that a Member of Parliament should receive an annual salary even though he never makes a speech?" the questioner has crossed the boundary between economics and ethics. Then the reaction from the *laissez-faire* of the nineteenth century has led the State to take an increasing interest in economic matters. Acceptance of responsibility for full employment has given the State a greater interest in economic affairs than ever before. The greater the extent of State planning, the greater is the intermingling of economics and politics. Since economics is a study of a certain aspect of human behaviour, it cannot help touching too upon psychology, itself a study of behaviour.

Thus economics, once merely incidental to philosophy, has become a separate social study, but, since all such study relates to Man and his environment, it cannot be rigidly marked off from the other social sciences.

IV. PURPOSE AND METHOD

(13) THE PURPOSE AND METHOD OF ECONOMICS

Indeed, many people come to economics to seek a solution of current problems, and feel a strong sense of disappointment when they realise the limitations of the subject. The economist cannot offer any final solution to the practical problems of everyday experience, though he may often be able to give advice or point out the economic advantages or disadvantages of a particular policy. A trained economist is, moreover, better equipped than others to understand these problems. This, however, is the sphere of applied economics, and before this branch of the subject is tackled the student of economics must know something of economic theory.

(14) ECONOMIC THEORY

There are really three branches of economics: (i) descriptive economics, which is concerned, as the name implies, with describing the working of economic institutions; (ii) economic theory or principles of economics; and (iii) applied economics, where theory is used to assist the study of actual economic problems.

Economic theory, or pure economics, consists of a body of principles, logically built up. It provides the tools of economic analysis, but it is pursued without any thought as to whether it is likely to yield practical results or not. Theory is developed, and reasoning is carried to its logical conclusion, irrespective of where this may lead. In this it is similar to other sciences, where the research worker pursues his investigations with the sole object of increasing the total of human knowledge. If there should prove to be some practical application of the theory that is something for others to develop. If, therefore, the new knowledge is misused the scientific worker engaged on fundamental research feels that he can disclaim all responsibility. Be that as it may, it would probably be beneficial to the world at large if some of the barriers between the theoretical sciences and the applied sciences were completely removed.

In the case of economics the misuse of pure theory is less likely to be attended by such disastrous results as, for example, the misuse of pure physics. In pure economics it is necessary to make so many assumptions that sometimes theory seems to bear only a slight relation to fact. It is assumed, for example, that men in their economic activities always behave quite rationally, whereas most people to some degree are creatures of habit or impulse. If two exactly similar commodities were offered for sale by different shops, the price at the first shop being 6d. and at the second $5\frac{1}{2}d$., a perfectly rational economic action would be for everybody to buy at the cheaper shop, whereas to most people it would be too much trouble to seek out the cheapest shop every time a purchase had to be made. Economics should not be condemned as "unrealistic" just because such unreal assumptions are made, for without making such assumptions it would not be possible to build up a body of economic principles at all, and a scientific approach to economic problems would be impossible. Nevertheless, there are times when one wonders whether some economists have not allowed themselves to be carried away by their enthusiasm for pure theory.

(15) ECONOMICS A SCIENCE

Frequent reference has been made above to economics as a social science. Does economics deserve the appellation science? Subjects such as physics, chemistry, botany, etc., are easily recognised as sciences, and though the Latin word *scientia* merely means knowledge, the modern term "science" has taken on a more restricted connotation. Characteristics of a science are the observation of certain facts, the selection and classification of relevant material, and the using of these as a basis for generalisation. It then becomes possible to formulate laws which are universally true under specified conditions, and which can be applied to the analysis of new situations. In this sense, economics can be considered to be a science, its fundamental facts being observations from everyday life. It is sometimes said to be a positive science because it considers things as they are, and not as they ought to be. As in other sciences, certain assumptions are made—though in the practical sciences these may be more realistic—and then, starting from a given hypothesis—some accepted fact of everyday experience—logical deductions follow. The most common assumption in economics is: other things being equal. The traditional method of pure economics has, therefore, been deductive, theories being deduced by logical reasoning. From these deductions economic laws are formulated which, as with other scientific laws, merely assert what takes place when certain conditions are fulfilled. Algebraic and geometrical methods developed from this because they show relationships, as for example, between demand and price, without actual quantities being required.

As an alternative to the *deductive* method, some economic problems are approached on *inductive* lines—that is, a mass of data is obtained from actual experience, and then used as a basis for generalisations. In the United States the inductive method has been used to check deductions of economic theory; for example, the effect of changes in wages on labour-saving inventions and on the employment of labour. In Great Britain the inductive method has been employed to discover business men's reactions to changes in the rate of interest and to obtain information on family expenditure as a basis for the index of retail prices. Economic statistics are compiled to supply economists with their raw material. Economics for a long time lacked accurate material, but each year now a vast amount of statistics is published on a wide range of economic subjects.

Compared with the practical sciences, economics is at a disadvantage, for the data obtained by a chemist from a succession of experiments are more precise than that acquired from the behaviour of human beings by the research worker in the field of economics. The deductive and the inductive methods, however, are appropriate to their own fields. The method of study in economics is, therefore, scientific, and there is no fundamental difference between it and other sciences.

(16) WHY STUDY ECONOMICS?

A student embarking upon a set course of study generally asks for a reason for his having to take a certain subject only if it is a subject that he finds distasteful. Few ask to know the use of physical training and games; many put the question, for example, in the case of history. The question seems unnecessary as regards applied economics, for it appears to be "useful" to understand economic problems, but economic theory may seem to many to be a "useless" subject. It would be a sufficient defence for the study of pure theory to assert that all knowledge is useful for its own sake, and so there is no need for a subject to have practical application for it to be useful. It is said that certain mathematicians used to toast pure mathematics with the words "May it never be of any use to anyone!"

If pure mathematics was merely an intellectual exercise it would still have its adherents, but it would hardly deserve the high place it now occupies as a subject of serious study. To allow theory to run riot, to the exclusion of all consideration of pressing economic problems such as confront the world today, would be sheer academic folly. It is the aim of pure economics to build up a body of principles, and to furnish the economist with tools of economic analysis that will enable him not only to understand current economic problems but also to see the economic consequences of pursuing a particular line of policy. Defects are to be found in any economic system or policy, and the economist should be able to say whether proposed changes are *likely* to be economically advantageous or not. Unfortunately, he cannot always say so with certainty, since the economic is only one of many aspects of actual problems; hence economists often disagree on such questions.

Against undue concentration on pure theory it may be argued that economists, of all people, should be imbued with a desire to increase the well-being of the community. Prof. Pigou believed that economics was worthy of study because it made it easier to institute practical measures to promote welfare—so that "statesmen may build upon the work of the economist." For, he says, "it is not in the ordinary business of life that man is most interesting, or inspiring." He concludes therefore that the study of economics is not worth while for its own sake but only "for the healing that knowledge may help to bring."[1]

As Sir Henry Clay has said, "Some study of economics is at once a practical necessity and a moral obligation,"[2] for economic questions touch the daily lives of all of us.

RECOMMENDATIONS FOR FURTHER READING

A. Marshall: *Principles of Economics*, Book I, Chapters 1–3.
A. C. Pigou: *Economics of Welfare*, Part I, Chapter 1.
L. C. Robbins: *The Nature and Significance of Economic Science*.
F. H. Knight: *Risk, Uncertainty and Profit*, Chapter 3.

QUESTIONS

1. Consider the subject-matter of economics by reference to any three definitions of the study. (R.S.A. Inter.)

2. "The problem of definition involves special difficulties to the economist." Discuss this statement. (R.S.A. Inter.)

3. What is meant by the statement that economics is a social science? (I.T.)

4. State carefully the scope of economic study. (I.T.)

5. Give a definition of economics and give an explanation justifying your definition. (Exp.)

6. For what purposes do we study economics? Of what value is the study of economics to a secretary? (C.I.S. Inter.)

7. Discuss the statement that modern economics is based upon a theory of scarcity and choice. (A.I.A.)

8. What are (a) the aims, (b) the advantages of a study of Economics? (C.C.S. Inter.)

9. Write a short essay on: "Economic laws." (I.M.T.A.)

10. Economics has been defined as (a) the Science of Wealth, (b) the Science of Scarcity. Discuss these definitions. (C.C.S. Final)

11. Economics has been described as the science that concerns itself, on the one hand, with *scarce means* and, on the other, with *wealth*. Do you consider this to be an adequate description? In your answer carefully analyse the use of the two terms, *scarce means* and *wealth*, in this context. (I.H.A.)

12. Give a definition of economics. Why do economists sometimes disagree with each other on matters of interpretation? (I.B.)

13. "Everything that occurs in economic life takes place in accordance with some law: it is the function of the economist to ascertain that law." Comment. (D.P.A.)

14. "The assumption of rational behaviour in modern economic theory is but a variant of the classical notion of economic man." Discuss. (Final Degree.)

[1] A. C. Pigou: *Economics of Welfare*, p. 10.
[2] H. Clay: *Economics for the General Reader*, p. 6.

PART TWO

PRODUCTION

CHAPTER II

PRODUCTION

I. THE PURPOSE OF PRODUCTION

(1) THE SATISFACTION OF WANTS

The aim of all production is to satisfy people's wants. When each family had to satisfy its wants by its own efforts the extent and strength of its wants decided the activities of the group. Man's earliest wants were for food, clothing and shelter, and in early days it might take all his time and energy to provide himself with even a bare minimum of these things. With the development of civilisation people's wants multiplied, but few people nowadays satisfy their wants directly. The use of money makes it possible for them to work for a money payment, and afterwards to use the money to buy the things they desire which other people have made. Under present conditions of economic organisation a vast range of goods is produced and new commodities are constantly being introduced. People engaged in production, then, in order to earn the means by which they will be able to satisfy their own wants, and at the same time they are helping to satisfy the wants of other people. The same people are thus at the same time both producers and consumers, and so production can be regarded either from the point of view of the effort involved or from the point of view of the satisfaction of wants.

(2) THE MEANING OF PRODUCTION

In everyday speech the word *production* is often used as if it were synonymous with *creating* something. A moment's thought will be sufficient to realise that the making or manufacture of some commodity —for example, a motor car—means no more than putting together quantities of many different kinds of materials. Even processes involving chemical action merely change the form of substances, and do not actually create anything. The economist, however, does not restrict production to the manufacture of commodities; he also takes the expression to include the provision of services, such as those of the lawyer, the accountant, the actor or musician, etc. Since all these people aim at satisfying other people's wants just as much as those working in a motor-car factory, their work can also be considered to be productive.

Similarly, the work of distribution—wholesale and retail trade, transport, etc.—can justifiably be considered to be part of the productive process, for production is not complete until the commodity that has been manufactured has actually reached the person who desires it.

As will be seen shortly, a larger total output is achieved when people specialise, but this makes exchange necessary, and so the extra cost of distribution must be set against the gain from specialisation. Production therefore means changing either the form of something or its situation in space or time, or the provision of a service of some kind.

(3) THE VOLUME OF PRODUCTION AND ECONOMIC WELFARE

The purpose of production therefore is to increase the economic welfare of a people, that is, to raise their standard of living by enabling them to satisfy more fully a greater number of their wants. Economic welfare clearly depends in the first place on the volume of production, and consequently to expand the volume of production will generally increase economic welfare, and make possible a rise in the standard of living. An expansion of the volume of production thus becomes one of the principal aims of economic policy, but this of itself will not increase the standard of living of the whole community if nearly all the additional goods and services produced go to a small section of the people. In the second place, therefore, a people's standard of living depends on how these goods and services are distributed among them, and generally the more nearly equal is this distribution, the greater will be the economic welfare of the community. This does not necessarily mean that in order to achieve the highest possible level of economic welfare the total product must be divided equally among all people, so that everyone has exactly the same income, but it does mean that extremes of very high or very low incomes should not exist side by side. In Great Britain in 1900 there was a much smaller volume of production and a very much greater inequality of income than there is today, and therefore for both these reasons economic welfare is greater and the standard of living higher at the present day than in 1900.

II. WEALTH

(4) WHAT IS WEALTH?

Production aims at producing both goods and services. Some goods are durable—for example, a church or a factory; some are wanted for immediate consumption—for example, food; and some are intermediate between these—for example, a radio set or an electric washer.

Services of many kinds—for example, those of doctors, solicitors, teachers, etc. At any given moment there is in existence in a country a definite quantity of goods of all types. These comprise the country's wealth at that time.

To the economist wealth is a stock of goods existing at a particular time that conform to certain requirements. Such goods must possess four qualities. In the first place, they must possess utility—that is, they must be capable of yielding satisfaction, or, as Marshall says, they must be desirable. Secondly, before goods can be considered as wealth they must have a money value. Thirdly, they must be limited in supply. Fourthly, the ownership of such goods must be capable of being transferred from one person to another. This fourth condition carries with it the assumption that all wealth is owned by someone. This definition of wealth is more precise than the meaning often attached to the word in ordinary speech, and would exclude intangible things such as acquired skills. Though an independent craftsman—*e.g.* a carpenter— would count his tools as part of his personal stock of wealth, he would not include his skill in using them, as skills are not transferable. In speaking of a country's wealth, one might include the quality of the labour (especially if there is a high standard of education, training, etc.) under this heading. In economics, however, it is essential to attach precise meanings to terms, and it is therefore better to restrict wealth to tangible things.

Attempts have been made to estimate the total national wealth of Great Britain at various times, but changing prices make comparisons of different periods difficult. Making allowance for the rise in prices, there is no doubt that the total wealth of this country is considerably greater today than in 1914.

(5) THE OWNERSHIP OF WEALTH

Three classes of ownership of wealth may be distinguished:

(i) *Personal wealth.* Firstly there is what may be called personal wealth. Personal wealth comprises personal belongings such as clothes, watches, jewellery, books, motor cars, household equipment and furniture, and the house one lives in. All these things presumably give satisfaction to their owner, or they would not have been acquired; all have a money value, all are limited in supply, and in all cases ownership is transferable from one person to another.

(ii) *Business wealth.* Secondly, there is business wealth—that is, such things as factory buildings, machinery, raw materials, railway systems, canals, roads, land. These things also possess all the attributes of wealth, although they do not yield satisfaction for their own sake. They are desired merely to assist the production of other things—for example, ultimately, personal wealth or social wealth. This kind of wealth is used as an agent of production, and, as will be seen below, economists differentiate it from other kinds of wealth by calling it land or capital.

(iii) *Social wealth.* This forms the third type of wealth. It consists of wealth owned collectively, and includes all property owned by the State or local authorities—schools, public libraries, art galleries and museums, gas and electricity undertakings, town halls, Government offices, etc. Since 1945, the coal-mines, railways, gas and electricity concerns previously in private ownership have all been added to the stock of social wealth. Some of this wealth (for example, art galleries) is similar to personal wealth, in being desirable for its own sake, but too costly for most people individually to afford; and some of it is collectively owned business wealth, as for example coal-mines and railways.

(6) THE WEALTH OF THE INDIVIDUAL AND THE WEALTH OF THE COMMUNITY

In calculating his personal wealth an individual would include any money he had in the bank, and the present value of any Saving Certificates, National Development Bonds, Savings Bonds or shares in companies that he possessed. An individual is justified in doing this, for he can turn his Government Stock or his shares into money, and with this money he can purchase actual, tangible goods that form real wealth.

In calculating the total wealth of the community as a whole, however, neither money nor Government Bonds must be included. Money is purely a claim to goods and services, and is worthless unless these goods and services are available when they are required. Government Bonds are generally claims to sums of money which the Government undertakes to pay to the holders at a future date, and the interest is paid to particular persons out of taxes collected from the whole community—that is, the interest is merely a transfer of purchasing power from one group of people to another. Further, these Government Bonds form part of the National Debt, most of which represents past Government borrowing, mainly in war-time, and therefore they represent no real assets. On the other hand, a share in a Company represents a definite fraction of the Company's business wealth, but the share certificate and the actual asset itself must not both be counted. In calculating a country's wealth it is necessary too to take into account its international assets and liabilities. A foreign debt must be deducted from the total, for it can be liquidated only by the export of actual goods or services. Similarly, any debts owing to it by other nations must be added to the total.

(7) THE FORM OF OWNERSHIP OF WEALTH DETERMINES THE FORM OF THE ECONOMIC SYSTEM

Three categories of ownership of wealth were noted above: personal, business and social. Business wealth or capital can, however, be owned by individuals or the State. The following diagram shows the ownership of wealth:

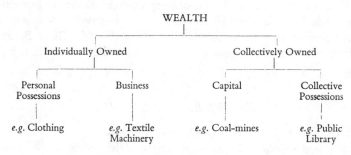

FIG. 1.—TYPES OF WEALTH.

Under private enterprise most wealth is owned by individuals, a minimum being collectively owned. Even under a communist system the individual would be allowed to own some personal possessions, though the ownership of most kinds of wealth would be forbidden to him, as also some personal possessions, especially those that are large and durable like houses. It is, however, the ownership of business capital that has given rise to different economic and political systems. The supporter of private or free enterprise (often called capitalism) believes that so far as possible business capital should be in private hands, whereas the collectivist believes that all means of production should be collectively owned by the State. In Great Britain there is a mixed system, the State owning a number of basic industries—coal-mining, railways, gas and electricity production—though most industries in this country are still carried on under private enterprise, though often subject to controls and restrictions imposed by the State. The present economic system of Great Britain is still therefore largely based on free enterprise and private property.

(8) POVERTY, WEALTH AND INCOME

Poverty may be defined as either (i) a lack of wealth, or (ii) insufficiency of income. Persons or countries therefore may be poor because they possess little wealth or because of the smallness of their incomes. Thus, the word is used in two senses. It can refer to one's stock of goods—for example, wealth—or it can refer to one's income. By income is meant a regular flow or addition to one's stock of wealth, and generally one considers a person to be poor if his income is small. Similarly, a poor country is one with a small income—that is, where the volume of production is small per head of the population. Poverty, therefore, means the ability to satisfy only a small proportion of one's wants. Though the output per head in countries such as Great Britain and the United States has been enormously increased over the past century, what, in these countries, is considered to be poverty today would have been thought to be comparative affluence in the Great Britain of 150 years ago, or by people in many parts of the world even today.

III. DIVISION OF LABOUR

(9) THE MEANING OF DIVISION OF LABOUR

If a man working alone undertook the entire production of some article there would be no division of labour. If, for example, he reared his own sheep, clipped the wool himself, cleaned and combed it, spun it into thread, and then himself wove it into cloth and dyed it, the manufacture of the cloth would have involved no division of labour. If, on the other hand, one man tended the sheep, another did the shearing, a third the scouring, a fourth the combing, a fifth the spinning, a sixth the weaving, and a seventh the dyeing, there would be considerable division of labour. Where a division of labour is by process, one person undertakes only a small part of the work, each specialising in a single process.

Development of division of labour. Even under the most primitive conditions of human existence there was some division of labour: the man spent his time fighting and hunting, while the woman looked after the home and the children. When agricultural pursuits were undertaken, work on the land often devolved upon the woman, the man regarding himself primarily as a warrior. Later, in village communities, some occupations required specialists, and so we find men working as millers, blacksmiths or carpenters. In the Middle Ages the number and variety of craft gilds in London, York and other cities indicates the extent of specialisation in those days—the goldsmiths, the merchant "taylors," the barber surgeons, the glovers, the mercers, the drapers, the haberdashers, the grocers, the smiths, the bakers and many more. Masters, journeymen and apprentices were members of the same gild, for no master employed more than a few journeymen, each of whom expected to be a master himself one day.

The development of the factory system led to a great extension of the principle of division of labour, and to the rise and development of capitalism. Under the domestic system the merchant-manufacturer financed production carried on in the homes of the workers; under the factory system there was an increasing use of capital in production, and this brought into existence the large-scale employer of labour.

Division of labour began, then, in the dividing of the day's work among the members of the family, extended with the growth of towns to the specialisation of individual trades, and with the development of the factory system it came to mean the splitting up of production into a number of separate processes, each being undertaken by a different worker. From the single firm the principle was eventually extended to the industry, for where an industry came to be concentrated in one area the individual firms could then specialise in single processes. The Lancashire cotton industry provides an excellent example of this, but this aspect of the division of labour—the localisation of industry—will be considered below.[1] From specialisation by districts to specialisation by countries is not a big step, and international trade is based on this principle.[2] Territorially, then, division of labour expanded from the family to the town, from town to the country, and from the country to the world.

(10) DIVISION OF LABOUR AND OUTPUT

The aim of division of labour is to increase output.

Adam Smith was greatly impressed by the increase in production resulting from division of labour, and he devotes the first three chapters of his book *The Wealth of Nations*[3] to a discussion of this topic. To illustrate how output is increased where division of labour is in operation he selected pin-making, which in his day involved eighteen separate operations. Without division of labour—that is, if one man performed every operation himself—a workman could produce no more than twenty pins in a day. In one small workshop that Adam Smith visited ten men were employed, and though some of them were apparently undertaking more than one operation, their total output often reached 48,000 pins per day, giving an average of 4,800 per workman, as against twenty each where there was no division of labour. A more modern example is provided by the manufacture of motor-car engines. At one

---

[1] See Chapter VIII.   [2] See Chapter XXVI.
[3] In full the title runs: *An Inquiry into the Nature and Causes of the Wealth of Nations.*

time the entire engine was assembled by one man. To speed up production Henry Ford divided the work into 84 operations, each performed by a different man, with the result that the total output of the 84 men was trebled.

It is perhaps necessary at this point to utter a cautionary word. The enormous expansion of production over the past two centuries has not been the result of division of labour alone. The most important influence has been the invention of new and better machines, that is, the increasing use of capital. Division of labour did, of course, make possible a greater use of machinery.

How, then, does division of labour increase output? We cannot do better than go to Adam Smith for our answer, since his analysis largely holds good today. Five reasons can be given:

(i) *Greater skill of the workers.* Division of labour results in workers acquiring greater skill at their jobs, for "by reducing every man's business to some simple operation, and by making this operation the sole employment of his life, necessarily increases very much the dexterity of the workman." The point is summed up in the phrase: "practice makes perfect." The constant repetition of a task makes its performance almost automatic. The importance of this sort of skill, however, was greatly reduced when machinery came to be used.

(ii) *A saving of time.* There is a "saving of the time which is often lost in passing from one sort of work to another, for a man commonly saunters a little in turning his hand from one sort of employment to another." By keeping to a single operation, a workman can accomplish a great deal more, since he wastes less time between operations. Less time, too, is required to learn how to perform a single operation than to learn a complete trade.

(iii) *Employment of specialists.* The carrying out of almost any piece of work requires the performance of many separate tasks, each often needing its own particular skill. Specialisation therefore makes it possible for each workman to specialise in the work for which he has the greatest aptitude.

(iv) *It makes possible the use of machinery.* Adam Smith, in listing the advantages of the division of labour, was thinking of it independently of the use of machinery. It may be put forward as a further advantage of the division of labour that it made possible a greater use of machinery. Once a piece of work was reduced to mere routine, it opened the way for the employment of a machine to carry out the operation, and so that output was still further increased. Though division of labour without the use of power-driven machinery is possible, yet specialisation of process is itself induced by machinery, and makes division of labour essential. Division of labour paved the way for the introduction of machinery and mass-production methods.

(v) *Less fatigue.* It is sometimes claimed that the worker, habituated to the repetition of simple tasks, becomes less fatigued by his work. But it is necessary for all workers to maintain the same pace if division of labour is to work smoothly, and so the fatigue of the slower workers may be increased by the effort required to keep up with the quicker. Machinery does not tire however long the day, and where it is used the workman cannot slow down, but must keep pace with it.

(ii) DISADVANTAGES OF DIVISION OF LABOUR

The increased output resulting from the division of labour is obtained, however, only at a certain cost, for it has brought with it its own problems. Consider some of its disadvantages:

(i) *Monotony of the work.* Minute specialisation of processes means that each workman performs only one small operation, perhaps thousands of times during each working day. His work therefore becomes very monotonous and tends to dull the intelligence. Well-meaning people are perhaps apt to over-sympathise with those who have to spend their working lives doing monotonous work. Such sympathy, however, is often wasted. Cases have been noted of workers transferred from routine tasks to work of a more varied kind calling for closer attention, and within a week asking to be allowed to return to their former jobs. It would seem that there are people—particularly it is said, young girls—who prefer purely routine work, because it makes so little demand upon them that they can chat with their fellow workers, or indulge in day-dreaming.

(ii) *The decline of craftsmanship.* It is said, too, that with the employment of machinery the workman ceases to be a craftsman and becomes just a tender of a machine. Though to a large extent this is true, it is also true that when all work was done by hand a good deal of it was both laborious and monotonous—as, for example, the planing by a carpenter of a large number of planks: work calling, no doubt, for a certain amount of skill, but hardly to be classed as craftsmanship. Many other forms of hand work were equally laborious and monotonous and not always well done. On the other hand, looking after some modern machines entails a considerable degree of skill and intelligence, and though the quality of the work may never approach the highest standards of the craftsman, it is generally well above that of the less efficient workers by hand.

(iii) *Greater risk of unemployment.* To a greater or less degree, the division of labour turns workers into specialists. The greater the skill

required in their work—that is, the more specific the labour—the
more difficult it becomes for the workers in a declining industry to
obtain alternative employment. Division of labour requires the co-
operation of a group of people in production, but this dependence on
others increases the risk of unemployment under modern conditions of
large-scale production, where goods have generally to be produced in
anticipation of demand, instead of in response to direct orders, as in the
days of small, independent craftsmen.

(12) DIVISION OF LABOUR NECESSITATES EXCHANGE

When a family provided for all its wants by its own efforts it was self-
supporting, and economically independent of other families. As soon
as division of labour was carried to the point where men began to
specialise in particular trades, it became necessary for them to make
exchanges with one another. Thus, exchange is a consequence of
specialisation. The carpenter, who spent all his time working in wood,
had to exchange some of the things he had made with the weaver for
cloth, or with the baker for bread. Specialisation and exchange make
all those taking part richer, since it increases their combined output.
An exchange of goods for goods is known as barter, but it is a clumsy
method of making exchanges, and at an early date some form of money
came to be used as a medium of exchange.

Division of labour increases output, but advantage can be taken of
specialisation only if the goods produced are distributed among all
those demanding them. The greater the degree of specialisation, therefore, the greater becomes the work of distribution and the larger the
number of people required in commerce. Thus, to some extent the
advantage of division of labour in making possible a great increase in
output is offset by the extra work of distribution.

Many people are engaged in the extractive industries, such as mining,
quarrying, farming, fishing; many more are employed in the various
branches of manufacture, in the textile, iron and steel, pottery industries, etc.; many others work at commercial occupations which assist
the distribution of raw materials and the manufacture of goods, such as
the retail and wholesale trades, import and export trades, transport,
banking and insurance. As a result of division of labour people engaged
in commercial occupations help to satisfy the wants of others indirectly.
A fourth category of workers perform more direct services. Among
these are doctors and dentists, lawyers and judges, teachers and parsons,
civil servants, and all employed in local government, and in the
Armed Services and police, musicians, sculptors and painters, and
actors, singers and entertainers of all kinds. The higher the standard of

living enjoyed by a community, the larger generally will be the proportion of its people in this group. Before 1939 about 20% of the working population of Britain was engaged in occupations supplying direct services; by 1965 the proportion of people in this group had increased to 27%. Division of labour thus makes it possible to have large numbers of persons employed in occupations not concerned with satisfying material wants.

The principle of comparative advantage. Both the individual and the community will benefit to the greatest extent if each person specialises in that occupation in which he has the greatest comparative advantage over others. A successful barrister may be at the same time an excellent interior decorator. Nevertheless, it will not be an economic proposition for him to decorate his own house if in order to give himself time in which to do this work he has to decline a valuable brief. He can earn much more as a barrister—the occupation in which he has the greatest comparative advantage over others—in the time it would take him to paint and decorate his house. Thus, he could indirectly accomplish this task of painting and decorating, by working only a fraction of the time as a barrister. Much work, therefore, that people do for themselves instead of employing others to do for them, is uneconomic and contrary to the principle of division of labour.

(13) DIVISION OF LABOUR IS LIMITED BY THE MARKET

The extent to which division of labour can be carried is determined by the demand for the commodity. Division of labour results in an increase in total output, and as division of labour is taken further, so output increases further. The greatest specialisation will occur, then, in the production of those commodities the cost of production of which can be reduced by division of labour and for which there is a wide market. For some things there is a very large demand if the price of the commodity is low enough, but however cheap some things became, the demand would remain small. Therefore, as Adam Smith pointed out, division of labour is limited by the market. In a densely populated area like Greater London division of labour can be carried to greater lengths than in a thinly populated area like the Highlands of Scotland, where a man must often of necessity be a jack of all trades. The extent of the market depends also on the facilities which exist for distributing commodities from the place of production. Division of labour was not possible therefore to any considerable extent before the middle of the eighteenth century because transport facilities were generally too poor before that time. The construction of roads, canals and railways made possible a wider distribution of manufactures, and the resulting extension of the market enabled greater specialisation of processes to be introduced.

RECOMMENDATIONS FOR FURTHER READING

A. Marshall: *Principles of Economics*, Book II, Chapters 1–3.
Adam Smith: *Wealth of Nations*, Book I, Chapters 1–3.

QUESTIONS

1. Consider the possible disadvantages to the individual and to the community which may arise from extreme specialisation. (R.S.A. Inter.)

2. Describe the conditions in industry which tend to encourage minute division of labour and mention the advantages and, if any, the disadvantages of minute division of labour. (L.C. Com. Econ.)

3. What do you understand by the term "wealth" in economics? Discuss the relationship between wealth and welfare. (C.I.S. Inter.)

4. Explain what is meant by "division of labour." How can the underlying principle be applied to increase production per man hour? (Exp.)

5. "Although machinery goes hand in hand with specialisation, the two things are obviously quite distinct, and each makes a separate contribution to industrial efficiency." (Cairncross.) Give a short account of the contribution to industrial efficiency of (a) specialisation and (b) machinery. (A.C.C.A. Inter.)

6. From what evidence would you argue that the extent of poverty has diminished in recent years? (C.C.S. Final.)

7. Distinguish carefully between the terms "income," "capital" and "wealth," and then show the possible relationship between them. (I.H.A.)

8. What is meant by the division of labour and what are its advantages? Show how the size of the market limits the degree of specialisation. (G.C.E. Adv.)

CHAPTER III

THE FACTORS OF PRODUCTION

I. THE PRODUCTIVE RESOURCES

(1) LAND, LABOUR AND CAPITAL

One of the principal influences on any country's total volume of production is the extent and quality of its resources of land, labour and capital. These productive resources are known as agents or factors of production, and are sometimes called inputs. The term *input* is perhaps to be preferred to *agent* or *factor* of production, for an agent implies the playing of an active rôle, whereas these three factors are better considered merely as resources at the disposal of the organisers of production. It is important to notice too that it is the services of the factor, rather than the factor itself, that contribute towards production.

The term *land* is used in the widest sense to include all kinds of natural (as distinct from man-made) resources: farm-lands, mineral wealth, such as coal and metal ores, and fishing-grounds. Perhaps the main service of the land is the provision of space where production can take place. *Capital* comprises an equally varied assortment of resources—factory buildings, tools and machinery, raw materials, partly finished goods, means of transport, but all these types of capital have one feature in common—namely, that they are things that are wanted not for their own sake but merely to assist the production of other commodities. Land consists of all resources provided by Nature; capital, on the other hand, has been accumulated as a result of Man's efforts in the past. "In a sense," says Marshall, "there are only two agents of production, nature and man."[1] By *labour* is meant the human effort employed in production. If land, labour and capital are considered as productive resources this has the advantage of emphasising their similarity rather than their differences.

Even for the most primitive method of production the co-operation of all three factors is required. Early Man, even in the Stone Age, made simple tools to assist him in his work. Some fruits—*e.g.* blackberries and bilberries—may grow wild, but nevertheless labour is needed to gather them and some form of capital required to transport them to

[1] A. Marshall: *Principles of Economics* (1890), IV. 1.

localities where consumers are to be found. In the extractive group of occupations—farming, hunting, fishing, mining, etc.—land is a predominant factor, but never to the complete exclusion of capital and labour.

II. THE ENTREPRENEUR AS A FACTOR OF PRODUCTION

(2) ARE THERE THREE FACTORS OF PRODUCTION OR FOUR?

The early nineteenth-century economists enumerated only three factors of production—land, labour and capital, as mentioned above—but Marshall[1] thought that *organisation* was sometimes worthy of being considered a separate factor. Since then many other economists have recognised the *entrepreneur* (or organiser) as an independent factor, though there are some who refuse to differentiate between labour and the organising function.

They argue that a certain amount of organising is required of all labour, though more in some cases than in others. The only difference, therefore, they say between the managing director and one of his lowest-ranking employees is that the managing director is primarily concerned with organisation and devotes nearly the whole of his time to it, whereas at the other end of the scale the organisation required of a workman is merely a preliminary to his ordinary work, and occupies only a small fraction of his time. In reply to such arguments it is pointed out that the organising undertaken by the entrepreneur is not merely on a wider scale but is also different in kind from that of the employee. The entrepreneur is responsible not only for arranging how a piece of work shall be carried out but also for organising the work of others—in fact, his organising covers all the factors he employs. He also has to make important decisions—determine what to produce, how much to produce and the production methods to be used. Further, as will be seen in Par. 3, it is regarded as the entrepeneur's primary function to bear the risk or uncertainty attaching to the enterprise, and this uncertainty is different economically from the risk run by labour in dangerous occupations, in that the entrepreneur cannot insure against the risk or uncertainty that he has to undertake. It is admitted by some critics of the entrepreneurial function that it is different in kind from the other three factors, but because of this difference they argue that it cannot be considered a factor of production, to which supporters of the entrepreneur as a separate factor reply: of what use, then, are land, labour and capital unless they have been organised for production?

[1] A. Marshall: *Principles of Economics*, p. 139.

To the entrepreneur land, labour and capital are just masses of resources, of no economic importance until they have been organised for the production of some commodity. How they shall be employed, and how much of each shall be used, are questions to be decided by the entrepreneur and not by the owners of the other factors. Land, labour and capital are passive factors, whereas the entrepreneur is the active factor and therefore a different type.

Where production is on a small scale and undertaken by a sole master-craftsman, the entrepreneurial function is easy to locate, for the factors—labour and organisation—are combined in the same person. The typical modern business unit is, however, the limited company, and in a company it is not easy to locate the entrepreneurial function, but though it is difficult to locate, it nevertheless exists.

The desire of some writers to eliminate the entrepreneur as a separate factor of production may be due to dislike of regarding labour as merely a productive resource. Labour is supplied by human beings, and as the entrepreneurial function also is carried out by human beings, they feel that there is no difference between them. This, however, is a social and not an economic argument, for economically labour is similar to land and capital. Two human beings may be similar to each other biologically, but their services to production may be of quite different kinds. There seems to be reasonable justification, then, for regarding the entrepreneur as a separate factor of production.

(3) FUNCTIONS OF THE ENTREPRENEUR

The following may be regarded as the main functions of the entrepreneur:

(i) *Uncertainty-bearing.* The bearing of uncertainty is the principal function of the entrepreneur. There are two kinds of risk which the entrepreneur has to face. (*a*) Many risks, such as fire, loss of goods in transit, etc., can be insured against because statistics are available which enable insurance companies to calculate the probability of loss arising from them. Such risks can therefore be pooled, and the business man, in exchange for the payment of a premium, shifts the responsibility for bearing them from his own shoulders to an insurance company. In addition to insurance, there are a number of ways by which risk can be reduced. Hedging is a sort of insurance against price fluctuation. The compilation of statistics, based on market research and providing the entrepreneur with more accurate information, reduce the risk he has to bear. But whenever risk is reduced in this way the pure entrepreneurial function is also lessened. (*b*) Some risks, however, cannot be insured against because their probability cannot be actuarily calculated.

It has been suggested the term "uncertainty" should be given, to this type of risk.

Entrepreneurs generally do not wait until they have received orders for a given quantity of goods before they undertake their production; instead, they first decide how much to produce and then try to sell the output later. In other words, production is carried on in anticipation of demand. Modern methods of production have become so complex that the time interval between the taking of the decision to produce and the marketing of the product has been considerably lengthened. The longer this interval, the greater is the opportunity for demand to change. Further, a single entrepreneur is never certain how much his rivals are going to produce. Because conditions affecting demand are constantly changing, future demand becomes difficult to predict. These are the kinds of uncertainty-bearing that devolve upon entrepreneurs. "The most fundamental fact in connection with organisation, it has been said is the meeting of uncertainty."[1] The importance of the entrepreneur has increased with the increasing complexity and uncertainty of production.

(ii) *Management control.* There are two important aspects of the entrepreneurial function—risk-bearing and management control. The responsibility for broad decisions of policy rests with the entrepreneur. He must be capable of delegating the carrying out of these decisions to his subordinates, and so must possess the ability to select the right kind of men to work with him. Thus a knowledge of men becomes more important than expert knowledge of the techniques of production. It is said that men with high entrepreneurial ability are few in number and this explains why the services of the most capable entrepreneurs are often in demand for widely different forms of production. There is, however, an increasing tendency at the present day for the functions of risk-bearing and control to be separated, and in the larger companies it is quite common for only a small proportion of the shares to be held by officials and directors.

(iii) *Other functions of the entrepreneur.* The other functions of the entrepreneur really arise from the first two. Having decided which industry to enter, the entrepreneur must next decide how much to produce and by what method to produce it—that is, in the language of economists, he has to decide his scale of production and in what proportion to combine the other factors of production that he employs. To a certain degree he can choose between employing more of one factor or more of another—more land, perhaps, and less labour—but if he is to produce most efficiently he will have to combine his factors in the best

---

[1] F. H. Knight: *Risk, Uncertainty and Profit*, p. 317.

or optimum proportion. On the combined decisions of entrepreneurs therefore depends the assortment of goods that will be available to consumers. In a free economy the entrepreneurs would try to produce those things for which there was a demand, and so it is sometimes said that consumers as a whole decide what things shall be produced. Finally, the entrepreneur is responsible for marketing the product.

From this account of the functions of the entrepreneur, it may appear that the entrepreneur must be an individual. This is true only of the one-man business, or possibly of the partnership or small private company, where the function is shared among a small group of people, all of whom take a direct interest in the management of the business. However, the large limited company is the typical business unit at the present day, and in this case it is very difficult to define the entrepreneurial function precisely, for risk is borne by the shareholders (many of whom never even attend a shareholders' meeting) and the day-by-day control of the business is generally in the hands of a salaried manager or managing director.

III. LAND

(4) DOES LAND DIFFER FROM THE OTHER FACTORS?

Formerly economists placed the factors of production in rigidly defined groups, and treated each of them as separate and distinct from the others. In particular, Ricardo and his followers considered that land differed fundamentally from the other factors. Three reasons were given for this:

(i) Land, they said, was "*a gift of Nature*"—that is, Man had done nothing to bring it into existence, whereas capital was accumulated only as a result of the employment of labour and other factors of production.

(ii) Unlike the other factors of production, land, they said, is strictly *limited in quantity*, so that even in the long period its supply cannot be increased.

(iii) It was said, further, that in those industries primarily dependent on land, production was subject to the *Law of Diminishing Returns*.

It can be shown without much difficulty that these alleged peculiarities of land do not entirely agree with the facts.

(i) The contention that land is a gift of Nature is of little economic significance. Man has certainly done nothing to bring into existence the

C

supplies of coal in South Yorkshire, but while the coal remains under-ground it can serve no economic purpose. Large stocks of coal, as yet unworked, exist several thousand feet below the surface near Selby, but until mining operations have been undertaken this coal is of no use to production. One aspect of land is outside the control of Man—namely, its situation—and this is a chief characteristic of land as a factor of production. Land, too, is said to have no cost of production, for no costs were incurred to produce it, but, as will be seen in the next para-graph, land has sometimes been reclaimed from the sea at enormous expense. Nevertheless, Man is in no way responsible for the location in particular places of minerals such as iron ore and oil, and for agricul-tural production he has to accept climate as a factor beyond his control.

(ii) Although it must be admitted that the total area of land on the earth's surface cannot be appreciably increased, it is nevertheless not strictly true to say that the supply of land is fixed. In the Netherlands, for example, land has been reclaimed from the sea; in Great Britain the Fenlands, formerly a mere swamp, have been transformed into one of the most fertile areas in the country; in the United States great irriga-tion schemes, such as that at Boulder Dam, have brought into cultiva-tion vast areas that were formerly desert.

Increasing the area under crops, as a result of improvements in farming technique, is really equivalent to an increase in the supply of land. This occurred in Great Britain in the mid-eighteenth century, when the cultivation of root crops made it possible to end the practice of leaving fallow each year one-third of all the agricultural land. Improving the fertility of existing land is also equivalent to increasing its supply, though the improvement is merely the result of the applica-tion of more capital and labour to the land. From the standpoint of a single country, to import additional supplies of food from abroad is similar in effect to increasing the supply of land at home, though clearly, all countries cannot do this.

The total amount of land can be reduced by such happenings as coast erosion, flooding or soil erosion. Whole villages have disap-peared into the sea on the Yorkshire coast; the Zuider Zee inundated a large area of the Netherlands during the thirteenth and fourteenth cen-turies. Soil erosion, considered by some people to be one of the most serious menaces confronting the human race, has resulted in a large area of the United States, once good grassland, becoming desert. Never-theless, even taken together, all the changes that have taken place in the land surface of the earth form a very small proportion of its total area.

(iii) At one period it was thought that agriculture was an industry peculiarly subject to the Law of Diminishing Returns, while manufacturing industry was carried out under conditions of increasing returns. The Law of Diminishing Returns, however, is not restricted to those forms of production in which land predominates. It can now be shown that in different circumstances both agriculture and manufacture can be subject to either law. It can be said therefore that economically land, though it has, of course, some special features of its own, is mainly similar to, and not different from, the other factors of production. Its distinguishing feature is that "the right to use a piece of land gives command over a certain area."

(5) THE LAW OF DIMINISHING RETURNS

It will be useful, however, at this stage to take a brief preliminary glance at the Law of Diminishing Returns as it applies to land. All that the law states is that after a certain point successive applications of equal amounts of resources to a given area of land produces a less than proportionate return. A simplified example will make this clearer. Consider a piece of land of a size larger than one man is capable of cultivating successfully by his own efforts alone. Assume that in successive years he takes into his employment one additional man, together with equal additional amounts of capital in the form of farming equipment. In the second year, if it is a large piece of land, the increased output may be greater than the amount produced in the first year, and in the third year the increase may possibly be even

TABLE I

Diminishing Returns to Land

Units of land	Number of men employed (each with equal amount of farming equipment)	Output per year (lb. of potatoes)	Addition to output	Average output per man
I	I	100	100	100
I	2	210	110	105
I	3	330	120	110
I	4	460	130	115
I	5	600	140	120
I	6	730	130	121·6
I	7	850	120	121·4
I	8	960	110	120
I	9	1,060	100	118
I	10	1,150	90	115
I	11	1,230	80	112
I	12	1,290	60	107
I	13	1,305	15	100
I	14	1,315	10	94

greater still. After some years, however, the additional output of one year will be smaller than the additional output of the previous year. In other words, the Law of Diminishing Returns will begin to operate. Obviously, this must occur sooner or later, otherwise it would be possible indefinitely to increase the output from a small piece of land merely by putting more men and equipment to work upon it. If this policy of setting more men to work on the same piece of land were continued, eventually the absurd situation would arise where the men would be so crowded together that they would find it physically impossible to move.

Table I illustrates the operation of the Law of Diminishing Returns when a fixed amount of land is cultivated.

This table shows that until the employment of five men there is a more than proportionate return—that is, there are *increasing returns*—whereas when the number of men employed is increased beyond five the successive additions to total output decrease—that is, there are diminishing returns. After the employment of eleven men there are steeply diminishing returns.

This can be illustrated by a diagram:

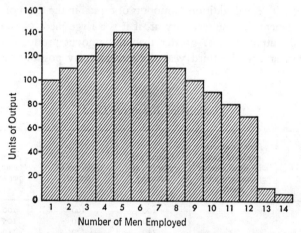

FIG. 2.—DIMINISHING RETURNS.

Each column represents the addition to total output resulting from the employment of an additional man. The shaded area shows the maximum output (under existing technical conditions) achieved by the employment of fourteen men. An improvement in technique—for example, the use of a new fertiliser—would increase output or achieve a similar output at less cost—that is, by the employment of fewer men.

The operation of the law can also be seen if one considers a self-sufficient country trying to produce more food to satisfy an expanding population. The most fertile land might be used first, and if this did not yield a sufficient output less fertile land would have to be brought into cultivation. If the same number of men and equipment were employed on each square mile of the less fertile land as on the more fertile land the output would be less. If the population increased further, and even less fertile land had to be cultivated, the additional output would be smaller than before. With each increase in population, even less fertile land would have to be cultivated, and so increased output would be achieved only under conditions of decreasing returns. During both the First and Second World Wars, Great Britain found it necessary to increase its output of food, but this could be done only by ploughing up inferior land, and so production was subject to diminishing returns. The operation of this Law of Diminishing Returns in relation to the expansion of population seriously perturbed Thomas Malthus in the late eighteenth century.

The law has also been applied to other extractive occupations, such as mining and fishing. In the case of mining the commodity is a wasting asset, that is, the total supply is fixed, and when this is exhausted the mine becomes worked out. As the area worked recedes farther from the shaft, each addition to output is obtained only at increasing cost in terms of time and labour. With fishing the position is somewhat similar, though replenishment of supply in this case is possible. The essential feature of the Law of Diminishing Returns as considered in this paragraph is that one factor of production is fixed and varying amounts of the other factors are combined with it. By its very character land is more likely to be fixed than other factors.

IV. LABOUR

(6) THE IMPORTANCE OF LABOUR

Some economists consider labour to be the most important factor of production. For the most part, such economists do not recognise the entrepreneur as a separate factor. There is no doubt that labour is absolutely indispensable to all forms of production, but under modern conditions of production so are the other factors, for production requires the co-operation of all of them. Labour differs from land and capital in that it is supplied by human beings, and because of that, ethical and moral considerations must be taken into account when dealing with labour. In applied economics this human aspect of labour cannot be ignored, but in pure economic theory labour is economically no different from land or capital. To the entrepreneur it is just one of the resources that are essential to the carrying out of production.

(7) THE SUPPLY OF LABOUR

There is some ambiguity in the term, supply of labour. The supply may be taken to mean the total number of people—men, women and children—of working age. Even the phrase "working age" is not precise and needs to be defined. Again, supply of labour may be taken to mean the supply of *labour service* available, and since it is the service of a factor, rather than the factor itself, that takes part in production, this is the more useful concept. The supply of labour service can be varied either by a change in the number of working population or by a change in the number of hours worked in a given period of time. The supply of labour available in a country depends, then, on three factors: (i) on the total population of the country; (ii) on the proportion of the population available for employment; and (iii) on the number of hours worked by each person per year.

(i) Economists have, therefore, always been interested in population changes. This question will be considered in Chapter V.

(ii) The proportion of the population available for employment will depend mainly on the standard of civilisation reached by the country concerned, the extent of its industrialisation, its social organisation and perhaps the attitude of its people to work. In a poor country it may require the maximum efforts of both men and women, young and old, to eke out even a bare existence, whereas in a highly industrialised State the provision of the necessities of life may require the employment of only a fraction of the total population. If the people consider all forms of productive work to be menial, as in the Athens of Aristotle, the size of the labour force will depend on the number of slaves the country possesses. In a highly civilised country the labour force will be reduced by keeping the children at school until a late age, though this loss may be more than counterbalanced by greater efficiency of labour. In a poor country both men and women may have to continue at work so long as they are physically capable of doing so; in a richer country fewer women may be expected to work, and the men may retire from work while still physically strong and mentally alert. It is something of an anomaly at the present day that in some occupations there should be compulsory retirement when many workers are mentally still at the height of their powers. The changing social attitude in Great Britain during the twentieth century to the employment of women, both unmarried and married, has had a considerable influence on the supply of labour in this country. At the beginning of the century it was considered to be degrading for young girls in middle-class families to go out to work, and married women went out to work only if their husbands' wages were very low. Two World Wars changed all this. By the 1960s half the women of working age in Great Britain were going out to work, forming a third of the total labour force.

(iii) The social development of the country may result in the adoption of a shorter working week, with a reduction in the number of hours worked per day, and with paid holidays. In Great Britain, in the early years of the industrial system, conditions prevailed similar to those existing when people either worked on the land or were independent craftsmen, when the hours of work were limited only by the hours of daylight, and holidays were confined to "holy days" such as Sundays and Saints' days, and perhaps an annual local "feast" day. Gradually working hours have been reduced, so that nowadays many workers in Great Britain enjoy a five-day week of eight hours per day, and are allowed public holidays and one to three weeks each year with full pay. If the hours of work are excessively long a reduction in hours may actually increase the amount of work done, but this countervailing effect quickly declines with each reduction in the number of hours worked.

(8) EFFICIENCY OF LABOUR

It has already been pointed out that two factors which reduce the supply of labour—the longer period of education and the shorter working week—might be offset to some extent by a consequent increase in the efficiency of labour. By increased efficiency is meant the ability to achieve a greater output in a shorter time without any falling off in the quality of the work—that is to say, increased productivity per man employed. The efficiency of a country's labour supply can be increased in a number of ways:

(i) *Social services.* An improvement in the physical welfare of the people by their being adequately fed, clothed and housed will raise the general standard of health and reduce the number of days lost through sickness. A national scheme of social security will help to achieve this purpose. Unemployment pay will enable a minimum standard of health to be maintained during unemployment, and retirement pensions will reduce the necessity to save at the expense of health during working life.

(ii) *Working conditions.* The general conditions under which people work affect their output. Minimum standards have been laid down under a long series of Factory Acts, and Factory Inspectors pay particular attention to such things as ventilation and overcrowding. Considerable research has been carried out into the problem of fatigue, and many firms have raised working conditions much above the legal minimum, believing it to be to their own advantage to do so. The provision of recreation facilities and canteens has the same objective.

(iii) *Education and training.* This factor has three aspects: general education, technical education and training within industry. A high standard of general education is essential for developing intelligence and providing a foundation upon which more specialised vocational training can be based. Technical education is available to most people only in their own time, generally by attendance at evening classes, though many firms are now willing to release employees from work for one or more half-days per week. Vocational education, which often continues beyond the age of twenty-one, consists chiefly of subjects of study related to the profession or trade of the student. The third type of training is known as training within industry, and this each firm must undertake for its own employees. To a greater or less extent each firm has to train its own employees in the way it desires its work to be done, for example, in the proper handling of the particular machines used.

(iv) *Efficiency and other factors.* The productivity of labour per man-hour will be increased if the quality of the other factors is high. The more fertile the land, the greater, other things being equal, will be the output per man. Similarly, the greater the amount and the better the quality of the capital employed, the greater will be the productivity of the labour. Perhaps even more important is the efficiency of the entrepreneur, upon whose organising ability depends the efficiency of the method of production adopted. It has already been noticed that division of labour increases the efficiency of labour. The greater the amount of specialisation, the more capitalistic the method of production, and the larger the output per man.

Economy of high wages. High wages may result in a high standard of efficiency, and this has often led employers to offer higher than the standard rates of pay to their employees. Efficiency will be increased if high wages increase the physical welfare of the workers. Generally low wages, as in Asia, are associated with a low standard of efficiency. The benefits of high wages cannot be obtained quickly as a result of increasing wages, for it takes people some time to adjust themselves to a higher standard of living, and there is a tendency for high wages to be dissipated at first in ways not conducive to higher efficiency.

(9) PRODUCTIVE AND NON-PRODUCTIVE LABOUR

Writers on economics formerly discussed at great length the question whether particular kinds of labour were productive or not. The group of economists known as physiocrats regard labour employed in agriculture as productive labour, and, though Adam Smith extended productive labour to all engaged in the production of goods, he classed domestic service and other direct services as non-productive. Only 54% of labour in Great Britain is at present engaged in industrial occupations, the rest being employed in commerce, or in supplying direct services. It has been shown above that the process of production is not complete until commodities have reached consumers, so that the distribution of goods becomes the final stage of production; and, further, production is now taken to include the production of services as well as goods. To class some labour as productive and some as non-productive is therefore not only pointless but inaccurate. The only labour that can be considered to be unproductive is misdirected labour, where effort has been wasted on the production of something that is incapable of fulfilling the function it was intended to serve.

V. CLASSIFICATION OF FACTORS OF PRODUCTION

(10) OBJECTIONS TO THE CONVENTIONAL METHOD OF CLASSIFICATION

There are two main objections to classifying factors of production into rigidly defined groups of land, labour and capital:

(i) *Substitution between units of the same factor is not always possible.* In the first place, the factors are not homogeneous—that is, each group does not consist of a number of units, each one of which is identical with each other, so that any one can be substituted for any other. All land is not alike—in fact, no two pieces of land are exactly alike, for no two pieces of land can have exactly the same situation. Land on which sheep are being grazed cannot necessarily be changed over to wheat-growing. Differences of climate and soil may prevent the substitution of one crop for another; minerals can be worked only where deposits are found. Similarly, raw wool has many alternative uses, but it cannot be substituted for any other kind of capital.

It is exactly the same with labour, many kinds of which are not interchangeable. A shortage of doctors cannot be made good by drafting lawyers, teachers and accountants into the medical profession. There are many kinds of land, many kinds of labour and many different kinds of capital. It would be more logical to recognise hundreds or even thousands of separate factors—each distinctive type of land, labour and capital being considered a factor in its own right—than to limit the number of factors to three or even four.

(ii) *Substitution between factors is often possible.* Although each unit of a factor like land is not a perfect substitute for any other unit of land, so that the purposes for which two pieces of land are required cannot be interchanged, yet it is frequently possible to substitute some land for either capital or labour, or some labour for capital or land, or again some capital for land or labour. Differences between these factors are merely superficial. The only factor for which there is no substitute is that of the entrepreneur. To use more land, or capital or labour does not make it possible to have less organisation.

Under present-day conditions of large-scale production the co-operation of all four factors of production is always required, and it is an important part of the business of the entrepreneur to decide how much of each of the other factors he needs. He cannot dispense with any of them, for he must employ a certain amount of each, but above this minimum he has a certain amount of choice. He cannot dispense with all his labour and substitute land or capital for it, but he can often, for example, employ a little less labour and more capital, or a little more labour and less land. This is known as the *Principle of Substitution*. His decision will depend on which method of production he considers to be the more efficient—that is, more economical. If labour is dear— that is, if wages are high—relatively to the cost of new machinery, then there will be a strong inducement to entrepreneurs to substitute machinery for labour wherever this is possible. Again, if land is cheap relatively to labour and capital, as in the United States in the nineteenth century, extensive rather than intensive farming will be practised.

Thus the older method of classifying factors of production is open to objection, first, because substitution between units of the same factor is not always possible, and secondly, because on the other hand, substitution between different factors is often possible.

(11) SPECIFIC FACTORS

A more useful distinction can be made between factors that are specific and those that are not. The great advantage of this method of classification it that it emphasises the similarity of the factors, for each of the two categories contains examples of land, labour and capital. A factor is said to be specific if it is of a specialised kind, and therefore cannot easily be used for some purpose other than that for which it was originally intended. There is probably very little land that was not in the first place open to alternative uses, for most land can either be built upon or devoted to some kind of farming. Once land has been built upon, however, it becomes more specific, for then the cost of trans-ferring it to some alternative use will be very considerably increased. Much of the sheep-grazing lands of the Pennine moorland lying between Lancashire and Yorkshire is, however, fairly specific, since most of it cannot be used for any other purpose.

Where a long period of study or training is required, or special aptitude is needed, labour may be highly specific. A dentist has to take a university course lasting several years and pass certain examinations before he becomes qualified to practise, while no amount of training will succeed in making a person into an artist unless he possesses some measure of natural talent. There are degrees of specificity depending on the ease or difficulty of transferring other labour into a particular occupation. The less skill and training required, the less specific will be the labour. Professional bodies and craft unions sometimes create artificial specificity by insisting upon unnecessarily long periods of training or apprenticeship, or by making their qualifying examinations competitive in order to restrict the number of successful candidates.

Many kinds of capital, too, are highly specific. A blast-furnace cannot be used for any other purpose, and some machinery is so intricate in character that likewise its use is limited to a single purpose. A railway system also would fall into this category. In the case of partly finished manufactured goods the nearer they are to the final stage of production, the more specific they are likely to be.

(12) NON-SPECIFIC FACTORS

Any factor of production that can fairly easily be transferred from one use to another can be considered to be non-specific.

It was noticed above that most land could be used either for building or farming. One kind of farmland can very often be used for some other type of farming. During the nineteenth century much wheat-land was turned over to grassland for grazing cattle or sheep. During the past twenty years a great deal of grassland has been brought under the plough again.

The easier it is to learn a job, the less specific is the labour required to undertake it. There are probably few occupations where nothing at all has to be learned, but whereas it may take years to acquire the knowledge or skill required for some occupations, there are others where probably half an hour's instruction or less may be sufficient. Unskilled labour is therefore non-specific. In good times and bad there are "rolling stones"—men who go from one type of job to another and never stay long at any, at one time a dustman, at another maybe a builder's labourer and later again perhaps a cleaner of motor omnibuses. With regard to labour, it is perhaps worthy of note that, though it may not be easy to increase the supply of a particular type of specific labour from the ranks of the non-specific, the reverse movement is possible: a shortage of unskilled labour could be made good by drawing on the supply of skilled labour, though this would obviously be economically wasteful.

Finally, there is non-specific capital. Most ordinary tools would fall into this category; a hammer could be used by workers in many totally different occupations. Machinery can frequently be adjusted to serve a different—though generally similar—purpose from that for which it was first intended. Buildings also can often be converted to other uses.

Raw materials are generally non-specific capital. For example, raw wool has many alternative uses—cloth, carpets, hosiery—while iron ore may eventually become one of a hundred different articles. With regard to partly finished goods, the nearer they are to the finished state, the more specific they are likely to be. Thus woollen cloth is more specific than raw wool.

VI. MOBILITY OF FACTORS

(13) THE MEANING OF MOBILITY

The term mobility, as applied to factors of production, is generally taken to include the concept of specificity considered above. There are, therefore, two aspects to the mobility of factors of production: mobility in the sense of specificity—movement from one employment to another, that is, occupational mobility—and mobility in the geographical sense of movement from one place to another, that is, geographical mobility. Thus, by mobility we mean the ease with which a factor can be transferred from one form of employment to another.

Geographical mobility and specificity, however, do not always go together. Some factors are highly specific, and it may be impossible or at least very difficult to transfer them from one form of production to another. These may be considered immobile in the first sense; on the other hand, non-specific factors are generally mobile in this sense. It is possible to apply the term "mobility" to both land and capital as well as to labour, though land and some forms of capital cannot be moved from one place to another. Capital, however, though durable, wears out, and the entrepreneur has the choice of replacing it or not, in the same place or elsewhere. The entrepreneur is probably the most mobile factor in either sense. He is non-specific, as he often moves from one industry to another of a very different kind on the technical side, as for example from road haulage to oil refining, or from one of the textile industries to motor-car manufacture.

(14) GEOGRAPHICAL MOBILITY OF LABOUR

At first thought it might be imagined that labour would be the most mobile factor in the geographical sense. Human beings have in themselves the power of physical movement, and in these days of excellent transport facilities people travel on an average many more miles each year than at any previous period of the world's history. In medieval England only a limited number of people ever spent even a few days away from the places where they were born. At an earlier period whole peoples, impelled by economic forces, moved away from their previous homeland in search of new places in which to live, and after the discovery of the New World emigration from Europe—sometimes for economic and sometimes for political or religious reasons—began as a mere trickle, but in the late nineteenth century became a flood. In Great Britain in the late eighteenth and early nineteenth centuries there was some movement of landless farm workers from the South of England to the new factory towns of the Midlands and the North.

In Great Britain, in the period between the two World Wars this tendency was reversed, and many people left Durham, Lancashire and South Wales to seek work in South-eastern England. Apart from emigration to the United States, which received people from nearly every country in Europe, people have often shown great reluctance to move from one country to another, even the possibility of higher wages often being an insufficient inducement. Differences of race, language and style of living, and a dislike of dwelling among foreigners, particularly inhabitants of neighbouring States, between which national rivalry has existed, have made most people prefer not to leave their native lands. Nevertheless, there are many examples of people who regularly cross national frontiers on their way to work every day, as for example from Italy to Switzerland and from the Netherlands to Germany.

Persecution for political, religious or racial reasons has generally proved a stronger impelling force to people's movements than economic reasons. French weavers came to England in the seventeenth century to escape the persecution that was being meted out to Protestants in France. During the later 1930s there were considerable movements of people in Europe for these reasons—Jews, liberal democrats, socialists and communists fleeing from Germany in the early part of the period, and refugees from communism later. The Second World War caused a gigantic upheaval of the people of Europe, and large numbers of "displaced persons" came to Great Britain. In the 1950s and 1960s many people came to this country from the West Indies and Pakistan, the reason in this case being economic. In spite of all these examples of movements of peoples, economists on the whole are still inclined to agree with Adam Smith that "a man is of all sorts of luggage the most difficult to be transported."

Even during the great depression of 1929–35, when unemployment was less severe in some parts of Great Britain than others, there was often unwillingness, especially among older workers, to leave the districts most severely affected to seek work elsewhere—a tendency for the unemployed labour to expect work of the desired kind to be brought to it. Direction of labour, however, is incompatible with democratic government.

The longer people live in one place, the more attached they become to it and the more reluctant they are to move elsewhere, for ties of friendship become stronger, and people become more closely associated with the social activities of the place. To move to another town means going among strangers and often losing one's old friends. After living a long time in one town a certain position of social importance may have been achieved, which may be completely lost by removal elsewhere. A job can be made uncomfortable by a man's immediate superiors, and if he is satisfied with the conditions under which he works he may prefer not to risk the unknown. All these may be considered as non-monetary advantages of staying in one place, and it may take quite considerable monetary inducement to overcome them. Another thing making for immobility of labour is the housing question. Whether a person rents or owns a house, removal to another town may involve considerable financial sacrifice. If a house is owned it will have to be sold and heavy legal charges incurred in addition to the cost of removal, and there are wide differences in the prices of similar houses in different parts of the country.

(15) OCCUPATIONAL MOBILITY OF LABOUR

Movement of labour from one occupation to another generally takes place indirectly. Though it might not be possible, for example, to expand the Civil Service by drafting people from textile mills, a redistribution of labour between these two occupations might be brought about through a number of intermediate stages. The Civil Service may attract people from other kinds of clerical work, these posts then being filled (say) by shop assistants, who in turn may perhaps be replaced by mill workers. Assuming the Civil Service to be offering the most attractive type of work and the mill the least attractive, an increase in the demand for workers in the former occupation will eventually lead to a reduction in the amount of labour available for the other, but this result will be achieved only after considerable changes have also taken place in the distribution of labour between other occupations.

The easiest method, however, of transferring labour from one industry to another is by the entry of boys and girls leaving school. A declining industry will attract few new entrants, and so vacancies brought about by retirement and other causes will not be filled, with the result that the total labour force in that industry will be reduced. On the other hand, an expanding industry will attract a larger proportion of new entrants, often by offering a higher rate of pay, and so will increase its labour force. Redistribution of labour among different occupations is gradually brought about in this way, but it is a method that is very slow in working itself out. Occupational mobility of labour is considered further in Chapter XVIII.

(16) THE MOST IMPORTANT FACTOR

At different times it has been asserted that labour is the most important factor of production. The classical economists in the early nineteenth century adopted this view. They wished to show that the value of a commodity depended on the amount of labour involved in its production. For political reasons this idea was again stressed later. Consequently, these economists emphasised the fact that land was a gift of Nature, while capital, they said, owed its origin to labour expended upon its production in the past. In their view, labour was an active factor, whereas land and capital were passive. It has, however, been one of the main purposes of this chapter to stress the point that all factors are merely resources at the disposal of the entrepreneur, and therefore, if the entrepreneur is accepted as a separate factor, labour is no more active economically than land or capital, the entrepreneur being the only factor. It was further pointed out by these early economists that some land was not worth cultivating, and therefore no one would pay anything for its use while there was no parallel of "wageless" labour. There are, however, a few people—their number fortunately being small—who on account of mental or physical disability are unable to undertake ordinary forms of employment. These "unemployables" are very similar economically to the "useless" kind of land. It was also stated that labour has some choice in the kind and amount of work it is willing to perform. There is probably a greater element of truth in the statement today than at the time when it was first made. Again, labour was declared to be the most important factor, because, if unemployed, it suffers a lower standard of living, whereas if land and capital are unemployed their owners merely suffer a loss of income. This appears to be a somewhat ingenuous argument. The services of all factors of production are owned by men and women, whether the factor be labour, land, capital or organisation, and whichever factors are unemployed (if labour is unemployed it is fairly certain that other factors also will be unemployed), the owners of those factors will suffer a decline in their incomes and a lowering of their standard of living.

A case can be made out on behalf of each of the other factors for considering it the most important in production. Take land, for example. It has been said that "the use of a certain area of the earth's surface is a primary condition of anything that man can do."[1] Of capital it can be argued that the greater the amount used in production, the greater the output, and the claim has been made that the increasing rate of recent economic progress has been due mainly to the application of more capital to production, the comparative poverty of those countries with little capital being contrasted with the greater wealth of those with a plentiful supply. On behalf of the entrepreneur it can be said that the other factors are of little economic importance unless production is efficiently organised. The fact is that all factors are important to production, for the co-operation of all is required, and no useful purpose is served by singling out any one of them for special commendation.

RECOMMENDATIONS FOR FURTHER READING

J. R. Hicks: *The Social Framework*, Chapters 6 and 7.
A. Marshall: *Principles of Economics*, Book IV, Chapters 1–6.

QUESTIONS

1. In what ways may the supply of labour be influenced by the State? (R.S.A. Adv.)

2. In what manner may the economic well-being of the community be affected by labour efficiency? How may the productivity of labour be increased? (R.S.A. Adv.)

3. Define the following terms and consider the relations between them: Wealth, Capital, Land. (C.I.S. Inter.)

4. "Land as a factor of production has lost much of its former importance." Comment on this statement. (A.C.C.A. Inter.)

5. Explain how insurance protects a business man against risks. Is there any type of risk that is not insurable? (I.T.)

6. It has been said that control must be vested in those who take the risk of enterprise. Comment on this statement. (I.B. Econ.)

[1] A. Marshall: *Principles of Economics*, IV, II, 2.

7. What factors influence the efficiency of labour? What steps can an employer take to increase the efficiency of the labour he employs? (C.C.S. Final.)

8. "It is the entrepreneur who bears most of the risks of industry." Examine this statement, bringing out the main functions of the entrepreneur in connection with the organisation of industry. (I.B.)

9. Explain the functions of the entrepreneur and show where he is to be found in modern industry. (C.I.S. Inter.)

10. What are the chief "business decisions" which an entrepreneur has to make? (A.C.C.A. Inter.)

11. What do you understand by the phrase: "*mobility* of factors of production"? To what extent are factors of production "mobile" in the sense in which you have defined the term? (D.P.A.)

12. What do you understand by "the law of diminishing returns?" Do you consider it to be universally applicable? (Exp.)

13. Explain the functions of the *entrepreneur* and describe how they are performed in the various forms of large-scale enterprise in the United Kingdom today. (G.C.E. Adv.)

14. Explain what is meant by the law of diminishing returns. (G.C.E. Adv.)

15. How can the mobility of labour be increased? Why is it important? (Final Degree.)

16. Examine the validity and usefulness of dividing the factors of production into the three broad categories of Land, Labour and Capital. (Final Degree.)

CHAPTER IV

CAPITAL

I. THE MEANING OF CAPITAL

(1) THE CAPITAL OF A RETAILER

Different people define capital in different ways. To those unacquainted with economic theory the term presents less difficulty, as they generally take it to mean money. If John Brown says that he would set up in business for himself if it were not for the fact that he possesses insufficient capital his hearers will take it to mean that he has not enough money for the purpose, and Brown would probably welcome a friend's offer to lend him money. A business man, however, does not want money for its own sake. If Brown contemplates opening a retail shop he will use his money-capital to secure suitable premises, fit them out suitably for the particular branch of the retail trade he intends to enter, purchase a certain amount of stock, and, if he is wise, keep some cash in reserve. Having now spent nearly all his money in this way, can it be said that Brown has less capital than he had at first? In fact, what has happened is that the form of Brown's capital has changed and now consists mainly of real things—a shop and its fittings, a quantity of stock together with only a small amount of cash.

The more durable part of his capital, that should require renewal only at fairly long intervals, is known as his *fixed* capital, and that part of his capital that he requires for the everyday running of his business, and which is constantly changing its form, is known as his *circulating* capital. The premises and fixtures comprise Brown's fixed capital, while his stock, cash in hand and any debts owing to him by customers to whom he has granted credit comprise his circulating capital. The form of this capital changes every time a transaction takes place: whenever he sells anything he depletes his stock and increases his cash; whenever he buys stock he increases his stock and reduces his cash. His cash in hand is known as liquid capital, because in this form it is capable of being converted into any variety of either fixed or circulating capital. In the case of the manufacturing business the fixed capital will consist of factory premises and machinery, while raw materials, partly finished goods and money set aside for the payment of wages form the circulating capital.

(2) CAPITAL TO AN ACCOUNTANT

The accountant, too, tends to consider capital as money, for he assigns money values to all the assets of a business—for example, when he draws up a balance sheet. Suppose that after being in business for a year Brown employs an accountant to draw up a balance sheet for him. It might read as follows:

TABLE II

John Brown's Balance Sheet at Dec. 31st, 19—

Liabilities	£	Assets	£
Sundry Creditors . . .	175	Premises	2,000
Loan	1,000	Fittings	350
Capital	2,610	Stock	1,030
		Sundry Debtors . . .	25
		Cash in hand and at Bank . .	380
	£3,785		£3,785

Here capital is taken to mean the excess of assets over liabilities, or the "net worth" of the trader, and so represents the capital owned by Brown as distinct from the capital he employs. The capital employed by him includes the whole of his assets, excepting debts owing to him— that is, £3,760 (£3,785 − £25).

(3) CAPITAL TO AN ECONOMIST

To the economist capital is a factor of production, or, as is sometimes said, wealth used for the production of further wealth. Confusion sometimes arises when capital is treated as if it were the same thing as wealth. In Chapter II wealth was defined as a stock of goods existing at a given time that yield utility, have a money value, are limited in supply and the ownership of which is transferable from one person to another. If capital is a factor of production it must be restricted to wealth used to assist production. Some wealth is used to assist production and some is not. Thus, all capital is wealth, but all wealth is not capital. The stained glass in York Minster is wealth—even though its money value cannot be assessed—but it is not capital. On the other hand, a blast-furnace is obviously an example of that particular type of wealth known as capital. Even when this distinction between wealth and capital is accepted, there is still considerable difference of opinion as to which goods are capital and which are not.

Before discussing this question further, however, it is necessary to define consumers' and producers' goods.

Consumers' goods. The ultimate aim of all production is to provide consumers with those goods which yield them satisfaction. These are goods in the form in which they are wanted by the people who actually wish to make use of them, and comprise such things as bread and other foods, clothing, household furniture, books, etc. Consumers' goods are sometimes called final products.

Producers' goods. Unlike consumers' goods, these things are not desired for their own sake, but only because of the assistance they render to the production of other goods. They comprise factory buildings and industrial plant, tools and machinery, raw materials (raw cotton, raw wool, iron ore, wood pulp, etc.), all goods that have not reached the final stage of manufacture (grey—that is, undyed—cloth, steel, newsprint, etc.) and means of transport (railway systems, roads, motor lorries, etc.). Producers' goods are sometimes called capital goods or intermediate products.

There is not, however, a hard-and-fast line of demarcation between these two types of goods. Cotton thread used by a tailor would be a producers' good, but if purchased by a housewife it might be considered a consumers' good. A motor car might be a producers' good to a commercial traveller who used it entirely for business purposes, but to a man who used his car solely for pleasure it would be a consumers' good. If the commercial traveller uses his car at the week-end to take his family for a day's outing in the country, does it then become a consumers' good? In this case the same article is at one time being used as a producers' good and at another as a consumers' good.

Some writers class stocks of consumers' goods held by manufacturers, middlemen or wholesalers, and retailers as capital. This can be justified on two grounds. It is consistent with accountancy practice, for a balance sheet includes the value of unsold stocks among the assets of the firm. To the economist, too, the act of production is not finally completed until the goods have actually been handed over to the people who desire to make use of them, and so wholesale and retail distribution are merely the latest stages in the process of production. By definition also goods that have not reached the final stage of production are producers' goods. It is probably more useful, however, to restrict capital as an economic term to the more generally accepted forms of producers' goods listed above, and to exclude unsold stocks of consumers' goods.

This does not quite resolve the difficulty, for some consumers' goods are durable, and at least strongly resemble capital goods, in that they yield services to their owners over a considerable period of time, though durability is not an essential attribute of capital goods. Houses come within this category, and nearly a quarter of the total wealth of

Great Britain is in this form. In the case of the landlord who owns a row of houses, which he has let to tenants in return for payment of rent, it would no doubt be felt that these houses comprise the landlord's capital, but there would be less certainty regarding a house occupied by the owner himself. Some writers resolve the difficulty by calling such things as houses personal or social capital, but this is more of a classification according to ownership than according to function.

In the modern world a good deal of production is devoted to the manufacture of armaments. Such things cannot be regarded as either consumers' goods or producers' goods. They resemble capital goods in one respect—their production withdraws factors of production from the manufacture of consumers' goods, but they certainly do not assist the production of other goods!

II. CAPITAL, MONEY AND INCOME

(4) CAPITAL YIELDS INCOME

There is another aspect of capital that is sometimes stressed—the fact that capital yields income. By income is meant an addition to an existing stock of wealth. Adam Smith said that a person's capital was "that part of his stock from which he expects to derive an income." Marshall made this definition more precise by expressly excluding land, which also yields income—a feature of all kinds of property. Capital is a factor of production, and the extent of a country's stock of it is an important influence on its volume of production. For the service capital renders to production its owner receives payment; a sort of hire-charge paid by those using it. The owner of shares in a company receives a share of the profits in the form of a dividend. Shares may be said to yield an income, but this income is earned by the real assets, the capital goods, which the shares represent. Capital is a stock of a certain kind of goods existing at a given time; income is an addition to a stock of goods over a period of time.

Capital considered as a stock of producers' goods used to assist in the production of other goods is the entrepreneur's approach to capital.

(5) MONEY AS CAPITAL

When Robinson Crusoe found a quantity of gold coins in the wrecked ship he was at first doubtful whether they were worth the trouble of taking ashore. Smiling at the sight of this money, he apostrophised it in this way: "What are thou good for? Thou art not worth to me, no, not the taking off the ground. One of these knives is worth all this heap." Being a prudent man, however, he took the gold with him.

To a solitary person in Crusoe's situation money was useless, and he could only hoard it. The tools he found on the ship and those he made were capital goods, factors of production capable of being used in the production either of further capital goods or of things to satisfy his immediate wants—that is, consumers' goods. The money was not capital to him, for it could not help in the satisfaction of his smallest want. Money is simply a means of exchange, and becomes capital only when it gives command over producers' goods.

Similarly, a modern community *as a whole* cannot regard money as either wealth or capital. To increase the quantity of money will not make that community one iota richer than it was before, for unless there is a corresponding increase in the quantity of goods, the value of money will fall—that is, prices will rise—and so the increased quantity of money will purchase no more than could be bought previously.

Money can, however, be exchanged for capital goods or any other kind of goods. An individual can, therefore, reasonably consider his money to be wealth. It has been seen that for this reason the accountant and the business man look upon money as capital, and when taking stock of the assets of the business, assess their value in terms of money. When a new company is formed the capital it requires is stated as a sum of money. When people save, they save money. When they "invest" by buying shares in a new company they purchase them for money, but the company desires the money only because it can be converted into real capital goods—factory buildings, machinery, raw materials, etc. In ordinary speech investment is usually regarded as a monetary action, but to the economist investment means the actual production of capital goods. Each share in a company represents a certain fraction of ownership of capital goods. In the strict economic sense, therefore, the shares themselves cannot be regarded as capital, but are merely titles to ownership. If an inventory were to be made of a country's stock of capital the inclusion of both the value of the shares and of the capital goods would result in double counting.

Can Government Stock ("gilt-edged") be regarded as capital? Some Government Stock is similar to the shares in a company; Transport Stock represents the money value of the real assets of the Transport Commission—railways, canals, docks, etc. The same applies to Gas Stock, Electricity Stock and all the other compensation Stocks issued to the former share-holders of nationalised industries. As with company shares, the real asset and the stock must not both be counted. The position is quite different, however, with most Government Stock, for this largely represents Government borrowing in the past to finance wars, and therefore it represents no tangible assets. Again, an individual who holds (say) £500 of 3% Savings Bonds may justifiably look upon this as personal capital, for it yields him an income of £15 per annum, but obviously the country as a whole is no richer because individuals and business firms hold some £28,500 million of Government Stock—that is, Government debt. By the same argument the country *as a whole* is really no poorer because of this huge National Debt.

III. CAPITAL AND OTHER FACTORS

(6) CAPITAL AND LABOUR

Capital, therefore, has to be produced, and some factors of production—land, labour and some capital itself, organised by the entrepreneur—have to be employed for this purpose. Karl Marx, author of *Das Kapital*, argued that all capital consisted entirely of labour that had been expended in the past. One of the first steps taken by Man in his climb up from savagery was to fashion for himself some simple tool, probably out of stone. This crude piece of capital would be made by hand, labour and land combining to produce a third factor—capital, and from this simple beginning ever more efficient types of capital have been developed. According to Marx, capital was nothing more than stored-up labour from the past ("crystallised" labour, as he called it), while land was a free gift of Nature, and so its ownership could not entitle anyone to an income from it. Since he did not recognise the entrepreneur as a separate factor, he argued, therefore, that there was really only one factor of production—labour—that was worthy of reward.

The accumulation of modern forms of capital, however, requires the co-operation of all factors of production. It also involves sacrifice; the sacrifice of present satisfaction in order to be able to enjoy a greater satisfaction in the future. An increased stock of capital makes it possible for a country to increase its volume of production and so raise the standard of living of its people.

(7) CAPITAL AND LAND

Some of the arguments formerly put forward to show that land was different in kind from the other factors have already been considered, and reasons given for their rejection. If capital is defined as wealth used in the production of further wealth, such a definition would logically include land. By land Ricardo meant the "original and inalienable powers of the soil," but these qualities are very difficult, if not impossible, to define or in practice separate from other qualities of land for there is little land (if any) of economic use that does not owe something to human effort and capital having been expended upon it. Land, in ordinary speech, is as much wealth as anything else, and down to comparatively recent times it was the principal form of wealth. It has been said that any distinction between land and capital is obviously arbitrary, for the conception of land as distinct from capital is "in flagrant and irreconcilable contradiction with the usages of language."[1] An accountant, compiling a balance sheet, would include land owned by a farmer or a railway as part of the capital of each. Similarly, it might be argued that in Aristotle's time the labour of slaves was capital.

The difficulty of framing mutually exclusive definitions of land, labour and capital, and the futility of many subtle distinctions often made between them, merely serve to emphasise once again the economic similarity of these factors. It is convenient to use the terms land, labour, capital, but it must be remembered that these names only broadly indicate certain groups of economic resources.

IV. CAPITALISTIC PRODUCTION

(8) CAPITAL AND DIVISION OF LABOUR

The essential feature, however, of capital as an agent of production is that its employment makes possible a "capitalistic" method of production. Division of labour makes possible the use of capital in the form of machinery. The essential feature of division of labour is specialisation of processes, and the greater the extent to which specialisation is taken, the more "capitalistic" is said to be the method of production. In this sense the word "capitalistic" merely means making use of more capital goods, and it would be applicable equally to production under communism, where capital is collectively owned, as to production under capitalism, where private ownership of capital exists. The term "roundabout" is also frequently used to describe a capitalistic form of production.

Division of labour, by giving each man a smaller task and allowing him to become more proficient in a single operation, leads to a large increase in output. How much greater, then, will output be if at each one of these stages of production a machine is employed to do the purely repetitive work. The greater the number of processes into which production is divided and the greater the amount of machinery (that is, capital) that can be employed, the greater will be the total output. The more capital that is employed (that is, the more capitalistic or more roundabout the method of production), the larger the output. Capital, then, makes possible even greater specialisation, with

[1] P. Wicksteed: *Common-sense of Political Economy*, Vol. I, p. 366.

the result that output is increased. Thus, the countries with the largest stocks of capital are those with the largest volumes of production, and the peoples living in these countries are those who enjoy the highest standards of living.

(9) "WAITING"

The use of capital therefore makes possible a larger output than could otherwise be achieved, but before a capitalistic method of production can be adopted the capital itself has to be made. It is usual to quote the case of Robinson Crusoe, alone, as he was at first, on his desert island. Having salvaged from the wrecked ship a certain amount of capital in the form of a chest of carpenter's tools, some nails and spikes, he made himself a raft. His earliest efforts towards providing himself with food, clothing and shelter depended principally on his own exertions. If in such circumstances he wished to speed up production of a commodity he considered necessary to his existence he would first have to make the capital required. To quote from his Journal: "The want of tools (a shovel or spade) made my work go on heavily . . . my other work *having stood still* because of my making these tools." This element of "waiting" is an important aspect of capital formation. During this period of waiting Crusoe had to sacrifice some present satisfaction; he may have had to curtail the amount of time he could afford to devote to hunting or fishing, or more probably, in his circumstances, he would have to sacrifice his leisure. His incentive to do so would be the knowledge that with the help of the machines he was making he would be able with less effort on his part to produce things more quickly and in greater quantity in the future.

An example from actual life closely akin to this was provided between the two World Wars by the U.S.S.R. In 1928, when the first Five-Year Plan was launched, it was a country with little capital in proportion to its area and the size of its population, though it possessed vast undeveloped mineral resources. For a period of five years, therefore, it was determined that production should be devoted chiefly to the making of capital goods, such as factory buildings, industrial plant, blast-furnaces, power-stations, machinery, etc. What the Russian people wanted, of course, was more consumers' goods, but they were told that they would have to *wait* until the necessary capital equipment with which to make them had been accumulated. The completion of the first Five-Year Plan in 1933 was succeeded by a second of similar duration. The first plan covered more particularly the production of heavy capital goods, the second being devoted to lighter capital goods. This meant that the people had to continue to wait a further period of five years, but with the hope of a vast flow of consumers' goods coming off the production lines in the future. The Second World War, however, broke out before this hope could be realised, and the consequent destruction of capital equipment was so great that a further period of waiting became necessary. A large increase in the output of consumers' goods at last appears to be possible as a result of the accumulation of capital during this long period of "waiting."

(10) THE STRUCTURE OF PRODUCTION

It is clear, therefore, that in order to make production more capitalistic, greater specialisation of processes is first required. The greater the degree of specialisation, the greater will be the number of processes. The larger the desired output, the more intermediate stages there will have to be in the process of production. According to the size of the required output, the entrepreneur will then be able to vary the length of the process. The more capitalistic the method of production, the longer will be the time interval between the moment when the decision to undertake a piece of production is taken and the time when the goods begin to flow out on to the market. Prof. Hayek[1] speaks of the lengthening or shortening of the period of production as altering the structure of production. To increase specialisation by introducing more intermediate stages, and so making production more capitalistic, is thus considered to be a lengthening of the structure of production. Similarly, to shorten the structure of production would mean making production less capitalistic. If the structure of production is lengthened, the period of "waiting" will be longer, but output will eventually be much greater.

V. CAPITAL FORMATION AND CONSUMPTION

(11) CAPITAL ACCUMULATION

It was possible for Robinson Crusoe to supply himself with a small quantity of capital only by giving up to its construction some of the time he would otherwise have devoted to other pursuits. In a non-monetary economy—that is, an economic system where no money was employed—the sacrifice involved in accumulating capital would be clear; production of goods desired for their own sake—that is, consumers' goods—would have to be curtailed in order that capital or producers' goods might be produced. Since each country has only limited resources of land, labour and capital, there will be no resources available for making producers' goods, if they are entirely given over

---

[1] F. A. Hayek: *Prices and Production*, Lecture II.

to the production of consumers' goods. A country's stock of capital at any given period of time is, then, the result of sacrifice by its people in the past, and any further increase in its stock of capital can be achieved only by forgoing the satisfaction of some present wants. Putting this in another way, it merely means that the quantity of goods consumed in a period must be less than the total produced if capital formation is to take place. For:

Capital formation = Production − Consumption

If the quality of a country's resources is so poor that it requires the application of nearly all of them to enable its people to provide themselves only with the bare necessities for existence, it will have little opportunity of increasing its store of capital, and the accumulation of capital will be a slow, painful process. In all countries the early stages in capital accumulation are slow, but once having acquired some stock of capital, this in turn can be used to assist further capital accumulation —that is to say, the rate of accumulation proceeds with cumulative effect. Thus, to provide a developing country with capital will speed up its economic progress.

Capital formation depends on saving. Money often tends to hide the real working of economic forces, and this is the "money veil" of which economists used to speak, but even in a monetary economy the accumulation of capital proceeds on similar lines to that outlined above. Abstention from consumption enables capital to be produced. Such abstention is called *saving.* Thus Robinson Crusoe was able to save even though his was a non-monetary economy. In a modern economic system where money is in use saving means refraining from spending on consumers' goods. If consumers spent their entire incomes on consumers' goods there could be no accumulation of capital goods, for the entire existing productive resources of land, labour and capital would be required to satisfy this demand. If, now, consumers decide to save a portion of their incomes—say, one-sixth—then one-sixth of the country's resources can be devoted to making capital goods. The following diagram will perhaps make this clearer:

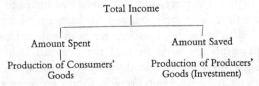

Thus the production of capital goods depends on saving. Economists use the term investment to mean the actual production of capital goods, and so it can be said that investment depends on saving. A more detailed consideration of saving and investment must be postponed till later, but it may be noted at this stage that mere saving does not guarantee that investment will take place—it simply makes investment possible. Saving reduces the demand for consumers' goods and frees resources that might otherwise have been used for their production, but if this results in these freed resources merely remaining idle it is quite clear that no capital formation ensues.

(12) CAPITAL ACCUMULATION IN GREAT BRITAIN

Capital accumulation is not likely to take place unless people are reasonably sure that their property will be secure, and so saving will be greater in a State where law and order are maintained. Saving, too, is a habit that takes time to develop. Unless opportunities for investment exist, there will be less inducement to save.

Before the eighteenth century there were few outlets for people's savings. The Government borrowed mainly to finance wars, and savings lent by people for this purpose were dissipated without their resulting in the production of real capital. Lending to the Government, however, developed the habit of saving, and in the eighteenth century enabled the new trading companies to obtain the funds with which to finance their activities. In spite of the losses incurred by many investors at the time of the South Sea Bubble (1720), people continued to put their savings into new ventures. During the second half of the eighteenth century the expansion of the turnpike-road system, with increasing expenditure on road improvements, presented people with new opportunities. The Industrial Revolution of the late eighteenth and nineteenth centuries provided further outlets for the investment of savings. The early factory businesses were small and generally financed by the savings of the small proprietors, their friends and relations, or, as in the case of the woollen industry, by merchants. Profits were rarely wasted in riotous living, but instead were put back into the business, the owners themselves often leading very frugal lives.

During the nineteenth century saving increased for a number of reasons. In the first place, the National Debt increased at a much slower rate than the population, and for long periods the debt was actually declining, so that taxation per head required to cover the interest payments declined. In 1815 the National Debt was £858 million, but by 1899 it had been reduced to £635 million. The building of railways offered further opportunities for the investment of savings. When joint-stock companies were permitted limited liability this reduced the risks of small investors, and so not only encouraged the formation of new companies, thereby increasing investment opportunities, but also increased the incentive to save, at a time when opportunities for this kind of investment were increasing. Not only did opportunities for investment increase but also with the rising standard of living there came increased ability to save.

(13) MAINTENANCE OF CAPITAL

Some capital is by its nature more durable than other forms of capital—a loom, for example, will last longer than the yarn fed into it. Raw materials and partly finished goods are forms of capital that are about to be converted into consumers' goods. In order to maintain stocks of these things, their supply must be constantly renewed. Even more durable forms of capital eventually wear out—though some of the machines used in the West Riding woollen industry have been in continuous use for over eighty years. Railway engines have often had very long lives, but motor buses and aircraft are less durable. Each year, however, some capital wears out and has to be replaced. All such capital has to be made good before any addition can be made to a country's total stock of capital. Therefore a certain amount of production each year must be devoted to the replacement of worn-out capital, for, if progress is to be maintained, new capital must be produced in excess of that required to cover depreciation.

Should old capital in good condition be scrapped? People are apt to boast of the durability of some of the capital goods produced in this country. They will point with pride to a machine that has given half a century of service and praise the workmanship that has made this possible. Economically, however, this may not be desirable. For economic progress to be maintained it is not merely necessary for worn-out capital to be renewed, but out-of-date capital also should be replaced. To scrap machinery, however old, that is still in good running order appears at first glance to be wasteful, but it is much more wasteful to continue to use obsolescent machinery when more efficient machinery is available. The extraordinary longevity of some of the machinery in both the cotton and woollen industries was one of the reasons for the long delay in re-equipping these industries with modern capital. One of the main arguments for the retention of old capital that is still in good condition is that it is wasteful to scrap it. The main question to be answered in such cases, however, is: will the newer capital be more efficient than the old? If the answer is in the affirmative, then the old capital should certainly be scrapped and replaced by new. The loss resulting from scrapping obsolete capital is easily outweighed by the increased efficiency of the new, up-to-date capital installed to replace it.

Therefore, in order to maintain capital intact a certain amount of production every year has to be given up to the replacement of worn-out and obsolete capital.

(14) CAPITAL CONSUMPTION

If a country ceases to add to its stock of capital it will fail to make economic progress; if it fails to make good depreciation of its capital—that is, if it does not replace worn-out capital—it is said to be consuming capital. Depreciation of capital can take two forms—the wearing out of machinery, etc., and the using up of stocks. Capital consumption may occur if too great a proportion of a country's resources are devoted to the production of consumers' goods, since it may mean that insufficient resources will be available for making producers' goods. This is really only another way of saying that the community as a whole is spending too much of its income on the satisfaction of current wants and that not enough saving is taking place. In such circumstances the stock of capital goods will be gradually reduced—that is, the country will become poorer, for as capital becomes worn out there will be no new capital to replace it. This will have a cumulative effect and after a short time the production of all kinds of goods will begin to decline. The condition will be very similar to that of an individual who is living beyond his means; he will be able to satisfy more of his wants for a time, but in the end he will be poorer.

Living on capital. A person is said to be "living on his capital" if he is having to supplement his current income by drawing on past savings in order to make both ends meet. When he has exhausted his "wealth" he will have to accept a lower standard of living. When a country is consuming capital the consequences will be very much the same. A country that fails to maintain its stock of capital is sometimes said to be "living on capital." Such a condition is now most likely to occur only in war-time. Some capital may be consumed as a direct result of enemy action; factories, machinery, roads, railways, harbours may be destroyed, but even if little or no loss is caused in this way, the nation's energies may be concentrated to such an extent on the effort to win the war that only a bare minimum of consumers' and producers' goods will be produced, most productive resources being given up to the manufacture of weapons of war, and as much labour as can be spared being drafted into the armed forces. At such times it may be necessary to run the risk that the war can be won before capital equipment at home deteriorates to such an extent that production begins to fall. Great Britain had to take this risk during the Second World War (1939–45), and for nearly six years the country was living on capital. When the war ended even the most casual observer could not fail to notice the deterioration of woodwork or ironwork for want of painting, the bad condition of many motor buses due to overloading and excessive use during the war and the frequency of breakdowns. Roads, too, were in need of repair. A growing population requires an increasing supply of capital goods. The population of Great Britain increased by over $1\frac{1}{2}$ million between 1939 and 1945, but because of the necessity to concentrate on the war effort there was no increased provision of schools, electric generating plant, gasworks or water supplies. Maintenance of the railways had also been neglected as much as was consistent with safety, and because they had been greatly over-worked during the war, they found themselves in 1945 with a shortage of rolling stock, coaches, wagons and engines, and with much equipment in need of repair. In factories also there was a great need of new machinery. Much capital, then, had been consumed in this way during six years of war, and had to be made good before further capital accumulation could take place.

Robinson Crusoe could increase his stock of capital only by reducing provision for his immediate needs; a modern State can increase its stock of capital in a short time only by severe sacrifice of current production and consumption of consumers' goods. Production normally has four objectives—to produce consumers' goods, to provide for depreciation, to accumulate capital and to produce for export. This can be shown diagrammatically as follows:

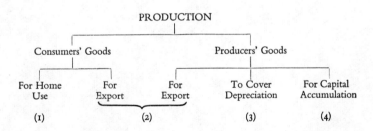

With the exception of the normal expansion of production arising from increased productivity, production for one of these four purposes can be increased only if there is curtailment of production for the other three purposes.

RECOMMENDATIONS FOR FURTHER READING

J. R. Hicks: *The Social Framework*, Chapters 8–10.
Irving Fisher: *The Nature of Capital and Income*, Chapters 4–6.

QUESTIONS

1. What do you understand by the term "capital?" (C.I.S. Inter.)

2. Discuss the various forms in which the capital of a country exists. (Exp.)

3. One of the major problems today is the replacement, renewal and extension of capital equipment. Discuss how this tends to be achieved in a system of private enterprise. (I.H.A.)

4. "Most economists agree that to secure a steadily expanding level of production in an industrial community 10 to 15 per cent. of the national income should be invested in new capital development." Comment on this statement and explain the relation between the production of Capital Goods and that of Consumption Goods. (A.C.C.A. Inter.)

5. "We shall define capital, then, as that sum of means which is available at any moment for transference to entrepreneurs." (Schumpeter.)
Discuss this statement. (A.C.C.A. Inter.)

6. Discuss the different aspects of the statement that a nation may be "living on its capital." (C.I.S. Final.)

7. What is meant by maintaining capital intact? (Final Degree.)

CHAPTER V

THE POPULATION PROBLEM

I. THE PAST

(1) THE CHANGING CHARACTER OF THE PROBLEM

For over a hundred and fifty years economists have been keenly interested in the population problem, but, says Marshall, "in a more or less vague form it has occupied the attention of thoughtful men in all ages of the world."[1] The form taken by the problem has varied with the particular conditions of place and time. At one period the aim might be to keep up the number of males, to make good the ravages of war; at another time, maybe, there was a fear lest the growth of population should outrun food supplies.

Linked up with the question of food production, the population problem was one of the earliest of Man's economic problems. Early peoples were keenly alive to it, and had their own methods of tackling it. The spread of Christianity, with its cultivation of respect for human life, aggravated the problem of peoples who had previously kept down numbers by such practices as infanticide. If a country is under-populated its people will be poor because they are too few in numbers to enjoy the advantages of large-scale production; if a country is over-populated in proportion to its stock of capital and land, again the people will be poor because output per head will be low.

In Great Britain in the late eighteenth and early nineteenth centuries the danger of over-population appeared to men like Malthus to be imminent, though apparently the march of events later in that century showed such fears to have been ill-founded. By the 1920s the whole character of the problem seemed to have changed from a fear of over-population to one of under-population. By the middle of the twentieth century, though the fear of a decline in population in Great Britain had not been entirely removed, some writers, taking a wider view and considering the world as a whole, were again becoming alarmed by the prospect of a population too vast for the resources of the world to feed.

(2) POPULATION CHANGES IN GREAT BRITAIN SINCE 1801

It is only since 1801, when the first census was taken in Great Britain, that accurate population statistics have been available. Though

[1] A. Marshall: *Principles of Economics*, IV, IV, 1.

particulars of the population of the country before that date must, therefore, of necessity be based only on estimates, it is generally agreed that
up to the year 1700, when it has been calculated that the population of
Great Britain was 7 million, population had been increasing at a very
slow rate. During the preceding six or seven centuries there had been
little difference between the birth rate and the death rate, both of which
were high, and for considerable periods the population barely replaced
itself, and in some years actually declined. Infant mortality was exceptionally high, and probably not more than half the children born
survived to the age of twenty-one. Famine, pestilence and war were
largely responsible for the high death rate.

By the time of the first census in 1801 the population of Great Britain
had reached a total of 10½ million, an estimated increase of 50% in the
course of a hundred years. During the following century growth was
even more rapid, the population increasing by three and a half times
between 1801 and 1901, to give a total of 37 million. After 1901 the
rate of growth slackened compared with the previous hundred and
fifty years, but the population continued to increase. The following
table shows the astounding expansion of population in Great Britain
during 1750–1961:

TABLE III

Growth of Population 1750–1965
(Census figures except for 1750 and 1965)

	Million						
	1750 (est.)	1801	1851	1901	1951	1961	1965 (est.)
England and Wales	6·3	8·9	17·9	32·5	43·9	45·7	47·2
Scotland . .	1·2	1·6	2·9	4·5	5·1	5·2	5·3
Ireland· . .	3·0	5·0	6·6	4·5	—	—	—

The change in the relative positions of the three areas is of interest.
In 1750 Ireland had a population only slightly less than half that of
England and Wales and more than two and a half times that of
Scotland. By 1901 England and Wales had a population nearly eight
times that of Ireland, while Scotland had drawn level with Ireland.
During the second half of the nineteenth century the population of
Ireland declined by one-third, largely as a result of famine and emigra-
tion.

A development somewhat similar to that in Great Britain took place
in most countries of Europe, the period 1801–1901 generally being the
one of greatest expansion, while during 1901–45 the rate of growth has

generally slackened. Since 1950 there has been an upsurge of population in most parts of the world so great as to be described as a "population explosion."

(3) CAUSES OF GROWTH OF POPULATION DURING THE NINE-TEENTH CENTURY

Why, then, did the population of Great Britain, after growing slowly for hundreds of years, increase at so rapid a rate in the late eighteenth and nineteenth centuries? The main cause was the steep fall in the death rate. In 1740 Great Britain had a death rate of 31·7 per thousand; by 1820 it had been reduced to 25·0 per thousand.[1] During this period the birth rate showed little change. In earlier centuries pestilences from time to time swept across Europe, and occurrences such as the Black Death of 1349 and the Great Plague of 1665 were only more serious examples of visitations that were not uncommon. The high death rate affected all classes, mortality being particularly high among children; only one of Queen Anne's seventeen children survived to ten years of age. Samuel Pepys, the famous diarist, was his parents' fifth child, but by the time he was seven years of age he had become the eldest, the four older children all having died. The big Victorian families were the result of a fall in the death rate among children rather than an increase in the size of the family. Development of medicine, where science replaced superstition, the opening of hospitals—new ones were opened in Great Britain at an average rate of one per year from 1700 to 1825—and improved sanitation lessened the incidence of epidemics, and many diseases that had previously been prevalent were completely or partially stamped out, as for example typhus, scurvy and small-pox.

It is no accident, however, that this decline in mortality coincided with the Agrarian and Industrial Revolutions. As a result of the cultivation of root-crops, it became possible to feed cattle during the winter, instead of having to kill off most of them during that season, as had previously been necessary. This meant that supplies of milk and fresh meat were maintained throughout the whole year. A second factor making for improved nutrition was that improved means of transport made a supply of green vegetables more generally available. Two of the main causes of the slow growth of population during the Middle Ages had been the frequency of epidemics and famine in years of bad harvests. As late as 1701 a succession of bad harvests in Scotland resulted in a famine that wiped out more than half the population in some areas. The improved milk supply and the wider distribution of green

[1] By 1957 it had fallen to 11·1; in 1965 it was 12·0. With an increasing number of old people it may be expected to rise in the future.

vegetables were largely responsible for removing the danger of famine from the countries of Western Europe.

Although the fall in the death rate was the chief factor, there was also some increase in the birth rate. Young people were marrying earlier, especially after it was no longer necessary to serve a lengthy period of apprenticeship, during which it had been forbidden to marry. The age of marriage was lowered also because of the increased demand for labour in new manufacturing areas; it became easier for young people to set up homes for themselves by moving to these places. The estab-lishment of the factory system enormously expanded the demand for the labour of both women and children. After marriage a woman could reasonably be expected to earn her own keep, and it was only a few years before children were old enough to work in the factories, and thereby add to the family income. Improved means of transport also made possible the movement to inland areas of bulky goods, including building materials, thus enabling more houses to be built. Fluctuations in the marriage rate in the early nineteenth century were linked to changes in the price of corn; later in that century the trade cycle became the chief influence.

(4) MALTHUS

Although in a vague sort of way his predecessors were aware of the population problem, T. R. Malthus (1766–1834) was the first economist to give it serious attention. Though quite a prolific writer on economic subjects, he is chiefly remembered for his work on what he called "the principle of population." First published in 1798 under the title of an "*Essay on the Principle of Population as it affects the Future improve-ment of Society,*" Malthus during the course of his lifetime revised his work five times, each of the later editions embodying additions and alterations both to the title and to the essay itself. Malthus was much abused by his contemporaries for his pessimistic outlook, but his pur-pose in writing his essay had been to refute the current idea that con-ditions of life were gradually moving towards an earthly paradise. At the time of the publication of the first edition it had become apparent that the population of Great Britain had begun to increase at a more rapid rate than previously. Such a growth of population was a new phenomenon, and led Malthus to speculate on the possible consequences of this new trend. At the same time wages were low and prices high, and there was real distress among the lower-paid workers. The Speen-hamland system (so-called because it was first introduced at the village of that name on the northern outskirts of Newbury in Berkshire) whereby the Poor Law Authorities supplemented the wages of agricultural workers according to the size of their families, soon spread to the rest of the country and encouraged large families.

Malthus declared that there was a "constant tendency in all animated life to increase beyond the nourishment for it." In the animal world the struggle for existence results in the survival of the fittest, whereas the greater the advance made by civilisation, the less is the effect of this tendency on the human race. No populous country, he said, could obtain the necessities of life so easily as a thinly peopled country. Peoples, according to Malthus, unless checked in some way, doubled their numbers every quarter of a century. During his own lifetime he noticed that the increased demand for wheat, consequent on the growth of the population, was causing wheat to be grown on inferior land where the yield per acre was low. This led him to state that while population increased in geometrical progression, food production could be increased only in arithmetical progression, a gross exaggeration of the situation, though he did not use these terms with mathematical precision. He sought, therefore, to show that the means of subsistence placed a limit on the growth of population, an increase in the means of subsistence bringing about an increase in the population, unless this was checked by "vice or misery" due to famine, war or pestilence. In the second edition of his work he added "moral restraint," by which he meant abstention from early marriage.

Malthus summed up his argument in three propositions:

(i) Population is necessarily limited by the means of subsistence.

(ii) Population invariably increases where the means of subsistence increase, unless prevented by some powerful and obvious check.

(iii) These checks are all resolvable into moral restraint, vice and misery.[1]

Malthus was impressed by two things: the rapid increase in population in Great Britain and the Law of Diminishing Returns as applied to food production in this country. Each successive increase in population, he thought, required the bringing into cultivation of ever less fertile land. "The best lands are taken up first, then the next best, then the inferior, at last the worst; at each stage the amount of food produced is less than before." If existing cultivated land were farmed more intensively the same inexorable law would operate, and again there would be diminishing returns. Consequently, it would be impossible to maintain an expansion of food production to keep pace with the increasing population. Great Britain could probably have supported a

[1] T. R. Malthus: *Essay on Population*, Book I, Chapter 2 (in the second and subsequent editions).

much larger population than it had at the time when he wrote his essay, but not a population increasing as rapidly as it was at the end of the eighteenth century. Unless this excessive growth of population were checked the standard of living of the people in this country would be bound to fall. Thus ran Malthus's argument. To him the only hope lay in checking the growth in population, and the remedy he suggested was moral restraint.

Malthus was not, however, unaware of the great improvements in farming methods that were taking place in his day. These improvements in both agricultural and pastoral farming made possible a much larger output than had previously seemed possible. He was not fully alive to the effects of this agrarian revolution, but considered it to be of temporary effect, merely postponing the day when food production would be insufficient for the population's needs.

(5) DID HISTORY PROVE MALTHUS WRONG?

For long it was usual to say that the history of the nineteenth century eventually proved Malthus's argument to be wrong. It was pointed out that although the population of Great Britain increased at a faster rate during the nineteenth century than it did in the fifty years preceding the publication of the first edition of his essay, yet the people enjoyed a higher standard of living at the end of the century than at the beginning. The explanation was to be found, (a) in the opening up during that period of many new lands—the United States of America, Australia, New Zealand, South Africa, and some of the countries of South America, and (b) in the improvement in transport, which made it possible to bring food from the New World to the Old. Most of these countries at this period were primarily producers of foodstuffs and raw materials, and were able to supply food to Great Britain, thus enabling this country to concentrate on the production of manufactured goods. As a result Great Britain could support a much larger population than would have been possible if it had had to feed itself directly from its own resources. Great Britain thus became an industrial country, dependent on the New World for the greater part of its food supply, which was paid for by the export of manufactured goods.

Malthus may perhaps have generalised too easily from the circumstances of the time in which he lived, but he could hardly have been expected to foresee the future tremendous economic development of the New World, though he appears to have been vaguely aware of this possibility. But does this opening up of the New World invalidate his arguments? Just as the effect of the Agrarian Revolution was, according to Malthus, merely to postpone the evil day, so in like manner might not the effect of the development of the New World be again of a temporary nature, its ultimate result merely being to cause the crisis to occur at a higher level of population? Nor can Malthus's critics altogether be blamed for being impressed by the economic development of the newer countries, which made the potential food production of the world appear almost limitless, and the picture painted by Malthus a pessimistic exaggeration. Around them there seemed to be ample evidence that industrial areas could support dense populations. In forecasting a severe decline in the standard of living in Great Britain by the end of the nineteenth century if population continued to increase, Malthus was undoubtedly wrong, for the population was greater and the standard of living much higher in 1900 than in 1800, but for the world as a whole the ideas of Malthus were revived with increased potency in the twentieth century.

II. THE PRESENT

(6) THE MODERN POPULATION PROBLEM: GREAT BRITAIN

The population problem of the twentieth century can be considered from two angles: (a) from the point of view of Great Britain, and (b) from the point of view of the world as a whole. In this country the Malthusian spectre of over-population was replaced for a time by fear of a declining population. In the early Victorian period the average family had between five and six children, but after 1870 the birth rate began to fall, and continued to do so for over half a century.

In the forty years 1801–41 the population of Great Britain increased by 76%, whereas in the forty years 1901–41 the increase was just under 26%. The average number of children per family fell from 5·5 in 1850 to 2·2 in 1930, and this is a more important factor than the birth rate. According to estimates made in the 1920s, the population of Great Britain would begin to decline after 1944, so that by 1956 it would show a reduction of 3 million, and by 1976 a reduction of 12 million as compared with 1944. This forecast proved to be completely wrong, but all such calculations are based on the assumption that "present tendencies continue." The fall in the birth rate slowed down in Great Britain in the later 1930s, but since 1945 it has tended to rise. Throughout the period when the birth rate was falling its effects were to some extent offset by a fall in the death rate. In 1870, for example, the expectation of life at birth was only 41 years for boys and 45 for for girls, but by 1965 it had risen to 68 years for boys and 74 for girls.

What, then, were the causes of this decline in the size of the family? Since there appears to be no evidence of any decline in reproductive capacity, it would seem that the reduction in size of families had been due to deliberate limitation on the part of the parents. It is generally agreed that birth control came to be widely practised. In the late nineteenth century there was increasing propaganda in favour of this practice, which received a rational basis from the Malthusian picture of the miseries of over-population if the expansion of population was not checked. The influence of Malthus is seen in the choice of name for the organisation founded by Annie Besant and Charles Bradlaugh for the propagation of their ideas—the Malthusian League.

TABLE IV

The birth rate in the United Kingdom per 1,000 of population	
1880	34·2
1885	32·9
1890	30·2
1895	30·3
1900	28·7
1905	27·3
1910	25·1
1915	21·9
1920	25·5
1925	18·3
1930	16·3
1935	15·2
1940	14·7
1945	16·3
1950	16·2
1955	15·4
1960	16·2
1965	18·6

Birth control, however, merely made possible the voluntary limitation of the size of the family. The reasons why parents desired smaller families are to be found in the social and economic changes of the period. In the opening years of the Industrial Revolution children became wage-earners at a very early age, and therefore soon ceased to be a burden on their parents. The Factory and Education Acts gradually raised the age at which children were permitted to work in factories, and by the end of the nineteenth century children were no longer a source of income to their parents, but instead had become an expense. There was a widespread desire about this time among people of all classes to raise their standard of living, and this was more difficult where the family was large. Trying to maintain a standard of life may lead to later marriages, and this of itself will reduce the average size of the family. There was, too, greater insecurity of industrial life under the factory system than under the former domestic system, and this insecurity appeared to become greater with the increasing complexity of industrial production, and before the days of social insurance a large family was a great hardship in times of unemployment or sickness. Parents, too, gradually came to desire to do better for their children— for example, to give them wider opportunities for education than they themselves had enjoyed—and this increased the cost of bringing up a family.

Another factor making for small families was the emancipation of women of the better-educated classes, the rearing of a large family being incompatible with their higher status or the pursuit of a career. Perhaps not least in importance was the fact that the small family became fashionable. These factors making for the smaller family influenced the educated classes to a greater extent than other people, so that the larger families tended to be among the less-cultured sections of the community. The following table shows the difference in size of the family in 1911 according to occupation (the figure indicates the variation from the average):

TABLE V

The Size of the Family According to Occupations

Occupation	Size of family as a percentage of average
1. Miners	110
2. Agricultural labourers	106
3. Unskilled labourers	105
4. Skilled workers	101
5. Textile workers	99
6. Employers in industry and retail trade . . .	98
7. Professional workers	86

Based on Table XVIII in the *Report of the Royal Commission on Population*, p. 27.

The average size of family of manual workers is still much greater than that of non-manual workers.

(7) THE "POPULATION EXPLOSION"

Although some of the countries of Western Europe perhaps still face the possibility of a declining population (but as a more distant prospect), for the world as a whole the problem is how to continue expansion of food production to keep pace with expanding population. In other words, Malthus may have been right, after all. His main point

had been the different ratios of increase for food and population, with
the latter tending to outrun the former. Recently, increased concern
has been expressed regarding the inability of food production to keep
up with the rapidly growing population of the world. Until about
1650 the population of the world increased very slowly. It has been
estimated that at that date the population of the world was approximately 540 million. Since then expansion has become increasingly
rapid. Even Western Europe, in spite of the slackening off in the rate
of growth, had 13 million more human beings in 1965 than in 1950.
By 1965 the world's population had reached 3,250 million, and it was
increasing at the stupendous rate of over 65 million a year. For a long
time the greatest numerical increase in population per year has occurred
in Asia, but in recent years both North and South America have shown
greater *rates* of increase. Between 1945 and 1965, for example, the
population of the United States increased from 140 to 194 million,
while that of India increased from 360 to 480 million. It has been
estimated that by the year 2000 the world may have a population of
upwards of 6000 million.

The huge increases in the population of Asia have been brought
about by a sharp fall in the death rate in that part of the world, expectation of life in India increasing from 32 to 54 years between 1945 and
1965. Largely as a result of the teachings of Christianity, a greater
respect for human life developed, and Christian missionaries were
usually accompanied by doctors and nurses. More recently, the
establishment of such institutions as the World Health Organisation
has assisted the decline in mortality in the countries of Asia. For
example, in India the death rate has fallen from 40·4 to 16·3 per thousand
during the past 40 years, but during that period the birth rate has fallen
only from 50·8 to 39·4 per thousand—more than doubling the excess
of births over deaths.

To feed the expanding population of the world it is necessary to
double the production of food every fifty years. Large numbers of
people in many parts of the world today are grossly under-nourished by
Western standards, and even if population were not increasing so
rapidly, it would still be desirable to expand food production. The
peoples of Asia, too, are beginning to demand a higher standard of
living, and countries like India, that were formerly exporters of food,
are becoming importers. The problem of increasing the world's food
supply has been aggravated in some parts of the world by neglect to
maintain the fertility of the topsoil. As a result of soil erosion, there has
been considerable loss of fertility, largely due to short-sighted farming
methods, adopted by "get-rich-quick" farmers looking for im-

mediate returns and with little thought for the future. Where natural vegetation exists soil formation takes place, but when brought under the plough the soil is easily carried away as a result of erosion. Good stock-rearing districts of the States of Kansas, Oklahoma and Texas in the United States have been turned into a great, infertile dust-bowl. During both war periods the high price of wheat led speculators to plough up much grassland in the hope of quick profits, the farms being abandoned as soon as profits fell. Such farmers care nothing for soil-conservation schemes. "Apart from the prevention of war," said Lord Boyd-Orr some years ago, "maintaining the fertility of the top few inches of soil is the biggest problem facing mankind."[1] This view was supported by the late Prof. Sir Dudley Stamp, who adds: "Unless soil erosion is checked the whole world is committing suicide."[2]

The fear of Malthus of over-population in relation to food supply and the consequent fall in the standard of living has, therefore, been revived, and this time, it is pointed out, there are now no new continents waiting to be opened up. Was Malthus right, after all?

(8) IS OVER-POPULATION OF THE WORLD IMMINENT?

Complaints that intensive farming is robbing the soil are no new thing, and they have been made from time to time during the past fifty to sixty years. No one would be so foolish as to deny the seriousness of the problem of soil erosion, but the work of men like Sir John Russell has drawn attention to this menace, and it may be possible to heed their warning. As long ago as 1935 the American Government established a soil-conservation service. In 1943, while the Second World War was still being fought, President Roosevelt called a conference, from which sprang the Food and Agricultural Organisation of the United Nations (the FAO). Under the auspices of this body research on an international scale is being carried out on all kinds of problems of food production. Immediately after the Second World War a general food shortage was experienced in Europe. This post-war food shortage perhaps tended to make people exaggerate the problem somewhat. Between 1939 and 1952 the population of the world increased by 13% while the production of food increased by only 9%, but between 1955 and 1965 food output increased by 14% and population by 10%.

Since 1955, however, as a result of increased mechanisation on the farms, and scientific research into farming problems, especially in the

[1] Lord Boyd-Orr: *University of London Sanderson-Wells Lecture*, 1948.
[2] L. Dudley Stamp: 'Feeding the World's Peoples' (article contributed to the *Westminster Bank Review*, February 1949).

developing countries, the world's output of food has been expanding at a slightly more rapid rate than population. Also, there are still considerable areas of land in the world as yet uncultivated on which food could be brought into cultivation, especially in Northern Canada and Northern Europe, and much additional land could be made suitable for agriculture by further irrigation schemes. In the New World farming is still mainly carried on "extensively," the output of many crops being much less per acre than in most countries of Western Europe. More intensive farming in these areas would increase the world's output of food. Then in the past half-century great progress has been made with the development of chemical fertilisers, and there seems to be no reason to think that progress in this direction cannot be continued. Successful experiments, too, have been made with quicker-ripening crops which makes possible their cultivation in places where there is only a short growing season. There is, too, the further possibility of obtaining more food from the sea. Efforts are being made in all these directions to expand the world's output of food.

There is no doubt that the output of food is capable of being very considerably increased. It has been estimated, for example, that India could produce twice the amount of food it does at present. If, however, the population of the world continues to increase it is not unreasonable to ask whether food production can keep pace with it. Unless the rate at which the population is increasing is checked a time must of necessity eventually arrive—even though every improvement in farming, of course, postpones it—when food output per head of the population will begin to decline. Thus, the problem propounded by Malthus might return in the future on a world rather than a national basis.

Thus, although the *rate* of increase of population is now highest in Latin America, the factor in the world population problem which is causing the greatest concern is the rapidly increasing population of the countries of South-East Asia. In 1965 the population of Asia was estimated at over 1,845 million, of whom approximately 720 million live in China. It is in Asia that there is the greatest annual increase in the number of people to feed.

The food produced in the world, however, is not evenly distributed among the whole of mankind. In the more advanced economies of Western Europe and North America there is ample food, but in many parts of the world the amount of food per head is less than is regarded as sufficient for the maintenance of health. China or any other densely populated country, faced by famine, can obtain food only from other countries either as a result of charity or in exchange for exports.

The other factor in the situation is the possibility of a fall in the birth rate. The industrial development of China, bringing with it a higher standard of living, might check the birth rate there, though that does not seem likely to occur in the immediate future. The Governments of both India and Japan, however, are taking active measures to check population increases. In India particularly it is realised by the Government that the present rate of increase must be checked if the standard of living of the people is to be raised, and since 1950 it has sponsored family limitation programmes.[1] In any case, a fall in the birth rate is likely to be slow to take effect; it is eighty years since the birth rate in Great Britain began to decline, and the population of this country is still increasing.

III. SOME FURTHER ECONOMIC CONSIDERATIONS

(9) THE OPTIMUM POPULATION

Mere numbers, however, do not show whether or not a country is under- or over-populated, and Malthus himself seems to have realised this. "A careful distinction," he says, "should always be made between a redundant population and a population actually great." He seems to have been vaguely aware that a certain density of population per square mile might be too large for one country but not for another. For the production of any good requires the employment of a number of factors of production, of which labour is only one, and these have to be combined in a certain proportion in order to obtain the maximum output.

The amount of labour which, combined with the other factors of production, yields the maximum output is the *optimum* population for that particular country. What is the optimum population for any country therefore depends on its natural resources and its stock of capital. If the population of a country falls short of the optimum it can then be considered to be under-populated; if its population exceeds the optimum it is clearly over-populated. Thus a country poor in natural resources and lacking capital might be economically over-populated, although in point of numbers its proportion was small. Similarly, a country is under-populated if there is insufficient labour relative to other factors of production to make the best use of them. The optimum, however, is not fixed, and even at a given time it would not be possible to state what was the optimum population for a particular country. Over a period of time, conditions are liable to change, and

[1] Details of the programme of the Indian Government were given in an article in the *Fund and Bank Review* of the I.M.F. and I.B. (September 1965).

what was formerly the optimum may cease to be so under changed conditions of production. If it were possible to increase the supply of other factors proportionately to the increase in population the optimum might be raised. The supply of land, however, cannot be appreciably increased, but the experience of Great Britain in the nineteenth century provides an example of how the optimum population can be raised if accompanied by an increase in capital.

(10) SOME CONSEQUENCES OF AN AGEING POPULATION

Though economists have often expressed concern at the possibility of the population of Great Britain beginning to decline in the near future, this attitude often surprises other people, who feel that these small islands are already overcrowded and that a little more elbow room would make for more comfortable living for all. Again, during periods of high unemployment—as for example 1929–35—the argument is sometimes put forward that a decrease in the population would reduce the numbers of the unemployed. In fact, this is far from being the case. With a decline in population there would probably come a falling off in total demand, and this would add to the difficulties of reducing unemployment. A small population would probably mean a reduction in productive capacity, thereby checking economic growth, and not merely a reduction in imports. It is possible too that any difficulties that might arise with the Balance of Payments would be aggravated, and not improved, by a reduction in population. A smaller population might both import and export less, and so there would be less need of shipping, an important source of income to Great Britain.

Whether or not a decrease in the population of a country is likely to be a good or a bad thing in the long run depends therefore on whether the present population is above or below the optimum for that country. Obviously, if the population is above the optimum a reduction in numbers will be an advantage, for this will increase output per head. A reduction, therefore, in the population of China, India or Japan would be economically advantageous to those countries. Clearly, if the present population is at or below the optimum any reduction in numbers will result in a fall in output per head. Even in those cases where it is agreed that a reduction in the population would be desirable, there would still be the disadvantages of a declining population to be faced during the period of decline.

There will be a tendency for structural unemployment—that is, unemployment due to changes in demand—to increase if a change occurs in the distribution of population among the different age-groups. A comparison of the distribution of population according to age in 1891 and 1965 will make this clear:

TABLE VIa

The Age Distribution of the Population (1891 and 1965)

Age	1891	1965
	%	%
0–19	45	30
20–49	31	27
40–59	17	25
60 and over	7	17

During this period there was a huge increase in the percentage of older people and a considerable fall in the percentage of young people. It has been estimated that, if existing tendencies continue, the percentage over sixty will reach 21% by 1971, with a corresponding fall in the number of people under twenty years of age. Between 1950 and 1965 the number of men and women in Great Britain over the age of sixty-five increased by 360,000 to a total of over 6 million. The number is likely to increase still further. The following table shows how the number of older people has been increasing in recent years:

TABLE VIb

The Number of People aged over 65 in the United Kingdom (in thousands)

	Aged 65–69	70–74	75–79	80 & over	Total
1945	←—————————	5,050	—————————→		5,050
1950	2,062	1,605	1,044	769	5,480
1955	2,102	1,657	1,125	832	5,716
1960	2,214	1,723	1,204	1,000	6,141
1965	2,348	1,798	1,287	1,102	6,535

To the extent, therefore, that the demand of the under-twenties differs from that of the over-sixties there will be a decline in employment in industries making goods for the young relative to employment in industries making things for the old. This will be additional to the normal changes in demand due to changing taste and fashion, and new commodities coming on to the market. Adjustments have regularly to be made to meet changes of demand, and if a country is making economic progress it will be found that at any given time some industries are expanding while others are declining. But labour is not very mobile, and cannot easily be switched from the declining to the expanding industries, and thus structural unemployment is likely to be aggravated.

In a short period some unemployment arises from technical progress, and this, as well as unemployment resulting from the ups and downs of the trade cycle, will be more difficult to bring to an end in a country with a declining population. Thus with a declining population the maintenance of full employment would become more difficult.

The burden of the National Debt and schemes of social insurance become heavier per head if the population is declining. Apart from increases due to the rising cost of living the cost of retirement pensions is likely to increase because of the increase in the proportion of beneficiaries to workers. To offset this, the Phillips Committee (1954) recommended that the retirement age for men should be raised from sixty-five to sixty-eight and for women from sixty to sixty-three, but there has been little support for this proposal.

Though the rise in the birth rate in the United Kingdom in recent years has at least postponed a decline in the population, this country is still faced with the problem of an ageing population, some of the consequences of which are very similar to—though perhaps rather less severe than those associated with a declining population.

IV. THE FUTURE

(ii) THE FUTURE TREND OF POPULATION

Though it is necessary to make the qualification "if present trends continue" in estimating the size of the population at a distant future date, fairly accurate estimates are possible of the numbers in particular age-groups some years ahead. For example, in 1965 there were 4½ million children aged four or less, and with this total as a basis it becomes possible to estimate the number of people aged twenty to twenty-four in 1985 or aged thirty to thirty-four in 1995. Similar calculations can be made for other age-groups at future dates. Estimates for the number of people under twenty years of age in 1985, or under thirty in 1995, are less accurate because these depend on the number of births in the intervening years.

The following table shows the distribution according to age-groups of the population of the United Kingdom at 30th June 1964:

TABLE VII

The Estimated Age Distribution of the Population (in thousands)[1]

30th June 1964

United Kingdom of Great Britain and Northern Ireland

Age-groups	Total	Males	Females
0– 4	4,648	2,384	2,264
5– 9	4,019	2,060	1,959
10–14	3,848	1,969	1,879
15–19	4,275	2,190	2,085
20–24	3,587	1,820	1,767
25–29	3,412	1,742	1,670
30–34	3,363	1,725	1,638
35–39	3,471	1,753	1,718
40–44	3,864	1,929	1,935
45–49	3,254	1,598	1,656
50–54	3,617	1,756	1,861
55–59	3,424	1,642	1,782
60–64	2,996	1,388	1,608
65–69	2,327	962	1,365
70 and over	4,110	1,474	2,636
Total:	54,213	26,398	27,815

From this table it can be seen how the number of children reaching working age in recent times has varied. When the numbers born in each quinquennial period vary considerably this presents other problems. In the years immediately after each of the two World Wars there was a big increase in the number of births. Accommodation in the schools of these larger numbers was difficult, as the first of these two large groups passed through the educational system in the 1920s and early 1930s. The large group of children of school age presented a similar problem to the education authorities during 1950–65.

From the numbers in the various age-groups at present it can be calculated that during the next fifteen years there is likely to be an increase of only 1½ million people of working age out of a probable total increase of 6¼ million. During the next thirty years there is likely to be an increase of more than 2¼ million in the number of people over 65. It is also of interest to notice that up to the age of 39 males are in excess of females; between the ages of 39 and 50 the sexes are fairly evenly balanced; over the age of fifty the preponderance of females becomes more pronounced.

As already noticed, birth-rate trends are more difficult to estimate. During 1937–39 the decline in the birth rate was checked, and during these years there was a slight increase over the previous period.

---

[1] From *Monthly Digest of Statistics* (H.M.S.O.).

During 1943–45, however, there was a considerable increase in the birth rate as compared with 1937–39, and a further increase during 1945–48. After the First World War there was also a sharp, but temporary, increase in the birth rate, but the remarkable thing about the recent rise in the birth rate is that it began before the Second World War, and though the rise was slight during 1937–39, it remained comparatively high for six years, and altogether has persisted for upwards of twenty years. Though still remaining well above the rate in 1937–39, the birth rate fell steadily during 1948–52, but then levelled out, but after 1955 began to rise again. The recent increase in the birth rate is largely a result of earlier marriages, for which a long period with little unemployment is probably chiefly responsible, further important contributory factors probably being the extension of the social services, the health service, family allowances, etc. Fifty % more people now marry under the age of 25 years than in 1931; 25% more marry under 30. The effect of the lowering of the average age at which men and women marry is likely to be ephemeral, though the shortening of the interval between generations will produce some increase in numbers. Earlier marriages, too, may lead to larger families.

(12) THE ROYAL COMMISSION ON POPULATION

As the *Report of the Royal Commission on Population* (1949) pointed out, the main factor determining the future trend of population is the size of the family. The average number of children per family in the years since the Second World War has been 2·13, a size below the level necessary for each generation to replace itself. The Commission forecast a fall in the number of births during the next fifteen years, whereas after 1955 the number increased. The Commission estimated that to prevent a future decline in the population of Great Britain required an annual total of at least 700,000 births. In fact, the average number of births since 1958 has been over 930,000 as compared with 722,000 during 1935–38.[1]

Every change in the birth rate or the average family size makes necessary a revision of estimates of the population at future dates. Thus at one time it was thought that the population of Great Britain would begin to decline in the 1940s; later forecasts put back the date of decline to the 1970s; now it is not thought unlikely to occur until well after the year 2000, if at all. The other chief influence on the future trend of population is the death rate, a rise in which may be expected in view of the increased number of people in the higher age groups.

In addition to being appointed "to examine the facts relating to the

[1] In 1964 the number of births for the first time since 1947 exceeded 1 million.

present population trends in Great Britain," the Royal Commission on Population also had to consider "what measures, if any, should be taken in the national interest to influence the future trend of population."

The Commission was concerned at the possibility of the population declining (unduly so as events turned out) and therefore proposed that means should be found to encourage parents to have larger families. It therefore recommended that parents should be given assistance in the form of cash and services:

(i) *Family allowances* should be increased, and eventually should be payable for the first child.

(ii) *Income Tax.* Allowances for children should be increased.

(iii) *Services* should be developed to give help to mothers of young children, such as home helps, sitters-in, day nurseries, etc.

It is doubtful whether money incentives will achieve the desired result, although the payment of very generous family allowances in France appears to have checked the decline in population in that country.

The Royal Commission further suggested that, as the number of people aged over 65 would increase, they should be encouraged to continue to work to a higher age than formerly. With increasing longevity some such change will eventually almost certainly be necessary. In order that this should not discourage younger people by delaying their promotion, the Commission recommended that those in high positions should not be permitted to remain at work beyond the normal age for retirement.

(13) EMIGRATION AND IMMIGRATION

During the nineteenth century the population of many countries in Western Europe increased more rapidly than ever before in spite of a greater volume of emigration than at any previous time to the countries of the New World. Much of the emigration was due to over-population in the conditions of the time in the countries from which the emigrants came—Ireland, Italy, the countries of Central Europe and the Balkans.

During the period of 1871–1931 Great Britain experienced average *net* emigration of over half a million persons per year. In the years immediately before the Second World War this country received many immigrants from Germany and Austria, including many people with high academic qualifications, and in post-war years many more immigrants came from Europe—the so-called "displaced persons."

During 1931–51, therefore this country had a *net* gain from immigration of an average of 60,000 persons per year.

At the present day Great Britain's population is affected by both emigration and immigration. During the ten years to 1961 a large number of people left this country to settle overseas, going mainly to Australia, Canada and New Zealand. During these same years large numbers of immigrants came here from the West Indies, India, Pakistan and Ceylon, The immigration totals include some people returning from Australia, etc., just as the emigration totals include some returning to the West Indies, etc. On balance, however, during this period Great Britain experienced a *net* gain of 131,000 persons.

Countries receiving large numbers of immigrants have often found it necessary to impose restrictions on entry. Between the two World Wars, for example, the Government of the United States had to restrict the number of immigrants it was prepared to accept from South-eastern Europe. More recently Great Britain has had to adopt measures to check immigration from the Commonwealth.

RECOMMENDATIONS FOR FURTHER READING

J. R. Hicks: *The Social Framework*, Chapters 4 and 5.
I. Bowen: *Population*.
Report of the Royal Commission on Population (1949).

QUESTIONS

1. Enunciate Malthus' theory of population and describe the conditions obtaining in England when he wrote which lent support to his theory and the changing views of economists since as to the soundness of his theory of population. (L.C. Com. Econ.)

2. "Cheap labour makes cheap food: cheap food stimulates population: the increase of population makes labour still cheaper." Would you accept any or all of these statements? Give reasons. (C.I.S. Inter.)

3. What theories did Malthus produce in regard to population? What truth, if any, do you think they contain? (A.C.C.A. Inter.)

4. If the birth rate showed a substantial and permanent rise would you regard the change as beneficial (*a*) in the present generation, (*b*) in the next generation? (I.B.)

5. What meanings can be attached to the statement that a country is over-populated? Can the statement be applied to Great Britain at the present day? (C.C.S. Final.)

6. Examine the economic effects of the present trend towards an ageing population in the United Kingdom. (G.C.E. Adv.)

PART THREE

THE ORGANISATION AND STRUCTURE OF PRODUCTION

CHAPTER VI

TYPES OF BUSINESS UNIT

I. THE SOLE PROPRIETOR

(1) THE FEATURES OF THE "ONE-MAN" BUSINESS

The oldest type of business unit is that of the sole proprietor—that is, the "one-man" business. As late as the end of the eighteenth and the beginning of the nineteenth centuries most manufacturing businesses were of this type, and even today, though large-scale production has made it increasingly difficult for individuals to set up in business for themselves, there are still some who manage to do so. Now, in the second half of the twentieth century the retail trade is probably the easiest to enter for the man with a little capital who wishes to be his own employer, though in the 1920s and 1930s many found scope for their entrepreneurial abilities in the development of road transport both for goods and passengers.

In the one-man business a single person undertakes the risks of production. He probably provides all the capital, though to enable him to start he may borrow from friends or relations. He is thus the owner of the business, undertaking all the functions of the entrepreneur, and shouldering the entire responsibility of management and operation. Success or failure depends primarily on his ability to produce things that other people want and at a price which they are prepared to pay—that is, upon the efficiency of his production methods. If he is successful he reaps his reward in the form of profits, which accrue solely to him, except so far as they are subject to taxation by the State; but if he is unsuccessful he must bear the entire loss himself. Businesses of this type are generally small at first, but many of them, operated by sole proprietors, have in the course of generations become quite large, though usually when that has come about the structure of the business has been changed to a form more suitable to large-scale production. A man with only a little capital can build up a business of fairly considerable size, by living frugally and devoting most of the profit to the expansion of the business. Many large old businesses in Great Britain today, covering a wide variety of trades, originated in this way.

(2) ADVANTAGES OF THE SOLE PROPRIETOR

The following are some of the advantages of this type of business:

(i) One of the chief advantages lies in the self-interest of the proprietor. He has every incentive to make his business as efficient as possible by minimising or preventing waste. He is his own "boss" and can devote as much of his time and energy to his business as he wishes.

(ii) There is no need for him to consult anyone else when embarking upon a new line of policy. His decisions can be put into effect immediately without the necessity of having to convince others that they are in the best interests of the business. Because of its smallness he can manage the whole business and so attain a high standard of efficiency.

(iii) Also, because of the smallness of the business he can maintain a closer and more personal contact with both his employees and his customers. Often he himself has worked for others and understands the employee's point of view. He is known personally to his employees and aware of their private problems, and as a result there often exists an intimacy between management and workers which is not easy to foster in large concerns, where the manager must of necessity remain somewhat aloof from the employees. Further, his personal knowledge of his customers' idiosyncrasies and financial standing makes it easy for him to meet their wishes and to be prudent in the granting of credit.

(iv) Sole proprietorship is a convenient type of business unit where special lines are being produced for a limited market. Where variety is to be preferred to standardisation of the product, the small firm can still hold its own.

(3) DISADVANTAGES OF THE SOLE PROPRIETOR

Of the disadvantages of this type of business the following may be noted:

(i) The smallness of his capital may hinder the expansion of his business.

(ii) His own personal abilities determine the success of the business, and on his death or retirement continued success depends on the ability of his son or whoever inherits the business, but there is no assurance that his successor will possess the necessary ability.

(iii) Since he bears all the risks, he is personally liable for the whole of the debts and obligations of the firm, that is, he does not have the advantage of limited liability.

(iv) This type of business is unsuitable for any form of production where economies of scale are available.

II. THE PARTNERSHIP

(4) THE ORDINARY PARTNERSHIP

One of the ways by which the sole proprietor can expand his business is to turn it into a partnership. There are two advantages to be derived from this method of expansion: it enables "new blood" to be introduced into the business, and it makes possible an increase in capital. There is a special kind of partnership known as a "Limited Partnership" (see below), but this type of partnership is not popular, since limitation of personal liability is more easily secured by the private company. The *Companies Acts* limit the number of partners in a firm to twenty, or in the case of a banking business, to ten. A Deed of Partnership, drawn up by a solicitor, should be entered into between the partners, and it should be sufficiently detailed and explicit to regulate every matter affecting the partners likely to arise during the continuation of the partnership, or on its dissolution. The provisions of the Deed can be varied subsequently only by agreement.

A partnership has many of the advantages and disadvantages of the sole proprietor, but there is greater continuity of existence for a partnership than for the business of a sole proprietor. Partners have equal powers and responsibilities, and each is jointly liable with the other partners for all the debts and obligations of the firm, and in a trading firm a partner can make a contract which is binding on his co-partners. Obviously, it would be sheer folly for anyone to enter into partnership with a person, unless convinced of his integrity, judgment and business acumen.

(5) THE LIMITED PARTNERSHIP

This kind of partnership was made possible by the *Limited Partnership Act*, 1907. Under that Act the liability of the limited partner is restricted to the amount of capital he has invested in the firm. His rights are also restricted. Though he may have access to the books of the firm, and offer advice to the ordinary partners, he may not take any part in the management of the firm and he cannot bind the firm, or withdraw any part of his capital. If he does take part in the management he becomes liable as an ordinary partner. Though there may be more than one limited partner, there must always be at least one ordinary partner. Limited Partnerships must be registered with the Registrar of Companies, and as stated above are not very popular. The private limited company of two or more persons has largely made this type of partnership unnecessary.

The entrepreneurial function of the partnership. Where there is more than one general partner this type of business has the advantage over that of the sole proprietor in that it is possible to share the function of management. For example, in a small manufacturing business one partner may assume responsibility for technical matters, and the other for administration and sales. In a partnership it is clear that *all* the entrepreneurial functions are shared among the partners—the risks of production, the work of management and the control of the business; and that the amount of their income from profits depends upon their efficiency in performing these functions.

III. THE LIMITED COMPANY

(6) THE DEVELOPMENT OF THE JOINT-STOCK COMPANY

The partnership owed its existence as a form of business enterprise to the need for greater capital than the sole proprietor could supply. The Joint-stock Company developed out of the partnership for precisely the same reason, and in fact the early Joint-stock Companies were legally nothing more than large partnerships. In ancient times works necessitating the employment of large amounts of capital could be undertaken only by rich, despotic rulers, with masses of slaves, or conscripted labour at their disposal, or from the tribute exacted of subject peoples. Such undertakings might be carried through as works of public necessity, or for the ruler's self-aggrandisement, or in honour of national gods. Of this the magnificent aqueducts, palaces, temples and tombs of the Ancient World bear eloquent witness. The Hebrews, for example, were heavily taxed to help pay for the temple built by Solomon, and Pericles defrayed the cost of the Parthenon at Athens out of funds contributed by subject allies.

Industry, in any case beneath the notice of ancient, despotic rulers, existed only on a small scale until the time of the Industrial Revolution, and required only limited amounts of capital. Overseas trade, however, required the building of ships, and, with the passage of time, these assumed larger dimensions and as a result became more expensive to build. The pioneer navigators of the fifteenth and sixteenth centuries had to seek the patronage of monarchs to defray the cost of their voyages. Columbus, though a Genoese, obtained the help of Ferdinand and Isabella of Spain; the Cabots of Bristol had some support from Henry VII.

As a substitute for this method of financing ventures, the Joint-stock

Company was developed. It is not surprising, therefore, to find that the earliest Joint-stock enterprises were trading companies, the British East India Company, founded in 1600, being one of the earliest.[1] The distinctive feature of the Joint-stock Company is that a large number of people provide the capital in varying amounts and receive shares in the profits (if any) in proportion to the amounts they have invested in the company. In this way it becomes possible to raise large sums, providing the sponsors of a proposed new company can persuade the public that its prospects are well founded. This development received strong impetus early in the eighteenth century when a number of these trading companies earned good profits for their shareholders. The early success of the South Sea Company led unscrupulous people to exploit the cupidity of an ignorant public by floating bogus companies. The collapse of the South Sea Company, after a period of frenzied speculation, brought about the bursting of the bubble in 1720 and led to the passing of an Act later in the year to control the establishment of Joint-stock Companies. In future there were to be two types: (a) Chartered Companies—that is, set up by Royal Charter—or (b) Statutory Companies, established by specific Acts of Parliament. The Bank of England was established by Royal Charter, and the building of railways in Great Britain was undertaken by companies established by Acts of Parliament. The increasing scale of production consequent on the Industrial Revolution increased the popularity of the Joint-stock Company, and in 1825 a third type of company was permitted— namely, the registered company. The control of a Joint-stock Company depends on the voting rights vested in the shares. The voting at shareholders' meetings is usually proportionate to the number of ordinary shares held, so that a shareholder owning over 50% of shares has the control of the company in his own hands.

At the present time there are over 3½ million people who hold shares in limited companies, the average holding being a little over £300.

(7) LIMITED LIABILITY

Probably the most important development in modern industrial organisation has been the evolution of the principle of limited liability. This simply means that the liability of the shareholder is limited to the fully paid up value of the shares he holds, and if the company should find itself in difficulties and unable to meet the demands of its creditors the shareholder may lose this, but no further amount, so that the rest of his property is free from any claims by the company's creditors.

[1] Two companies had, however, been incorporated in 1565 for the mining of copper and zinc. (See A. L. Rowse: *The England of Elizabeth*, Ch. IV.)

Where there is no limited liability the unfortunate shareholder may have to sell his possessions to meet the debts of the Company, as occurred in the case of some bank failures in the early nineteenth century. In such circumstances cautious people hesitate to become shareholders in companies, whereas with limited liability the maximum possible loss is known in advance, so that people are more willing to subscribe to an issue of shares.

The Act of 1720 allowed limited liability to chartered and statutory companies, but the Act of 1825, which permitted the registration of new companies, abolished limited liability. This privilege was not fully restored for thirty-seven years, an Act of 1855 permitting limited liability where the shares were of a nominal value of £10 or over, and an Act of 1862 allowing it for all companies, whatever the nominal value of the shares. Banks were expressly excluded from the Act of 1855, but limited liability was extended to them in 1858. Companies may be of limited or unlimited liability, but the latter are now extremely rare. Indeed, the Act of 1948 refers only to limited companies.

(8) CLOSE AND PUBLIC COMPANIES

Companies are of two types—close and public. The close company has three important features: the number of shareholders may be as few as two, but the maximum must not exceed fifty, not counting past and present employees of the company; a shareholder cannot transfer his shares without the consent of the company nor can any invitation be made to the general public to subscribe for shares. This type of company is very similar in many ways to a partnership, but it has the advantage that all the members enjoy limited liability.

In the public company there must be at least seven shareholders, but no maximum number is fixed. Seven persons or more wishing to form such a company draw up a *Memorandum of Association* giving particulars of the type of business to be undertaken, the amount of its nominal or authorised capital and the kinds of shares to be issued. A second document, known as the *Articles of Association*, has then to be compiled, giving particulars of the internal working of the proposed company, including such things as voting rights of shareholders, powers and duties of directors, etc. The next step is to secure the *registration* of the company with the Registrar of Companies, after which it becomes possible for a *Prospectus* to be issued and an appeal to be made to the general public to subscribe for its shares.

The public Limited Company is thus able to raise very large amounts of capital from small investors, and gigantic undertakings, involving many millions of pounds sterling in capital, become possible. The construction of railways is an outstanding example of the kind of enterprise which the public Limited Company made possible.

The raising of large amounts of capital is further assisted by the easy transferability of shares on the Stock Exchanges. Limited Companies are also an advantage to the large investor, who is enabled to spread his investments over many companies, and not have all his eggs in one basket. The *Companies Acts* of 1869, 1929, 1948 and 1967 were principally designed to protect the people from unscrupulous company promoters. For example, the annual Balance Sheet has to be made public as a safeguard against fraud, the Act of 1948 declaring that it must be "a fair and true record."

(9) TYPES OF SHARES

The capital of a Limited Company is divided into shares. These may be in units of 1s., 2s. 6d., 5s., 10s., £1, £5, £100, etc., but small denominations are usually preferred. There are a number of different kinds of shares, some of the commoner ones being considered below, and a single company may issue two or three different types in order to attract different classes of investors, some of whom may be willing to undertake greater risks than others. Shares are not always fully paid up—for example, only 12s 6d. may have been paid for a £1 share— but the company can call up the balance if required.

(i) *Ordinary shares.* Generally these shares carry no fixed rate of dividend (unless Deferred Ordinary Shares are issued), and receive a share of the profit only after all other claims have been met. The dividends paid by firms producing goods for which there is a steady demand may not vary much from one year to another, and even the difference between trade boom and slump may not be very great. Other firms may be greatly influenced by general conditions of trade, and in a boom dividends on ordinary shares may rise to 100% or more, but in a slump may fall to as low as $\frac{1}{2}$%, or even to nothing at all. Clearly, those people who invest in ordinary shares are bearing the principal risk, but in the hope of a commensurate reward.

(ii) *Preference shares.* These shares usually have a fixed rate of dividend, and their holders are paid in full before the ordinary shareholders receive anything. To persuade people to invest in preference shares a higher rate of dividend has to be offered than the yield on Government Stock.

There are several varieties of preference shares, and hybrid types which combine features of both the ordinary and the preference shares. Two may be mentioned: (*a*) Cumulative Preference Shares, which are entitled to receive arrears of dividend owing from previous years before any allocation of profit is made to the ordinary shares; (b) Participating Preference Shares, where, in addition to the fixed dividend, a bonus depending on the amount of profit is payable.

(iii) *Debentures.* In addition to the issue of various types of shares, a company may obtain further capital by applying to the public for a loan. This loan capital is obtained by the issue of debentures. Debentures are not shares, and the holders are creditors, and not members of the company, like the shareholders. They are therefore entitled to receive interest whether the company makes a profit or a loss. Debentures carry a fixed rate of interest, usually a little lower than that paid on the preference shares. They are generally redeemable—that is, repayable at par at some future date. Mortgage debentures are those issued on the security of the firm's assets.

An example will illustrate the method of distributing the profits of a company. Assume that the Northern Manufacturing Co. Ltd. has a share capital of £400,000 divided into £300,000 in ordinary shares of 10s. each and £100,000 in 7% cumulative preference shares of £1 each, with a loan capital of £50,000 in 6% debentures of £1 each. It will require £3,000 per annum to pay the interest on the debentures and £7,000 to cover the dividend on the preference shares. If one year the company makes a profit of £6,000, after the debenture-holders have been paid, the preference shareholders will have to be satisfied with 6% instead of the 7% to which they are entitled, and there will be no dividend at all for the ordinary shareholders. If next year the profits total £12,500, after the debenture-holders have been paid, the cumulative preference shareholders will receive £8,000 (£7,000 + £1,000 arrears) and the ordinary shareholders £2,000, giving them a dividend of $1\frac{1}{2}$%. If at a later date the company makes a profit of, say, £43,000 the cumulative preference shareholders receive the 7% to which they are entitled, and the ordinary shareholders will receive a dividend of 12%.

Entrepreneurial functions in the Limited Company. In a Limited Company, therefore, it is the shareholders who bear the risk or uncertainty, the principal function of the entrepreneur. At the shareholders' meeting they elect a Management Committee, known as the Board of Directors, who in their turn may elect one of themselves as Managing Director, or appoint a salaried General Manager from outside. If a Managing Director is appointed he will probably be one of the large shareholders, and so will bear some risk as well as being responsible for the management of the business. The salaried manager may owe his appointment entirely to the Board's confidence in his managerial abilities, though it is said that few managers' salaries are independent of profits, some being given a block of shares, while others are paid a bonus based on profits.[1] In any case, a paid manager's tenure of office is, however, likely to be short unless satisfactory profits are earned.

In the Limited Company, therefore, it becomes difficult to locate precisely the entrepreneurial function. It has been suggested that wherever the making of decisions is to be found, there is the entrepreneur, but practice differs between one company and another, and all that can be said is that the function is divided between the shareholders and the executive, the ownership of capital and its control thus being separated.

IV. THE CO-OPERATIVE MOVEMENT

(10) CO-OPERATION IN PRODUCTION

Producers' co-operatives have had little success in Great Britain. Under this form of business unit the workers themselves own the business and elect some of their number to manage it, the profit then being divided among them. The chief difficulty, however has been to secure efficient management, for popular election is not the best method of securing the most able managers, nor is appointment by election conducive to the maintenance of discipline in the factory. A number of co-operative societies of this type have been established at different times in England and elsewhere, but they have generally been small concerns, because the workers have been able to supply only a small amount of capital.

At the present time there are 21 firms in membership of the Co-operative Production Federation, with total combined assets of over £3 million. Most of these firms are engaged in the manufacture of boots and shoes and clothing, over 80% of their output being purchased by co-operative societies. Profits are divided between dividends on sales, bonuses to employees and interest on share capital.

Co-operation among farmers, however, has been steadily gaining ground, so that today farmers' co-operatives in Europe cover nearly 60% of the farming population. For long, the dairy industry has been organised on a co-operative system in Denmark, where the farmers combine to purchase and manage the dairies, to which they send the milk from their farms. The proportion of the total quantity of milk supplied by each farmer is recorded, and he is then credited with a proportion of the dairy's output of butter, cheese, etc. The profits of the enterprise are divided among the farmers in the same proportion.

---

[1] F. H. Knight: *Risk, Uncertainty and Profit.*

During the past twenty-five years there has been a great extension of co-operation in farming in Great Britain. Most farmers in England and Wales are members of purchasing societies and marketing schemes, which lead to more effective buying and selling. There are, for example, farmers' co-operative societies for the purchase of fertilisers, seeds and feeding stuffs, for the sale of wool and for the operation of bacon factories. Marketing Boards have been established for a number of farm products, including hops, potatoes, milk, tomatoes and eggs.

(II) CONSUMERS' CO-OPERATIVE SOCIETIES

A much greater measure of success has attended the development of consumers' co-operative societies, though most of the early co-operative ventures even of this type failed. The success of the movement really dates from 1844, when twenty-eight weavers provided the capital to open a shop at Rochdale. Thus it began as a working-class movement. Progress was slow at first, but after 1918 development became more rapid. In 1880 there were only just over half a million members and in 1918 only 3 million, but by 1965 the total membership had risen to 13 million. On account of the tendency towards larger societies there has been a decline in their number, mainly as a result of the amalgamation of societies. In 1901 there were 1,438 societies, but by 1967 the number had fallen to 467, and the number is expected to fall still further. There are still many small societies—117 in 1965 with fewer than a thousand members—but at the other extreme there were nineteen each with over 100,000 members, the largest being the London society, with over a million and a quarter members. The latest Census of Distribution shows that in Great Britain co-operative societies were responsible for 11% of all retail trade, although for the sale of groceries their share was nearly 25% of the total.

An entrance fee of 1s. is usually required of members, who are generally allowed to purchase only one £1 share each, though they may invest up to £1,000 in their society. Each member, therefore, has only one vote at members' meetings, which elect the Committee of Management and a President. There are some similarities between a co-operative society and a limited company. The members' meeting of the co-operative society corresponds to the shareholders' meetings of the limited company, but whereas each shareholder has a number of votes proportional to his holding of shares, each member of the co-operative society has only one vote. The shareholders of the limited company elect a Board of Directors, and the members of the co-operative elect their Committee of Management. Each of these bodies is responsible for general policy, and each appoint paid officials to be responsible for the day-to-day management of the business. The co-operative society appoints a General Secretary or Secretary-Manager, and the limited company a General Manager or Managing Director. The profits of a limited company are distributed among the share-holders according to the type of shares held (*see* **9**), whereas in the co-operative society profits are distributed among members in pro-portion to the value of their purchases, a dividend being declared of so much in the pound on all purchases. In recent years there has been a tendency for the dividends of most societies to fall.

The Co-operative Wholesale Society and the Scottish Co-operative Wholesale Society were founded to supply the retail societies. Their organisation is similar to that of the retail societies, except that at general meetings the voting power of the member societies, like their share of profits, is proportionate to their purchases from the wholesale societies. In their turn the wholesale societies own many factories and tea-plantations, and this type of co-operation on the productive side has been more successful than earlier efforts.

Both the C.W.S. and the S.C.W.S. are also interested in retailing through Co-operative Retail Services Ltd., which in 1965 had forty branches, each with its own group of shops. The aim of the C.R.S. has been two-fold: (*a*) to establish retail societies in areas where this could not be accomplished by local effort; and (*b*) to assist established societies.

(12) ADVANTAGES AND DISADVANTAGES OF CO-OPERATIVE SOCIETIES

An advantage of the Co-operative Society has been the stability of trade that results from the loyalty of the members, this loyalty being sustained in some cases because the dividend is based on purchases, and in others from a desire to support the movement for its own sake. Secondly, it is claimed to be democratically managed. This, however, may be more apparent than real, especially in the larger societies, where many members are as apathetic as the average shareholder of a limited company, so that, as in limited companies, the management tends to fall into the hands of a small group. It is said that since the customers and the profit receivers are one and the same, there is not the same con-flict of interest between them as, for example, in the case of a multiple-shop type of business. But men whose lives have been spent as em-ployees often make hard taskmasters when they themselves become managers, and are often reluctant to pay their secretaries and branch managers very highly.

Criticism is often levelled against the co-operative societies regarding

E

the lack of business experience of the majority of the members of the Committees, and it is often said that the method of promotion is not conducive to efficiency. It is a frequent complaint that the co-operative societies are able to compete unfairly against the other retail traders, because their profits are exempt from profits tax which falls on the profits of other business undertakings, the dividend on purchases being regarded as a discount rather than a distribution of profit. Another objection frequently made is that some co-operative societies (which include among their members people of all shades of political opinion) use some of their funds for political purposes, the Co-operative Party associating itself with the Labour Party. Co-operation, however, is a social movement, and each society allots a certain sum every year for the propagation of its ideals.

V. STATE AND MUNICIPAL UNDERTAKINGS

(13) MUNICIPAL ENTERPRISE

In Great Britain many local services—more particularly where competition would be wasteful—have been provided by the municipalities. Chief among these services have been markets, local transport—horse, steam and electric trams, petrol-driven buses, trolley-buses—the supply of water, gas and electricity, restaurants, in Birmingham a savings bank, and in Hull the telephone. An increasing number of local authorities too, are establishing municipal airports. The owners of these various undertakings are the ratepayers, but, unlike the shareholders of a limited company or the members of a co-operative society, they are not allowed to decide for themselves whether they are willing to accept the risks of ownership, nor, as in the other two forms of business organisation, are they allowed to vote directly for the Management Committee. The management of a municipal passenger transport undertaking is vested in a committee of the local Council, who appoint a salaried manager. So again the entrepreneurial function is divided, profits or losses in this case falling upon the ratepayers, who bear the risk. The nationalisation of gas and electricity removed two of the main types of business from municipal control.

(14) STATE UNDERTAKINGS

The Post Office. For a long time the principal undertaking in Great Britain operated by the State was the Post Office. In this case the Postmaster-General, a member of the Government of the day, is at the head of the administrative system, and is responsible to Parliament. He is assisted by a Board, with purely advisory powers. The permanent head of the undertaking is the Director-General. The Postmaster-General occupies a position somewhat similar to that of the Chairman of a public corporation, and the Director-General corresponds to the paid General Manager of a company. Taxpayers can thus be considered to correspond to the shareholders, except that their control over policy is even more indirect and slender. Until recently the revenue and expenditure of the Post Office appeared in the Budget, but nowadays it is run as a commercial undertaking like the nationalised industries. In 1969 it became a public corporation.

The public corporation. Before 1939 it was considered that municipal or State ownership was most suitable in the case of monopolies, the municipality for local services, the State for national services. In the years before 1939 the public corporation developed as a new type of business unit in those cases where it was felt that an undertaking should not to be left to private enterprise at a time when Parliament was not favourably disposed to outright nationalisation. Among these were the Port of London Authority, established in 1908, the Central Electricity Board (1926), the British Broadcasting Corporation (1927), the London Passenger Transport Board (1933) and a number of other undertakings. The B.B.C. was granted a Charter that had to be renewed at intervals, the application for renewal providing an opportunity for a debate in Parliament upon the previous policy of the Corporation. Once a Charter has been granted, a corporation has freedom of operation for a prescribed period. Similar public corporations were set up for British Overseas Airways (1940), the North of Scotland Hydro-electric Board (1943) and the National Film Finance Corporation (1948). The taxpayers bear the risk, for any losses will have to be made good from taxes, and control rests with paid officials.

Nationalised industries. The nationalisation policy of the Government of 1945–51 brought the Bank of England, the coal, gas, electricity production and some forms of transport under State control. To operate them several new public corporations were established, as, for example, the National Gas Board, the Gas Council and the Central Electricity Generating Board. The nationalised section of transport has been under the control of four Boards—Railways (British Rail), London Transport, British Transport Docks and British Waterways—and the Transport Holding Company, the latter body holding shares in road haulage (British Road Services), many bus companies, some shipping companies and travel agencies. The form of organisation of these industries differs in detail, but in each case there is at the head a Minister of the Crown who is responsible to Parliament. In all the public corporations it is Parliament that is responsible for general policy, but day-to-day management is generally free from parliamentary influence, though there is usually some ministerial control. The management of a public corporation is in the hands of a committee, the chairman and members of which are appointed for fixed periods by the appropriate Minister, subject to parliamentary approval. The financial side of a public corporation is operated independently of the Treasury. There are no shares and no shareholders. The nationalised industries are considered in Chapter XXVIII.

QUESTIONS

1. Discuss the principles and the organisation of a co-operative society. In what ways do they differ from a nationalised industry? (R.S.A. Adv.)

2. "The victory of the co-operative store movement has not been overwhelming even among the working classes; and it has left the more prosperous classes almost untouched." Give a careful account of the co-operative movement in Great Britain, and account if you can for the fact stated above. (R.S.A. Adv. Com.)

3. What are the advantages of the limited liability company over other types of business organisation? (C.I.S. Inter.)

4. What are the characteristic features of:

(a) Co-operative retail trading societies;
(b) Public limited joint stock companies; and
(c) Partnerships? (Exp.)

5. Analyse the main economic features of the co-operative movement? (C.I.S. Inter.)

6. Distinguish between a joint-stock company and a co-operative society. (I.B.)

7. Consider the main economic effects of the introduction of the system of limited liability. (B.S. Final.)

8. What is meant by a joint-stock company? What are the advantages of this type of organisation? (G.C.E. Adv.)

9. "The public corporation can be controlled neither by the consumer nor by Parliament." Consider, having regard to this criticism, the part that this form of organisation could usefully be made to play in the economic sphere. (Final Degree.)

CHAPTER VII

THE SCALE OF PRODUCTION

I. THE TENDENCY TOWARDS EXPANSION

(1) THE FIRM AND THE INDUSTRY

Production, then, is carried on by a large number of firms of different types and sizes, ranging from the smallest of one-man businesses with very little capital to huge limited companies with hundreds of thousands of shareholders and issued capital of several hundred million pounds sterling. An industry may be large or small, and may consist of both large and small firms. The firm may be defined as an independently administered business unit. An industry consists of a number of firms producing broadly similar commodities, though it is not always easy to differentiate all industries completely one from another. It is usual to speak, for example, of the woollen industry, the cotton industry, the motor-car industry, the shipbuilding industry, and these terms give a broad indication of the branch of production to which reference is being made.

If the entire output of a whole industry is produced by a single firm, then the firm and the industry are clearly one and the same. Nationalised industries in Great Britain, such as coal-mining, are of this type. In some forms of production the average size of the business unit is small and the number of firms large. This is true of the retail trade, where the sole proprietor is still the most common type of organisation. In other kinds of production the average business unit tends to be large—railways, the chemical industry (I.C.I., for example, is responsible for a quarter of the total output of this industry in Great Britain), while in the wool-textile industry the firms are mostly of medium size, together with quite a few small and a few very large ones. What, then, determines the size of the firm and the industry? It is the purpose of this chapter to consider some of the factors affecting the size of the firm.

(2) THE MOTIVE FOR EXPANSION

In the first place, it has to be assumed that it is the aim of every entrepreneur to make maximum profits. If this is so, he will adopt that form of production in which his costs are lowest, and take all measures open to him to effect economies. It is probably not true in all cases that the entrepreneur will always seek to maximise his profits. To do so may require an increase in his scale of production and involve obtaining additional capital, and he may prefer not to do this. He may prefer the more personal relationship between employer and employee that is possible in a small firm, or he may shrink from the responsibility of controlling a larger firm, feeling himself not competent to undertake such work. For any one of these reasons he may prefer not to try to maximise his profits. Generally, however, entrepreneurs will strive to maximise their profits, and unless this assumption is made it is impossible to build up a theory of the firm. The entrepreneur will, then, increase the size of his firm if there are any economies of scale to be obtained by his doing so.

(3) THE GROWTH OF LARGE-SCALE PRODUCTION

First, it will be worth considering briefly some of the reasons for the growth of large-scale industry, for one of the main features of industrial development during the last century and a half has been the increasing size of the business unit. Specialisation or division of labour has gone hand in hand with the progress of transport, and the past one hundred and fifty years have seen an enormous extension of cheap transport. Without adequate transport facilities large-scale production would be impossible. The development of the limited company has been an important factor making possible large-scale production involving huge amounts of capital. Then there has been a great expansion in the demand for all kinds of things consequent on the rise in the standard of living that has taken place during the past century and a half. When most people were living near subsistence level they could afford to buy little other than necessaries, and in such circumstances there was no market for mass-produced goods.

These developments made large-scale production possible. There were also definite incentives to the entrepreneur to expand his scale of production in the prospect of higher profits, for certain economies were open to the large firm that gave it the advantage over its smaller competitors of lower costs. In some cases the hope of securing some measure of monopoly power, and so being able to keep up prices, may have been the spur to expansion. Growth was often gradual, entrepreneurs frequently putting back into the firm a large proportion of their profits. In this way many large businesses were built up. Another way was by the amalgamation of two or more existing firms to form a new larger undertaking. The British railways grew from small local companies to great national systems in this way before nationalisation turned them into one huge concern. Many railways contributed to the making of the London, Midland and Scottish Railway, the largest being the Midland Railway and the London and North-Western Railway, but many of the constituent companies were themselves the result of the amalgamation of a number of small companies. The five big English banks came into existence in similar fashion, partly by expansion and partly by amalgamation.

II. ECONOMIES OF SCALE

(4) INTERNAL AND EXTERNAL ECONOMIES OF LARGE-SCALE PRODUCTION

The economies to be derived from large-scale production are of two kinds: those which any single firm by its own individual policy can enjoy, and those open to an industry as a whole. Economies that are possible to a single firm are called internal economies. Economies of this kind are considered in this chapter. Further economies are possible to an industry as a whole when most of the firms comprising it are concentrated in one area. Economies arising from localisation of industry are known as external economies, and these are considered in Chapter VIII.

(5) ECONOMIES OF LARGE-SCALE PRODUCTION

The following are some of the principal internal economies of scale:

(i) *Economies in the use of factors of production.* To produce a large output at a lower cost per unit of production than a smaller output clearly means that total cost must increase less than proportionately to output. Consider the case of a small firm that has decided to build a new factory in order to double its output. It will probably not be necessary to double the plant, raw materials and labour to gain this greater volume of production. It would be rare, for example, for the new factory to require twice the area of the old, and therefore the cost of the land per unit of output will fall. Nor is it likely that it will be necessary to double its labour force, for greater division of labour may become possible with the result that average output per man-hour will increase. It will also be possible to employ fully qualified specialists. If the small firm employs such people they will have to spend part of their time doing work requiring less skill, for which the large firm can employ lower-paid labour. As a result, the larger firm will attract more efficient labour to itself merely because it is able to offer its employees better prospects of promotion, since it has a larger number of better-paid posts to fill. The greater division of labour will make possible a more capitalistic method of production and the employment of more specialised machinery. Some types of capital are of necessity very large, and can be used, therefore, only by the larger firms, for the small firm has not sufficient work to keep such big "indivisible" units of capital fully employed. These large units of capital are, however, often more economical in their use of power and generally require fewer men to tend them. It would, therefore, be uneconomic for the small producer to use such capital, for the small firm would find the cost of such plant or machinery too great for its resources. The large undertaking can make a more economical use of its materials, for what might be waste to a small firm can often be used in the manufacture of by-products. Chemical manufacturers particularly are constantly developing new lines of production in this way.

(ii) *Economies in administration.* In the earlier stages of its growth it is unlikely that the costs of administration of the firm will keep pace with increasing output. While the firm is still of medium size, to double the output will not require a doubling of the office staff, for here again the large firm may be able to enjoy the benefits to be derived from division of labour, and more specialised office machinery may be introduced. One advantage of greater specialisation will probably be that the entrepreneur will be able to devote himself purely to administrative and managerial duties. With growth in size, administrative economies, however, generally cease, and in the later stages of expansion the cost of administration may rise quite steeply. As will be seen shortly, the increasing complexity of management is in fact the main factor that sets a limit to the growth in the size of the firm.

(iii) *Marketing economies.* A large firm can generally buy more cheaply than a small one, for it can buy its raw material in bulk, and so obtain it at a lower price. The small firm has to pay some merchant for "breaking bulk" and selling in smaller quantities. Similarly, in distribution the large retailer can buy direct from the producer at a lower price than that charged by the wholesaler. The merchant or manufacturer who has a large order to place usually finds himself in a strong bargaining position, for suppliers are anxious to secure his orders, and will generally cut their prices to obtain them. In proportion to output the selling costs of the large undertaking are lower than those of the small. A firm with a nation-wide market can afford to advertise in the national daily papers, and so bring its products to the notice of potential buyers in all parts of the country. The cost of such advertising would be prohibitive to the small firm. Expansion of a firm's output, say by 50%, does not necessitate a proportionate increase in the number of its commercial travellers. The large firm, therefore, enjoys economies in both buying and selling.

(iv) *Other economies of large scale: (a) Finance.* The large firm often also has an advantage over the small on the financial side. Many firms borrow their working capital from the banks. There is not, however, a standard rate at which banks lend to business men, the rate of interest that will be charged depending on the standing of the borrower, the security offered, the amount borrowed, the purpose for which the loan is required and the bank's estimate of the risk involved. Generally large firms are considered to be the safer borrowers, and there is a tendency for the rate of interest charged by banks to vary with the size of the firm. The less-favoured firms usually pay 1% more than Bank rate, with a minimum of 5%, and the more favoured firms $\frac{1}{2}\%$ above Bank rate, while nationalised industries pay a rate equal to Bank rate, with a minimum of 4%.

(b) *Research.* At one time it was chiefly the chemical and allied industries that spent money on research, but nowadays most industries are alive to its importance. Again the large firm has advantages over the small, for it can have its own laboratories and employ a large number of trained research workers. Since they are in the full employ of the firm, any discoveries they make become the property of their employers. Imperial Chemical Industries, Ltd., makes research one of its most important activities, and on the Board is a Director with the special function of co-ordinating the research work carried out in the firm's various laboratories. In the wool-textile industry very few of even the larger firms have their own laboratories, and, as in other industries where the average size of the firm is not large, there is a Research Association which draws its funds partly from the industry and partly from Government grants and fees. Realising that economic progress and growth depend to a large extent on technical advance, the British Government itself sponsors research in many fields of activity, since 1964 under the surveillance of the Ministry of Technology. In such cases research must be for the advantage of the industry as a whole, and though this may be desirable from the point of view of the community, the individual firm assesses its value less highly than research carried out entirely for its own benefit.

(c) *Welfare.* The efficiency of the workers can be increased by improving the conditions under which they work, and by the provision of canteens and other welfare facilities. These can more easily be provided by the large firms, most of which nowadays make some such provision. Any benefits to be derived from this service are possible only for the larger firms, for the expense is too heavy for the smaller ones.

III. LIMITS TO EXPANSION

(6) LIMITS TO THE SCALE OF PRODUCTION

If by expanding the scale of production certain economies can be obtained it might be asked why firms do not go on expanding indefinitely. A number of things, however, limit the scale of production:

(i) *The extent of the market*. The scale of production is, obviously, dependent in the first place on the demand for the commodity. Production on a large scale cannot be undertaken unless there is sufficient demand to warrant it, though it is often possible to stimulate the demand for a commodity, However, the extent of the demand for a commodity is probably more likely to affect the size of the industry than the size of the individual firms comprising it.

(ii) *Individuality* versus *standardisation*. Mass production means the standardisation of the product, or at least restriction of production to a limited number of varieties. The extent to which variety of product is required will have a limiting effect on the scale of production. In order to create as wide a market as possible for their products, British motor-car manufacturers, for example, each produce a wide range of models, the largest turning out more than fifty models, each slightly different from the other. By the standardisation or semi-standardisation of their models the scale of production has been increased and the average cost of production reduced. Standardisation is possible, however, only if buyers are prepared to accept this restriction of their choice. Consumers may be willing to accept a degree of standardisation in the case of motor cars (the different styles of the various manufacturers giving sufficient variety), but it is doubtful whether they would accept greater standardisation in textiles—especially of the material for women's clothes. Indeed, standardisation of pattern and quality might be fatal to the export trade in woollens and worsteds, where variety and high quality have been the main considerations. This therefore, offsets the disadvantage of smallness of size of the average firm in the woollen industry. Standardisation of the product may cheapen production, but it is liable to check progress, on account of the expense of altering the plant for a new style of product. It has, for example, become an extremely expensive business to alter the design of a mass-produced motor car of today.

(iii) *Increasing cost and complexity of organisation*. Even if there is a sufficiently wide market to make large-scale production practicable, there are other things that check the growth of the firm. First among these is the increasing cost and complexity of organisation as it expands. Imperial Chemical Industries, Ltd., for example, have found it necessary to have fourteen operational divisions, each with a divisional chairman and Board of Directors, and seven functional departments (covering such things as research, personnel, development), each presided over by a director with a seat on the main Board, to co-ordinate and control policy in regard to these matters throughout the firm.[1] When the railways were nationalised all the old area divisions were retained, and a co-ordinating body had to be created to link them together. Another problem that the very large firm has to face is to find someone with the ability to manage it. It is said that the supply of competent managers is limited, and perhaps the difficulty of securing capable and efficient managers is the chief brake on the expansion of firms. In this connection it is of interest to note that I.C.I., Ltd., dispensed with the post of managing director because the duties of this office had become too onerous, and replaced him by a number of executive directors, in charge of the operational divisions of the firm.

(iv) *Increasing costs and falling price.* It has been seen that substitution between factors of production is possible after a certain point. How much of each of the factors the entrepreneur will employ depends on how much he has to pay for them. If a particular entrepreneur wishes to increase his scale of production he will have to engage more factors. It will be seen later that an increased demand for a factor tends to raise its price. Assuming that when the entrepreneur makes his decision to expand production all factors are fully employed, he will be able to increase his supply of them only by drawing some away from other employments, and to do this he will have to offer them higher payments. Consequently, the entrepreneur's costs of production will begin to increase. At the same time, unless there is a change in demand, a larger output can be sold only by lowering the price. Under perfect competition each firm produces only a small proportion of total output, and so an increase in the output of one firm will not substantially affect total supply or price. In actual conditions of imperfect competition, however, this is not so. Suppose, however, that total cost to the entrepreneur (including his own reward each week and "normal profit") is £100 per week at an output of some commodity of 100 units, and assuming all these are sold each week for £120 (that is, at 24s. each), then the profit will be £20 per week. If by increasing his output to 150 per week he increases his costs to £140, but has to reduce his price to 23s. each, his total receipts will be £172 10s., giving a profit of £32 10s. per week. Obviously in this case there were economies of large-scale production. If, however, beyond an output of 150

---

[1] See *Large-Scale Organisation*, edited by G. E. Milward, pp. 144 et seq.

per week costs begin to rise more steeply and total receipts increase less than proportionately owing to the falling price of the commodity, a time will arrive when to increase output by one unit more will raise total costs as much as total receipts. Clearly, it will not pay an entrepreneur to expand production beyond this point. In this case an output of 175 might represent the most profitable output of the firm, and so further expansion would not take place.

(v) *Increased risk.* As the scale of production increases, so do the risks of production. The greater the output, the greater, therefore, will be the loss from an error of judgment. Unwillingness to bear greater risks may be another limitation on the growth of firms.

(7) DISADVANTAGES OF LARGE-SCALE PRODUCTION

The large firm suffers from the following drawbacks:

(i) *Bureaucratic control.* The larger the firm, the more bureaucratic its organisation tends to be. In order to ensure the carrying out of the policy that the management has decided upon, rules and regulations are necessary and must be strictly adhered to. The large firm is more impersonal than the small, and contact between management and staff is therefore less easy.

(ii) *Sluggish response to changes.* However important the decision a sole proprietor has to take, he alone is responsible for making it. If he is a man who rapidly makes up his mind he can decide at once and quickly put his ideas into effect, for he is under no obligation to consult anyone else. In his case changes in policy or organisation can be introduced without delay. In a large firm, however, only decisions on minor matters can be left to subordinates, and important questions have to be referred to superiors. For example, the manager has to convince his board of the soundness of his policy before he is allowed to carry it out.

(iii) *Loss of motive of self-interest.* It is claimed on behalf of the sole proprietor that his own interests and those of the firm are one, with the result that there is less waste and greater efficiency. Nevertheless, the interests of most managers of large firms are bound up with those of the firms that employ them. Even if they are not shareholders, their own remuneration is probably closely linked with the success of the business, and should a manager fail to make progress, his tenure of office will probably be cut short. However, even if due allowance is made for this, the man who owns his business is often spurred on by a pride of achievement that is unlikely to influence the salaried manager to quite the same extent.

(8) THE SURVIVAL OF THE SMALL FIRM

The growth in size of the firm has not prevented the survival of the small firm, in spite of the fact that, though there are some disadvantages of large size, these are more than counterbalanced by the advantages of large-scale production. The size of the business unit tends to be small if the work involves the provision of direct services, such as those of the doctor, the dentist, the solicitor, the accountant, or where the work can be done only by craftsmen, as in bespoke tailoring, or where a personal service is provided, such as that of the domestic plumber or electrician. Similarly, the small retailer survives, in spite of the competition of multiple shops, co-operative societies and department stores, because he can give personal attention to the particular requirements of his own group of customers who are willing to pay a little extra for this service. It has been pointed out that large-scale production is possible only where there is a wide market for the commodity. Obviously, where there is only a limited demand for a commodity, or where standardisation of the product is not desirable, small firms can produce sufficient to satisfy it. It may be, too, that, in some forms of production, costs quickly begin to rise as production expands, and so the most economical unit is the small firm—that is, the optimum size of the firm is small. Similarly, when the technical side of a large firm has grown beyond this optimum it may be more economical for it to put some processes to small firms rather than undertake them itself.

IV. THE OPTIMUM FIRM

(9) WHAT IS THE OPTIMUM FIRM?

At a certain size the costs of production of a firm per unit of output will be at a minimum. At that size there will be no motive for further expansion, for at any other size, either larger or smaller, it would be less efficient. Such a firm is known as the optimum firm—that is, *the best or most efficient size of firm*.[1] Between one industry and another the optimum size will vary, for, as has already been seen, the small firm is most efficient for some purposes and the large one for others. It is fairly easy in theory to conceive of an optimum size of firm in any particular industry, though in practice it would be difficult—if not impossible—to decide in an actual case whether a firm had reached the optimum or not. It has been further suggested that there may be more than one optimum, a low and a high, expansion from the lower to the higher position being difficult because at any intermediate point between the two optima the firm would be less efficient.

[1] See E. A. G. Robinson: *The Structure of Competitive Industry*.

For example, a survey of the Lancashire cotton industry in 1945[1] showed the firms engaged in cotton-spinning to be distributed according to size as follows:

TABLE VIII

Cotton-spinning Firms

Number of spindles	Number of firms
Less than 20,000	23
20,000–40,000	38
40,000–80,000	78
80,000–200,000	110
200,000–1,000,000	26
Over 1,000,000	5

Of 280 firms, 188 (that is, 67%) fell within the third and fourth groups. If it can be taken that the majority of firms will be clustered round the optimum, then in cotton-spinning the optimum at that time might be taken to be the firm with between 80,000 and 200,000 spindles.

In cotton-weaving the position was as follows:

TABLE IX

Cotton-weaving Firms

Number of looms	Number of firms
Less than 200	438
200–400	194
400–800	253
800–2,000	153
Over 2,000	25

The distribution of firms in this section of the industry indicates the possibility of there being a minor optimum (the firm with under 200 looms) and a major optimum (the firm with between 400 and 800 looms). A comparison of the two lists seems to show that the optimum in the spinning section of the industry was larger than the optimum in the weaving section.

Again, the optimum in any industry may itself vary from one period to another. Under perfect competition there would probably be a tendency for all firms to expand towards the optimum. The optimum, too, may change as a result of changing conditions and the development of new techniques. Changes in the relative prices and efficiency of

[1] *Working Party Report on Cotton*, p. 38.

factors will affect the optimum proportion in which factors are combined; a rise in the price of labour may reduce the amount of labour
in the optimum proportion. In a society where economic progress is
rapid these changes will be constantly taking place, with the result that,
though firms are always tending towards the optimum, they never
reach it. The actual size may, however, be near what was previously
thought to be the optimum. The idea of the optimum firm is a useful
concept; at any given moment there must be a certain size of firm at
which production will be most efficient.

(10) THE RECONCILIATION OF DIFFERING OPTIMA

The chief difficulty confronting any firm striving to reach the optimum is the possibility that the different divisions of the firm may have
different optima. For example, the optimum administrative division
may not suit the optimum technical division, which may require an
administrative department either greater or less than the optimum of
the other department. In the heavy industries, where the most economical technical unit is very large, an administrative unit much greater
than the optimum may be required. In firms where the technical unit
is relatively small (for example, woollen weaving) the required administrative unit may be much smaller than the optimum. From the point
of view of finance it has been seen that the large firm can borrow more
cheaply than the small, and so the optimum firm from the standpoint of finance is large. The big firm, too, can obtain additional permanent capital more easily than the small firm. Similarly, there may
be again a different optimum for the marketing side of the firm. Large-
scale buying enables expert buyers to be employed and lower prices
to be paid, and large-scale selling also yields economies, for example,
in the employment of commercial travellers. The entrepreneur is
thus faced by the problem of reconciling these different optima.

If the technical unit is too great for the administration, one way out
of the difficulty in some cases might be to reduce the size of the technical
unit, for example, by limiting production to fewer varieties of the
commodity. Or, it may be possible to reduce the size of the technical
side by putting out some processes to small firms, as has occurred in the
motor industry. Or again, it may be possible to split up the technical
unit into a number of productive departments, each with its own Board
of Management. A central board would then be required to formulate
general policy and to co-ordinate the activities of the departmental or
divisional boards. Thus, although the nationalisation of British railways increased the complexity of management, this may have been
counterbalanced by technical economies.

If the technical optimum is small and the administrative optimum is large reconciliation may be achieved by duplicating the technical unit. In a weaving-shed this would merely require the addition of more looms. If there is insufficient demand for the product to make this course feasible the firm might widen its range of products. However great may be the difficulty of achieving this objective, the entrepreneur has the incentive of lower costs to spur him on.

V. THE LAWS OF RETURNS

(II) THE PROBLEM OF PROPORTIONS

The first mention of the *Law of Diminishing Returns* was made when considering the factor of production, *Land*. It was noticed then that early in the nineteenth century economists thought that one of the special features of land was that production in which it played an important part was peculiarly subject to this law. Modern economists no longer restrict the application of the law to land, but apply it in similar circumstances to all factors of production.

The Law of Diminishing Returns states that if the amount of one or more factors used in a particular form of production is fixed, and increasing amounts of other factors are combined with the fixed factor or factors, then both the average output in relation to the variable factor and successive additions to total output will eventually diminish. If this were not so there would be no limit to the yield of one small area of land.

Suppose first, for example, that land and capital are fixed in amount and that varying amounts of labour are used with them, then, as the following table shows, there may be increasing returns up to the employment of four men, but after that diminishing returns may set in:

TABLE X

Diminishing Returns with Labour the only Variable Factor

Number of men	Fixed amount of land units	Fixed amount of capital units	Output units	Average physical product per man
1	2	8	10	10
2	2	8	30	15
3	2	8	60	20
4	2	8	100	25
5	2	8	120	24
6	2	8	132	22
7	2	8	140	20
8	2	8	146	18

It should be noted that the above table shows the output and average product per man for eight different firms, working with a different combination of factors, and not for a single firm recruiting additional men at varying stages of production. The table shows that after a certain point the employment of more men reduces the average output per man, and so illustrates the Law of Diminishing Returns with reference to labour.

The following production table shows how diminishing returns will eventually set in if the amounts of labour and land are fixed and capital is the variable factor.

TABLE XI

Diminishing Returns with Capital the only Variable Factor

Units of capital	Area of land fixed	Number of men fixed units	Output units	Average physical product per unit of capital
1	6	2	3	3
2	6	2	14	7
3	6	2	30	10
4	6	2	52	13
5	6	2	75	15
6	6	2	96	16
7	6	2	119	17
8	6	2	132	16·5
9	6	2	144	16
10	6	2	150	15

The table shows that in this case the Law of Diminishing Returns begins to operate when the amount of capital employed reaches seven units, after which the average output per unit of capital declines. Here, then, is an illustration of the Law of Diminishing Returns in relation to capital.

A third table could be constructed to show the operation of the law with land as the variable factor—a very unlikely occurrence. In these examples two factors have been taken as fixed and only one as variable. In actual conditions it is more likely that two of the factors would be variable and only one fixed or scarce.

If this law is stated as the Law of Eventually Diminishing Returns it becomes applicable to any kind of production. There may be increasing returns in the early stages as a result of increasing the amount of the variable factor, but sooner or later the Law of Diminishing Returns will begin to operate. In all cases, when this law comes into play as a result of varying the proportion between the factors generally on account of the difficulty of increasing the factors to equal proportions. Indeed, it has been suggested that a better name for it would be the *Law of Proportions*.

Within certain limits, the entrepreneur can vary the proportion between the factors he employs. It has previously been noticed that, though the entrepreneur requires a certain minimum amount of each factor, he can to some extent choose between employing more of one factor or more of another—for example, more capital and less labour, or more labour and less capital. In other words, it is often possible to substitute one factor for another. This is known as the *Principle of Substitution*. If, therefore, one factor is scarce it becomes possible to use more of the other factors. If one factor is fixed output can be increased only by using proportionately more of the other factors.

(12) RETURNS TO SCALE

If the factors land, labour and capital had to be combined in a fixed proportion in order to carry out any particular kind of production there would be no problem of proportions for the entrepreneur to solve, though he would still have to decide his scale of production, for the factors can be combined in the same proportion to make firms of many different sizes, for example:

TABLE XII

Change of Scale with Fixed Proportions

Firm	Area of land	Number of men	Units of capital
A	1	20	8
B	5	100	40
C	10	200	80

All three firms, A, B, C, have their factors combined in the same proportion, but B is larger than A, and C much larger than B. It may be that merely to expand the firm from size A to size B will yield increasing returns. If so, there would be said to be *increasing returns to scale*. Perhaps if the firm expands from size B to size C diminishing returns will set in. In some cases the expansion of a firm may be accompanied by constant returns.

It will be seen, therefore, that there are really two sets of laws relating to returns, one resulting from varying the proportions in which the factors are combined, and the other arising from increasing the scale of production.

It is not easy, however, to conceive of either increasing or diminishing returns being purely the result of an increase in the size of the firm. Indeed, some economists are inclined to doubt whether "pure" returns to scale are possible at all. If the reader cares to glance back at the economies of large-scale production listed above[1] he will see that most of the advantages of large-scale production arise because it is not always necessary or even possible to increase all the factors of the firm proportionately with output. He might find it of interest to pick out those economies which he regards as being "pure" returns to scale. In such cases increasing returns appear to be due to varying the proportions between the factors, though obviously this can be achieved only by increasing the size of the firm.

To produce a small output a small firm is required, and at this size it may not be possible to combine the factors in the "best" proportion. In actual conditions the *indivisibility* of some factors prevents the optimum proportion being achieved, for some factors are not divisible into small units. Capital, for example, often consists of large indivisible units such as blast-furnaces; and labour can be employed only in exact units, for fractions are not possible. Thus over a wide range of output the same amount of one of the factors may have to be employed. At a small output, therefore, there will be excess capacity, the large, indivisible factor not being fully employed, but if output is increased there will be increasing returns until this factor is working at full capacity. Any further expansion of output will require the duplication of this large indivisible factor, and this may check further expansion.

(13) APPLICATION OF LAWS OF RETURNS TO AGRICULTURE AND MANUFACTURE

Ricardo and his followers related the Law of Diminishing Returns solely to land, and it used to be said that this Law operated principally in agriculture, while the Law of Increasing Returns related more particularly to manufacturing industry. It is clear, however, that at different times and in different circumstances each law could apply either to agriculture or to manufacturing. In the early stages of the opening up of a new country the factors may be disproportionately combined—a large amount of land, but comparatively small quantities of labour and capital. The addition of more labour and capital will probably result for a time in a more proportionate increase in output, and so increasing returns will occur. In most old countries, however, land is "scarce" relative to other factors, and if it is desired to produce more food at home this can be accomplished only under conditions of diminishing returns. Any attempt to increase agricultural output in

[1] See pp. 107–109.

Great Britain today can be carried out only under such conditions, but though it may appear to be uneconomic to do so, it may be justified on other grounds, for example, because of an expanding world population or possibly for strategic reasons.

Similarly, in manufacture either law can operate. In manufacture, expansion is more likely to stop short of this point where diminishing returns set in. Defective proportions between the factors, due to the indivisibility of large units of some factors, will give diminishing returns; expansion, due to improving the proportion in which factors are combined, will be accompanied by increasing returns. But eventually diminishing returns will set in both in manufacture and in agriculture, though expansion will generally proceed much farther in manufacture than in agriculture before this occurs. There may also be increasing returns resulting strictly from an increase in the scale of operations—that is, "pure" returns to scale—in either branch of production, mere size of itself producing greater efficiency. Similarly, expansion of both manufacture and agriculture may be accompanied by constant returns or by diminishing returns, in the latter case the unwieldy size of the firm resulting in a loss of efficiency.

(14) THE LAWS OF RETURNS AND THE OPTIMUM FIRM

By definition the optimum firm in any industry is the most efficient size of firm possible, the one where the average cost of production per unit of output is at the minimum. Upon what does this standard of efficiency depend? The concept of the optimum firm can be linked up with the Laws of Returns, and it can therefore be considered from two angles. The optimum firm must first have its factors of production combined in the "best" proportion; secondly, it must have reached the size where it can enjoy the maximum advantages of scale. In other words, the expansion of the firm must be pressed forward so long as it continues to work under conditions of increasing returns, whether these conditions arise from improved proportions or economies of scale; and expansion will cease at the point immediately before diminishing returns, from either cause, set in. The firm then will have reached the optimum for the industry at that particular moment of time, for it must be remembered that what are the best proportions at one period of time may not be the best at another, since new conditions may arise and new methods of production be developed, or the relative prices of factors of production may change.

The development of the optimum firm may take place in the following manner: assume that y represents the variable factor and x the combination of fixed factors; the first stage in the firm's growth is towards the optimum proportion of factors, increasing amounts of y being combined with fixed amounts of x:

TABLE XIII

Variation of Proportions

	Factors x	y	Total product	Average product per unit of y	
	5	1	10	10	Increasing returns to proportions
	5	2	24	12	
Optimum proportion } →	5	3	39	13	
	5	4	52	13	
	5	5	63	12·6	Decreasing returns to proportions
	5	6	74	12·3	
	5	7	82	11·2	

With the combination $5x + 4y$ factors the average output per unit of y employed reaches a maximum. This is therefore the optimum proportion in which to combine the factors.

The second stage in the development of the firm is its growth of scale. In the following table the optimum combination of factors is maintained at different scales of production:

TABLE XIV

Returns to Scale

	Factors x	y	Total	Average production per unit of y	
	5	4	52	13	Constant returns to scale
	10	8	104	13	
	15	12	156	13	
Optimum scale } →	30	24	320	13·6	Increasing returns to scale
	60	48	600	12·5	Decreasing returns to scale

At first, doubling or trebling the amount of each factor employed results in a proportionate increase in output, and so there are constant returns to scale. If the scale of production is increased (the same proportions being maintained between the factors) until $30x + 24y$ factors are employed there are increasing returns to scale, but the firm will not expand beyond this size, for after this point decreasing returns to scale set in. At this size the firm is at its optimum both as regards the proportion between its factors and also with regard to its scale of production.

Until the optimum is reached the firm will be working under conditions of increasing returns, and if it expands beyond the optimum there will be diminishing returns. Similarly, any reduction from the optimum will produce diminishing returns, just as any reduction from a point beyond the optimum will give increasing returns. Using the production table given below, expansion of output up to 100 units of

TABLE XV

The Optimum Firm and the Laws of Returns

Number of men (land and capital being fixed)	Output units	Average physical product per man		
1	10	10		Returns
2	30	15	Returns	
3	60	20		
4	100	25	→OPTIMUM	
5	120	24	Increasing	Diminishing
6	132	22		
7	140	20		
8	146	18		

the commodity is accompanied by Increasing Returns, as also is any reduction of output from any amount over 100 down to 100; there will be diminishing returns if output is reduced below 100 or increased beyond that amount.

This can be shown graphically:

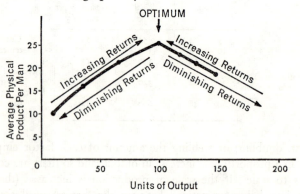

Fig. 3.—The Optimum Firm and the Laws of Returns.

The optimum firm can thus be related to the Laws of Returns, with Diminishing Returns occurring when moving away from optimum, and Increasing Returns occurring as the optimum is approached. In actual conditions it may be impossible for a firm to reach optimum size, since it may be unable to employ the factors of production in the optimum proportion. This is likely to occur especially where large "indivisible" units of capital are employed.

RECOMMENDATIONS FOR FURTHER READING

F. H. Knight: *Risk, Uncertainty and Profit*, Chapter 7.
E. A. G. Robinson: *The Structure of Competitive Industry*.

For the Laws of Returns:
G. J. Stigler: *The Theory of Price*, Chapter 8.

QUESTIONS

1. What are the conditions which determine the degree of specialisation in an industry? (R.S.A. Inter.)

2. Discuss the economic factors which promote the growth in the size of some business undertakings, while others remain small. (R.S.A. Adv.)

3. Describe the growth of joint-stock enterprise in Great Britain and account for the continued survival of small firms in particular types of industry. (L.C. Com. Econ.)

4. Discuss the economies of large-scale production. Explain why some small firms still exist. (I.T.)

5. Describe some of the economies which can be achieved through large-scale production. In view of these economies, how is it that, in the same industry, small firms can flourish side by side with big firms? (Exp.)

6. "The bigger the better." Under what conditions is this true of industrial undertakings? (C.I.S. Inter.)

7. Distinguish between internal and external economies and indicate the main economies of large-scale production. (I.B.)

8. It was at one time thought that the small business would not be able to survive the competition of the large-scale enterprise, but this has proved to be incorrect. To what do you attribute the continuance of the small business and what do you consider to be the most favourable conditions? (L.C. Com. C. & F.)

9. In what sense is it true to say that the large firm has become the representative business unit in the advanced industrial countries? (C.I.S. Final.)

10. Explain the meaning of Increasing Returns. For what reasons may an industry be subject to increasing returns? (C.C.S. Final.)

11. Is it true to say that agriculture is peculiarly subject to a law of diminishing returns? (C.I.S. Inter.)

12. What do you understand by the optimum size of a firm? What are the principal factors which determine it? (C.C.S. Final.)

13. The way in which the factors of production may be substituted one for the other is an important element in deciding the economic policy of an employer. Explain why this is so. (I.H.A.)

14. Why are the main British and American producers of motor cars large and few? (C.I.S. Final.)

15. Outline precisely what is meant by the *economies of large-scale production* and show how these may lead to the growth of monopoly in an industry. (G.C.E. Adv.)

16. Discuss the factors affecting the size of firms and the degree of vertical integration in any *one* industry with which you are familiar. (G.C.E. Adv.)

17. "Conditions of increasing returns can be regarded as exceptions to the operation of the law of diminishing returns." Discuss. (Final Degree.)

18. On what factors does the size of an industry and the number of firms comprising it depend? (Final Degree.)

CHAPTER VIII

THE LOCATION OF INDUSTRY

I. ADVANTAGES OF LOCALISATION OF INDUSTRY

(1) EXTERNAL ECONOMIES OF LARGE-SCALE PRODUCTION

In Great Britain many industries are highly localised. The main centre of the cotton industry, for example, is concentrated in South Lancashire, over 90% of worsteds are made in the West Riding of Yorkshire, most boots and shoes come from the Northampton and Leicester district, pottery manufacture is almost entirely confined to North Staffordshire, the Black Country is the chief seat of the motor-car industry, most cutlery is made at Sheffield, tin-plate at Swansea and shipbuilding is confined to three or four centres. Why, then, should business men who are contemplating setting up a particular industry generally prefer to do so in areas where others similarly engaged are already established? Under competitive conditions production has to be carried on at the lowest possible cost, and so firms in the same industry are found together because it was discovered that it was cheaper to carry on production in certain areas and that there are often economies to be enjoyed where industries are concentrated in particular areas. Economies resulting from the expansion of a single firm are called internal economies, and these have already been considered; economies resulting from the localisation of an industry are termed external economies of large-scale production.

(2) ADVANTAGES OF LOCALISATION OF INDUSTRY

A number of advantages accrue to an industry when it is concentrated in one area:

(i) *Regional division of labour.* It has already been seen that division of labour within the firm increases output and cheapens production. When an industry is highly concentrated in an area this principle can be extended to a whole industry, for when firms are located close together it becomes possible for individual firms to specialise in single processes or in particular varieties of a commodity. This has been called territorial division of labour. In the cotton industry and the worsted section of the woollen industry, for example, some firms are engaged solely in spinning, weaving, dyeing or some other process, and this has brought about even greater specialisation within these industries. In Lancashire the spinning section of the cotton industry is concentrated in the south-east of the county, and the weaving section chiefly in the Preston, Blackburn and Burnley area. In the West Riding specialisation is according to the type of product, fine worsteds being made in Huddersfield, cheap tweeds in the Colne Valley, carpets in Halifax and shoddy and heavy woollens in Dewsbury and the Spen Valley. Such specialisation, whether of process or of product, is dependent on adequate and cheap transport being available.

(ii) *A supply of skilled labour.* Another advantage of localisation of industry is to be found in the development of a reservoir of skilled labour for the local industry. A new firm might establish itself in a particular area because the appropriately skilled labour was available there. This factor is probably less important at the present time than formerly, when it was more usual for children to follow the same occupation as their parents, for the greater use of machinery makes general alertness of more importance than special skill.

(iii) *Development of subsidiary industries.* When an industry is highly localised subsidiary industries grow up that cater for the needs of the major industry, and so textile machinery for the cotton industry is made in Lancashire, and for the woollen industry in the West Riding of Yorkshire. The financing of industry, too, can be more easily undertaken where bank managers have specialised knowledge of the local industry. Though small local banks have disappeared, the larger institutions that have succeeded them are aware of this, and generally appoint as managers of their branches men who have had previous experience of the economic problems of the area.

(iv) *Organised markets.* Finally, localisation of industry often leads to the establishment in the area of highly organised markets, such as the Liverpool and Manchester[1] Cotton Exchanges. The existence of these facilities acts as a magnet to new firms desiring to enter the industry.

(3) WHERE LOCALISATION IS NOT POSSIBLE

In the case of the production of some cheap or bulky goods the relatively heavy cost of transport outweighs any advantages to be derived from localisation, and their production is consequently more widely distributed. Building materials are of this kind. Stone houses are to be found only in districts where there are local supplies of stone, and brick-making is carried on near most large towns. Public utility services have to be provided in the places that require them, though the electricity grid scheme has made it possible to concentrate the generation of electricity at a few large centres. Retail distribution cannot very

[1] The Manchester Royal Exchange closed in 1968.

tion of electricity at a few large centres. Retail distribution cannot very easily be concentrated, as most consumers prefer to use shops near their homes, though improved transport services from the country to the towns have compelled many village shops to close, and the development of mail-order business has widened the market for the large city stores. Where direct services of a personal kind are provided, concentration is not possible, and doctors, dentists, teachers, etc., are distributed over the country generally according to the density of population.

II. FACTORS INFLUENCING INDUSTRIAL LOCATION

In considering the factors influencing industrial location it is necessary to distinguish between three historical periods: (i) the years before 1914; (ii) the period between the two World Wars, 1919–39; and (iii) the period since 1945.

(4) THE PERIOD BEFORE 1914

A number of influences affected the location of industry before 1914, of which the following were the most important:

(i) *Nearness to coal.* During the nineteenth century the main influence was proximity to power. In the early days of the Industrial Revolution water-power was employed, and the first factories were built near fast-flowing streams, as for example, on the eastern and western slopes of the Pennines. When steam power was introduced nearness to coal became the chief localising influence, as means of transport were limited and the price of coal increased steeply the farther it had to be carried from the mines. As a result, costs of production were lowest on or near the coalfields. Coal also replaced charcoal in the smelting of iron ore. The result was that all the basic industries— cotton, wool, iron and steel—were established on or near coalfields. Woollen manufacture—the oldest industry in Great Britain, and dating from the Middle Ages—had been fairly widely distributed down to the eighteenth century, but the effect of the Industrial Revolution was to concentrate it in the West Riding of Yorkshire, though one or two small centres managed to survive.

(ii) *Nearness to raw materials.* Second in importance of the influences on the location of industry in the nineteenth century was proximity to raw materials. This was especially the case where the cost of the raw materials formed a large proportion of the total costs of production. Nearness to supplies of iron ore, limestone and (for Sheffield) millstone grit influenced the location of iron-smelting. Middlesbrough owed its growth to its nearness both to the coal and to the Cleveland iron-mines, just as in more recent times Scunthorpe and Corby have grown rapidly as a result of their nearness to supplies of iron ore, now that less coal than formerly is used in iron-smelting. Boots and shoes came to be manufactured in Northampton and neighbouring towns because of nearness to supplies of leather.

(iii) *Minor influences.* The presence in the Pennines of ample supplies of soft water for cleaning the fibres was an important influence on the location of the Yorkshire and Lancashire textile industries. The use of soft water reduced the cost of this process. Another minor influence on the location of the cotton industry was the humid atmosphere of Lancashire. A feature, therefore, of the late eighteenth and early nineteenth centuries was the drift of population to the coalfields of the North and Midlands, London eventually being the only great centre of population not close to a coalfield. The effect of every one of these influences was to make costs of production lower in some places.

(5) THE PERIOD BETWEEN THE TWO WORLD WARS (1919–39)

Between the two World Wars the coalfields ceased to attract new industries. Nearness to coal, however, still remained the principal influence on the location of heavy industries, where the cost of power forms a high proportion of the total cost of the product. Thus the main centres of the motor-car industry came to be established near the coalfields of the West Midlands. Even where the original advantages of their situation had passed away, it was difficult for such industries to move because of the large amount of fixed capital involved. It was the new industries which tended to be established away from the coalfields, mainly because they were light in character, that is, the cost of power was not their principal cost. The new industries of this period included the manufacture of electrical equipment and accessories, because of the expanding use of electricity, wireless sets and components. There was, too, a great increase in the number and variety of packaged branded goods and patented foodstuffs. In spite of heavy unemployment, the standard of living was rising, and that meant an expansion of the production of consumers' goods. Heavy industry is primarily occupied with the production of capital goods; light industry is to a great extent mainly concerned with consumers' goods. Capital goods generally do not require to be as widely distributed as consumers' goods. The products of the light industries, too, were mainly intended for the home market. Thus the new industries of the period between the two World Wars were different in character from the older industries, and this had great influence on their location. During this period the main influences on industrial location were:

(i) *New means of transport.* In the nineteenth century the development of canals and railways encouraged localisation of industry and regional specialisation; the rapid development of road transport during the 1920s, more mobile and for many goods cheaper than the railways, tended towards a wider dispersal of both population and industry.

(ii) *New forms of power.* Throughout the nineteenth century, once it had superseded water power, coal became the sole source of power. By the third decade of the twentieth century alternative forms of power—gas, electricity and oil—had been developed, and these were capable of being transmitted to all parts of the country more cheaply than coal, so that industry became no longer restricted in its location to the coalfields.

(iii) *Nearness to large centres of population.* Large conurbations came into existence during the nineteenth century as a result of people being attracted to the new industries then developing on the coalfields. During the 1920s and 1930s a large centre of population became of itself an attraction to the new consumer-goods industries, as a market for their products. Where production was undertaken mainly for the home market a firm setting up near London for example, could have a fifth or more of its potential customers almost on its doorstep. London could also deal with exports. Few new industries were established on the coalfields, where unemployment was heaviest, because of other dis-advantages, such as the unsuitability of much of the labour and the high local rates levied in most of these areas. As a result, labour tended to go to the new industries instead of the new industries moving to the labour.

The drift to the South. The inter-war period, then, showed some reversal of the nineteenth-century tendency of population to increase more rapidly in the North. London, South-east England and, to a lesser extent, the Midlands, attracted the newer industries, and since the heavy industries of the older manufacturing areas felt the impact of the Great Depression more severely than the rest of the country, there was some drift of population from Northern England and South Wales to the expanding industrial areas of the Midlands and the South-East. The extent of this change in the distribution of population is shown by the fact that there was an increase in the number of insured workers in the London area of over half a million, while a loss of 176,000 workers was experienced by South Wales, 100,000 by Durham and 94,000 by South Lancashire.[1] Many towns in Lancashire declined in popula-tion between the census of 1921 and that of 1931.

[1] See S. R. Dennison: *The Location of Industry.*

In view of the extent of unemployment, the number of people who actually moved to the South was perhaps not very great, but undoubtedly there was some shift of population, and when mobility of labour is under discussion this movement is worthy of note. As a result, London began to eat up the countryside on its outer fringes, the further growth of a population already vast accentuating the problem of large conurbations. In the West Midlands the effects of the Great Depression on the older industries was counterbalanced by the extraordinary growth of the motor-car industry during this period, and there was also some drift of population into this region.

III. PLANNED LOCATION OF INDUSTRY

The period since 1945 has been one of planned location of industry.

(6) DISADVANTAGES OF LOCALISATION OF INDUSTRY

There is, however, one serious drawback to a district being dependent on a single basic industry. Even if full employment is successfully maintained, there will still be the risk of structural unemployment resulting from a change in demand. At any given time there are always some industries that are expanding because of an increasing demand for their products, and other industries that are declining owing to decreasing demand. Such changes are a feature of a progressive economy. If the declining industry is highly localised mass unemployment in that area may result, even though the rest of the country is enjoying a trade boom. This has been the experience of Belfast, parts of Scotland, South Wales and North-east England during the later 1950s and the 1960s. There was unemployment in these areas while the rest of the country was enjoying full employment.

Similarly, during a depression some industries will be found to be expanding; even during the Great Depression in Great Britain (1929-35) the motor-car industry, the manufacture of electrical apparatus and of artificial silk were all expanding industries. On the other hand, the cotton industry became a declining industry after 1929, largely due to the contraction of the export trade—the result of increased foreign competition—and even if there had not been a general trade slump at that time, it is possible that there would have been high unemployment in Lancashire. The coincidence of cyclical and structural unemployment during the Great Depression produced the so-called "distressed areas"—those parts of the country where the level of unemployment was well above the national average. Another disadvantage of extreme localisation is the growth of great conurbations, where one town merges into another, with consequent overcrowding, lack of open spaces and traffic congestion.

(7) PLANNED LOCATION OF INDUSTRY

Areas of localised industries are then liable to more severe unemployment than areas with greater variety of industry. This was apparent in the Great Depression, when 35% of insured workers in the various "Distressed Areas" were out of work (in the cases of Jarrow and Merthyr the percentage was 75), while unemployment in Bedfordshire, Hertfordshire and Middlesex never rose above 6%. The aim of planned location of industry, therefore, was to give greater variety of industry to the former distressed areas, and at the same time to check the industrial expansion of the London area, as recommended by the Barlow Report of 1940.

Special Areas. There had been an attempt in the 1930s to encourage new industries to be set up in places where there was heavy unemployment, the Acts of 1934 and 1937 giving the Government powers to assist these areas, which were given the name of Special Areas. Trading estates were established in Durham, West Cumberland, South Wales and Central Scotland, factories at low rentals being available to firms willing to go there, and the Government undertaking to train workers for new occupations. Although some measure of success was achieved, it was difficult at that time to persuade firms to establish themselves in places to which they did not wish to go, and with heavy unemployment in the country it was not possible to refuse to allow firms to set up elsewhere. After the outbreak of war in 1939 the Government itself established over a hundred new factories in the Special Areas.

After 1945. The planning of economic activity was regarded as imperative in both World Wars, but it received greater emphasis in the years following 1945. The maintenance of full employment was accepted as an objective by all political parties in Great Britain. Lord Beveridge declared that control by the State of the location of industry was the alternative to the creation of distressed areas. Controlled location of industry was in fact his second condition for a successful full-employment policy.[1]

It has already been noticed that at any given time some industries are expanding while others are declining, as a result of changes in demand. In such cases, though some unemployment may occur in the declining industries, it may be balanced by the additional employment created in those that are expanding. If labour could be transferred from one occupation to the other without economic friction no unemployment would arise, but labour is not sufficiently mobile to make this possible. In 1945, therefore, Parliament passed the *Distribution of Industries Act*, which made the Board of Trade responsible for the location of industry.

[1] Lord Beveridge: *Full Employment in a Free Society*, p. 32.

This was followed in 1946 by the *New Towns Act*, which aimed at checking the further expansion of large conurbations.

(8) THE DEVELOPMENT AREAS

The first step towards planned location of industry was the passing of the *Distribution of Industries Act* in 1945. This Act designated certain parts of the country as Development Areas, and the Board of Trade was empowered to add to this number when circumstances warranted it. The first four districts to be designated as Development Areas comprised the pre-1939 Special Areas, generally with enlarged boundaries:

(i) the North-East, that is, most of the Durham coalfield together with neighbouring portions of southern Northumberland and the North Riding of Yorkshire, and including the towns of Newcastle-upon-Tyne, Sunderland and Middlesbrough;

(ii) West Cumberland, comprising the coalfield and the towns of Workington and Whitehaven;

(iii) South Wales and Monmouthshire, with the towns of Cardiff, Swansea and Newport with in addition a small area around Milford Haven;

(iv) Clydeside and the Lanarkshire coalfields of West Scotland together with the district around Dundee.

All these regions were mainly dependent on coal-mining and iron and steel, industries offering little scope for the employment of women. In 1946 two more Development Areas were designated:

(v) the cotton-spinning area of south-east Lancashire, situated to the north and east of Manchester, but excluding that city;

(vi) the coal-mining district of North Wales, centred around Wrexham.

Two years later there were two further additions to the list of Development Areas, these differing from earlier creations in that neither included a coalfield:

(vii) Merseyside;

(viii) the district round Inverness in northern Scotland, including in addition to Inverness itself, the towns of Dingwall, Tain and Invergordon.

The aim in northern Scotland was to check the drift of population to the South by the development of a new industrial area dependent on hydro-electric power.

Finally, in 1953, the total number of Development Areas was increased to nine by the addition of:

(ix) North-east Lancashire, including the cotton-weaving towns of Burnley, Nelson and Colne.

It will be noticed that portions of Lancashire fell within three different Development Areas. The contraction of the cotton industry has made essential the attraction of new industries to Lancashire.

During the fifteen years, 1950–1965, even though in the country at large full employment was generally maintained pockets of unemployment often arose in districts outside the Development Areas, as, for example, in Hull, the Furness district of Lancashire, Belfast and in the winter in the seaside resorts. Encouragement was given to firms to set up in these districts as well as in the Development Areas. The Government also assisted the contraction and reorganisation of the cotton industry in 1958–59. Then the position was regularised by the passing of the *Local Employment Act* in 1959 which empowered the Government to assist any part of the country where there was unemployment above the national average, the Development Areas being replaced by Development Districts.[1] Under this new scheme motor-car manufacturing firms have been assisted in the building of branch factories on Merseyside, in South Wales and on Clydeside.

(9) FOR AND AGAINST PLANNED LOCATION OF INDUSTRY

For a number of reasons a greater measure of success was achieved after 1945 than before 1939 in giving greater variety to areas where industries were highly localised. In the first place the Special Areas were established only a few years before the outbreak of the Second World War, whereas the Development Areas had a much longer existence of over fourteen years. Most important of all was the difference between the two periods, the earlier one being a time of severe unemployment, the later one of full or over-full employment. Before 1939 new industries were for this reason welcome everywhere. During most of the time since 1945 there have been insufficient factors of production to satisfy the demand for them, and in such circumstances it becomes easier to steer new firms to particular areas, the firms themselves being willing to set up almost anywhere where labour was available.

Down to 1959 control of investment was the most powerful instrument available to the Government in carrying out its policy of planned location of industry. When to raise new capital required the sanction of the Capital Issues Committee it could be made conditional on the new

[1] *See* p. 134.

F

firm or branch being established in a Development Area. The *Town and Country Planning Act* still further assisted Government policy. In many parts of the country there were serious shortages of labour, and this made it necessary for firms to go elsewhere. At one time high local rates made firms shun certain towns, but a measure of equalisation has been achieved through differential Government grants.

During the first ten years of their existence the Development Areas received most of the new firms established during that period, but during recent years the proportion of new firms going to these areas has gradually declined. With the passing of the *Local Employment Act*, 1959 and the activities of the Capital Issues Committee almost coming to an end in 1959, planned location of industry has taken a slightly new form.

Is dispersal of industry sound on economic grounds? Most firms that have been encouraged to set up in the Development Areas, if they had been left to decide for themselves, would probably have gone elsewhere, and in the case of highly localised industries, to the region where their particular industry was concentrated. It must be remembered that when industries became localised it was for economic reasons— that is, because production could be carried on more efficiently in those areas, and external economies associated with localisation could be enjoyed. Any scheme of dispersal will rob the firms settling in other areas of these external economies, and in a trade depression these firms may be the first to be affected, especially since more than half the new firms are only branches of firms with headquarters elsewhere. Most of the newer industries in the Development Areas, however, are of the light type engaged in the production of consumers' goods, and these have less to gain from localisation.

If the scheme for greater local diversification of industry is based on the assumption that full employment will be permanently maintained the effect should be to spread structural unemployment over a wider area and so prevent serious pockets of mass unemployment arising. For such a policy to be really effective a much more ambitious scheme is probably required. There is no doubt, however, that the decline of the cotton industry had less effect on the level of employment in South Lancashire on account of the Government's policy in encouraging new industries to establish themselves in that area. The greater variety of industry has made it easier for many workers previously employed in the cotton industry to obtain alternative employment. With the development of road transport and the newer forms of power, the advantages of localisation are less strong today than they were in the nineteenth century.

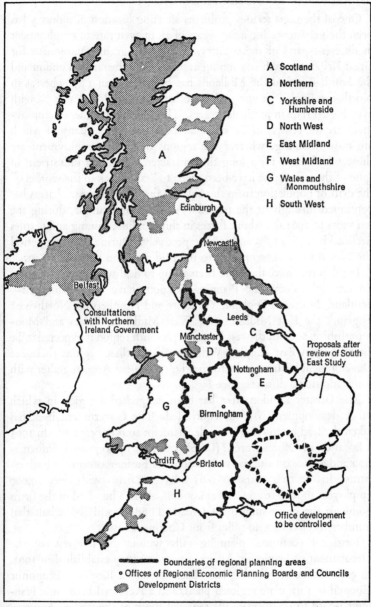

A Scotland
B Northern
C Yorkshire and Humberside
D North West
E East Midland
F West Midland
G Wales and Monmouthshire
H South West

Boundaries of regional planning areas
○ Offices of Regional Economic Planning Boards and Councils
Development Districts

Reproduced from Progress Report No. 1 (Department of Economic Affairs) by permission of the Controller of H.M. Stationery Office.

FIG. 4.—ECONOMIC PLANNING REGIONS

Note that: (1) The Northern Ireland Government has set up an Economic Council;
(2) Orkney and Shetlands (not shown) are development districts.
(3) East Anglia, comprising mainly Norfolk and Suffolk has now been separated from the South East Region.

(10) REGIONAL ECONOMIC PLANNING

One of the most serious problems affecting location of industry has been the persistence for many years of an uneven rate of employment in different parts of the country. With average unemployment for Great Britain as a whole running at only 1·5%, the rate in London and the South-East and the Midlands has been less than 1%, whereas in North-east England it was 3·0%, Scotland 3·4% and Wales 2·7%, with even higher rates in particular places. The regions of higher unemployment are the centres of the old-established industries, many of which are now declining, whereas the regions of low unemployment are those which have for a long time attracted expanding industries. In spite of the efforts that have been made to "take work to the workers," the drift of population from the older to the newer industrial areas has continued throughout the period 1945–65. For example, during the ten years to 1964 the labour forces in shipbuilding, mining and textiles declined by 27%, 25% and 19% respectively. During the same period the North lost 600,000 people to the Midlands and the South-East.

Local bodies have therefore been set up to deal with these problems. So far eight Economic Planning Regions have been delineated— Scotland, Northern England, Yorkshire and Humberside, North-west England, the East Midlands, the West Midlands, Wales and Monmouthshire, and South-west England. A ninth region is expected to be established in East Anglia. Within some of these regions there are Development Districts—the former Development Areas together with some additional districts. (See Fig. 4).

The Greater London Area has been designated a region in which office development is to be controlled. The Government itself has taken the lead by moving some departments to other regions. In 1963 a Location of Offices Bureau (L.O.B.) was set up to provide information and advice on alternative locations for business offices for business firms. In the two years 1963–65 over 200 firms with over 20,000 employees moved from Central London, about a hundred of the firms going to the outer suburbs of Greater London, and about half that number to places 20–40 miles from Charing Cross.

Regional economic planning falls within the purview of the Department of Economic Affairs, a new ministry established in 1964. In each region two bodies have been set up—a Regional Economic Council to formulate regional plans, and a Regional Economic Planning Board to co-ordinate the regional work of the various Government Departments concerned. The aim of regional planning is to bring about a more balanced economic development of the country as a whole.

(11) THE NEW TOWNS

To check the unregulated growth of London and other large conurbations, the building of a number of new towns was undertaken. Five small towns were originally selected as nuclei for this purpose, four within easy reach of London, and one in Durham. The *New Towns Act* (1946) set up a Development Corporation for each town. Loans from the Treasury provided the initial finance for the undertakings. Crawley in Sussex (population 8,000), Harlow in Essex (pop. 4,500), Hemel Hempstead (pop. 21,000) and Stevenage (pop. 7,000), both in Hertfordshire, were the southern places selected. The fifth town was Newton Aycliffe, in County Durham, lying west of the Great North Road seven miles north of Darlington and situated in a Development Area. Immediately to the south of the new town is the Aycliffe Trading Estate, housing 50 firms employing over 3,000 people.

In 1949 and 1950 additions were made to the list of new towns. The plan for checking the expansion of London aims at eventually rehousing half a million people in eight new towns, people to move from congested parts of London to the new towns nearest to them. The building of four more new towns within reach of London was undertaken—Basildon in Essex, Bracknell in Berkshire, Hatfield and Welwyn Garden City in Hertfordshire.

Other places being developed as new towns are Corby (Northants), Peterlee and Washington (Durham), Skelmersdale and Runcorn (Lancashire), Redditch (Worcester), Dawley (Shropshire), Cwmbran (Monmouth), together with four in Scotland, East Kilbride (Lanark), Glenrothes (Fife), Cumbernauld and Livingston (W. Lothian), making a total of 21. Other new towns may be added to the list later. Between the two World Wars Corby grew from a village to a town of 14,500 inhabitants, and the extension of the ironworks there made it necessary to plan for a population of 40,000. Peterlee, in south-east Durham, is a miners' town housing 30,000 people who previously lived in scattered villages. Under the *New Towns Act* (*Northern Ireland*) of 1965 a new city of Craigavon, with a population of 100,000–150,000, has been planned. A number of other new towns has been suggested, including a large new city south of the River Humber. In 1965 it was proposed, too, to expand Ipswich from a population of nearly 120,000 to 190,000, and similar proposals were made for the expansion of Northampton and Peterborough.

Most of the towns were planned to have populations between 50,000 and 80,000. Progress was slow at first, but by 1960 most of them had passed the half-way stage in their development, and by 1965 most of the first group of towns had reached the size originally planned for them. The eight towns in the London area were to be self-sufficient and not merely dormitory towns for people working in London, and to ensure this development housing accommodation was guaranteed to all employees of firms moving into these places from London. Since mainly young people have been attracted to these towns, the average age of the inhabitants of the New Towns is low.

The *New Towns Act* (1959) set up a Commission of the New Towns to take over the property and liabilities of the individual Development Corporations when they reached a certain stage of development, Crawley and Stevenage being the first to be treated in this way.

RECOMMENDATIONS FOR FURTHER READING

W. H. Beveridge: *Full Employment in a Free Society*, Part IV.
S. R. Dennison: *The Location of Industry*.

QUESTIONS

1. An industry will tend to become localised in the place where it can be carried on most profitably. What are some of the main causes of localisation? (R.S.A. Inter.)

2. What do you understand by the localisation of industry? What causes it and what economic and social results accrue as a result of it? (A.I.A.)

3. What do you understand by localisation of industry? What problems may be caused by changes in location? (Exp.)

4. Discuss the economic factors that are modifying the distribution of industry and population in your own country. (I.T.)

5. What are the forces that tend to bring particular industries to particular areas? (C.I.S. Inter.)

6. What are the main factors determining the location of industry? In the light of your analysis consider the inter-war growth of the industrial population in London and the Home Counties. (I.B.)

7. Explain with examples why some industries are highly localised while others are carried on in small units scattered throughout the country. (G.C.E. Adv.)

8. Explain how changes in the occupational distribution have affected the geographical distribution of population in the United Kingdom during the last fifty years. (G.C.E. Adv.)

9. Argue the case for and against a policy of local diversification of industry in Great Britain. (Final Degree.)

10. What forces determine the localisation of industry? In what ways may the localisation of industry be influenced by the State? (C.C.S. Final.)

THE TOOLS OF ECONOMIC ANALYSIS

(i) Supply and Demand

CHAPTER IX

MARKETS

Part IV of this book is devoted entirely to a consideration of two important tools of economic analysis—namely, (i) the supply and demand technique, and (ii) the concept of the margin. By means of these tools many problems in applied economics can be investigated.

First, however, it is necessary to notice the environment in which the forces of supply and demand operate—the market.

I. PERFECT AND IMPERFECT MARKETS

(1) WHAT IS A MARKET?

It is the function of a market to enable exchange to take place, and in an economy using money this means the business of buying and selling of goods or services of some kind. In ordinary speech the word *market* appears to have two meanings: it may denote a particular place, possibly a special building, where a market is held, such as Covent Garden Market in London; or it may indicate the extent of the sale for some commodity, as in the phrase: "There is a wide market for cheap paper-backed books." Many examples are still to be found of markets in the narrower sense of the term. Most small country towns have market days, when stalls are erected in the market-place and business is transacted in the open air. In some of the larger towns there are permanent covered retail markets, and there are many wholesale markets of this type too. The right to hold markets was at first granted to Lords of the Manors, to monasteries or Municipal Corporations by Royal Charter, but since 1858 a number of Acts of Parliament have been passed giving local authorities power to establish markets. An area, large or small, can be considered as a market if within it buyers and sellers are in easy contact with one another.

The development of communications—means of transport, postal telephone and telegraph services—banking and the scientific grading of commodities have all helped to widen markets. Dealings in some commodities are now world-wide, and for these there may be said to be a world market. The essential feature of a market, however, whatever its extent, is that buyers should be able to strike bargains with sellers, and so a market becomes a sum total of such dealings. "The market," says Wicksteed, "is the characteristic phenomenon of economic life," and "the constitution of markets and market prices is the central problem of Economics."[1] The reason for the economic importance of the market is that it is the place where prices are determined.

(2) PERFECT MARKETS

One of the most frequent assumptions made in economics is that of the perfect market, the following conditions would have to be fulfilled: for a market to be perfect:

(i) *Homogeneous commodity.* In the first place, the commodity dealt in must be such that any one unit of it is exactly like any other—that is, that the commodity is homogeneous. It is of no consequence then from which seller a buyer makes his purchase, for there will be no name or trade-mark to distinguish the supply of one seller from that of another. If the commodity offered for sale is tea all the sellers will be simply selling tea, and not one Brown's Tea, and another Black's Tea, and a third Green's Tea. Formerly a great many more commodities than at present would very nearly fulfil this condition, but the past thirty years have seen a vast extension in the "branding" of all kinds of things—jam, tea, tinned goods, even fresh fruit. By dint of extensive advertising the producer tries to convince consumers that his brand is different (that is, better in some way) from those of other producers, and so the commodity ceases to be homogeneous. In fact, different brands are, strictly, different commodities, though close substitutes for one another.

(ii) *A large number of buyers and sellers.* This is the second condition for a perfect market. If there are only a few suppliers it may be possible for one of them to increase his profits by curtailing his supply, and so keeping up the price. If, on the other hand, there is a large number of sellers no one of them will be able materially to influence total supply, and so each will have an incentive to put as big a supply on the market as possible. Similarly, if there are many buyers one of them cannot hope to reduce price by curtailing his purchases. Combinations of buyers are difficult to form, and even when they are formed easily tend to break up. For one thing, it is difficult to persuade a sufficient number of them to combine, and for another, there is no strong community of interest among buyers.

(iii) *Buyers and sellers must be in close touch with one another.* In early days when communication was difficult the only way in which this

---

[1] P. Wicksteed: *Common-sense of Political Economy*, Book I, Chapter VI.

condition could be fulfilled was for the buyers and sellers to be present together in the same place. By telegraph and telephone buyers and sellers can now be brought into easy contact with one another, even though they may be thousands of miles apart. Thus, improved communications have widened the extent of markets. For a market to be perfect it is essential that all buyers and sellers should be immediately aware of what is happening in any part of the market. In this way an increased supply or a change in demand in one part of the market will affect price throughout the market.

(iv) *No preferential treatment.* In a perfect market there must be no preferential treatment of favoured customers, or discrimination against a group of either buyers or sellers. By imposing tariffs on foreign imports countries can break up the world market for a commodity into a number of smaller markets. What happens in one part of the world market will not then necessarily affect to the fullest extent all parts of that market. If a market is perfect, similar goods will command the same price in all parts of the market, for if one seller offered to sell at a price higher than the market price he would have no sales, for, the commodity being homogeneous, there would be no inducement to buyers to pay one seller a higher price than others were charging.

(v) *Portability or transferability of commodity.* Finally, it is necessary that the commodity dealt in on a perfect market should be capable of being easily transported from one part of the market to another.

(3) IMPERFECT MARKETS

It will be clear that the conditions required for a perfect market are of a kind to make the development of such markets under actual conditions very difficult, if not impossible, to achieve. Indeed, an absolutely perfect market exists only as a theoretical concept though some markets approach fairly near to perfection. Examples of these are the markets for foreign exchange (especially in the days of "free" exchange rates), the securities markets (Stock Exchanges) and some of the highly organised wholesale produce markets, such as those for cotton, wool and wheat. In the real world markets are to a lesser or greater extent imperfect.

Some retail markets are notoriously imperfect, for most people will not spend the time necessary to go round all the shops to find where prices are lowest. In the retail trade it is impossible for all buyers to be in close touch with the sellers. Generally, communication between retail buyers is poor, and many who would buy at the cheapest shops do not do so merely because they do not know where these particular shops are to be found. Then, many people continue to buy at certain shops, even though well aware that they are charging higher prices than some others. This may be due simply to a dislike of changing their suppliers, or it may be that the dearer shop is more conveniently situated, or perhaps they like the shopkeeper because he is always pleasant and cheerful or it may be too much trouble to look elsewhere, especially if the saving is likely to be small. The cheaper the article to be purchased the less is the consumer likely to worry about its price, and the more imperfect, therefore, will the market probably be. Preference for one shop rather than another may be due to a belief that the dearer shop sells a better quality of goods, so that the commodity is not, therefore, regarded as homogeneous.

Where there are only a few buyers and sellers, as in the case of the market in antiques, the market tends to be imperfect, though in this case imperfection may be caused by buyers and sellers lacking knowledge of what is happening in other parts of the market. Also, where the commodity cannot be transported from one place to another the market is almost certain to be imperfect. Houses probably provide the best example of such a commodity. Houses of similar type may differ widely in price between one town and another, or even between different districts in the same town; but however great the inducement of difference in price, the commodity cannot be moved from the cheaper to the dearer part of the market. If there are great differences in the prices of similar houses in different towns this can have considerable influence on the mobility of labour. A government, too, by import duties, taxes or subsidies, can increase the imperfection of a market.

Only if a market is imperfect can similar commodities be sold at different prices after allowance has been made for cost of transport.

(4) TYPES OF MARKET

It has so far been assumed that markets exist only for the buying and selling of commodities. This, however, depends on what we mean by a commodity. One can speak of a labour market, in which case the "commodity" dealt in is labour, the "buyers" being the entrepreneurs, the "sellers" the workers, and the "price" being the wage or salary. Entrepreneurs require some of each of the factors of production—land, labour and capital—before they can undertake any form of production, and the services of each factor are purchased in a market. Such markets are known as factor markets.

It is important also to distinguish between different kinds of commodities, and to differentiate between the markets for consumer goods —sometimes called markets for final products—and the markets for producer goods or intermediate products. The market for consumer goods can be further subdivided into wholesale and retail markets. Then there are the various financial markets—the Capital Market (the market for new securities), the Stock Exchange (mainly the market for the transfer of securities), the Money Market (the market for short-term loans), the Discount Market (the market for bills of exchange), and the Foreign Exchange Market (the market for foreign currencies). In all these markets the buyers and sellers of a commodity or service are brought together.

The determination of price in the market becomes, therefore, one of the most important problems of economics. In fact, it is so fundamental a part of the subject that one economist[1] has defined economics as "a study in prices." Before considering how price is determined it will be useful to continue our survey of the various kinds of market by a consideration of wholesale markets.

III. WHOLESALE MARKETING

(5) MIDDLEMEN

Formerly the normal channel by which commodities passed from the producer to the consumer was by way of wholesaler and retailer. Nowadays there is great diversity in methods of distribution, in some cases the goods being handled by a single wholesaler, in other cases by several middlemen and in others the goods passing direct from producer to retailer, or even to the consumer. The wholesaler is frequently described, almost as a term of reproach, as a middleman. He is often looked upon almost as a parasite, his intervention in distribution merely serving, it is thought, to make goods dearer to the consumer. The fact that "distribution costs" are sometimes greater than "production costs" encourages this view. If, however, the wholesaler performed no useful function, would not all producers and retailers by-pass him and divide his reward between them? The fact that this is not generally done seems to indicate that the wholesaler is of use to producer and retailer. In fact, where the wholesaler is cut out it generally merely means that someone else—producer or retailer—has to do his work. Only if wholesalers receive excessive payment for their services, or if it can be shown that goods are passing through too many hands, do middlemen lay themselves open to criticism.

The number of middlemen between producer and retailer varies from one trade to another, according to the particular needs of each

---

[1] H. J. Davenport: *Economics of Enterprise*, Chapter II.

trade. Sometimes the employment of a large number of middlemen is due to the existence of greater division of labour in the wholesaling function, especially where an intermediate process requires special knowledge or skill, or where distribution is complicated by irregularity of supply, or the existence of a large number of small producers, or the absence of any method of standardising the commodity. In such cases the intervention of a greater number of middlemen may result in fact in more efficient distribution, just as in industry greater division of labour achieves more efficient production. In foreign trade distribution is more complex, and so clearly more middlemen are required.

(6) FUNCTIONS OF THE WHOLESALER

What, then, are the services that the wholesaler performs in the work of distribution? Some of his main functions may be briefly mentioned:

(i) *The "breaking of bulk."* The manufacturer generally does not wish to have to undertake the distribution of his product, preferring to dispose of it in large quantities as produced. In order to have greater variety of stock, most retailers, on the other hand, buy in small quantities. The wholesaler forms a link between them, and attempts to satisfy the needs of both. It is possible too that if the wholesaler were omitted, transport costs might be even higher, for the manufacturer might have to send a larger number of parcels, each a long distance if he supplied retailers direct. Wholesalers are more conveniently situated for particular districts; each receives a large parcel from the manufacturer, and then splits it up into smaller parcels with only short distances to travel. The following diagram will make this clear:

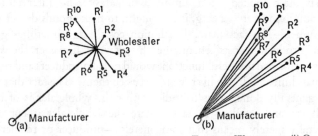

FIG. 5.—THE BREAKING OF BULK. (*a*) DISTRIBUTION THROUGH WHOLESALER (*b*) OMISSION OF WHOLESALER. R^1 TO R^{10} = RETAILERS

The wholesaler's more convenient situation also enables the retailer to obtain additional supplies more readily than he could from the manufacturer.

(ii) *Warehousing.* Manufacturers produce in large quantities, which they want to dispose of quickly in order to keep their factory space clear for further production. The wholesaler can relieve the manufacturer of the trouble and expense of holding large stocks. By allowing a regular supply to enter the market, especially where production is irregular, the wholesaler helps to prevent prices fluctuating unduly. The holding of stocks by the wholesaler is a valuable service, as it acts as a lubricant to the economic system, enabling distribution to work smoothly and preventing the development of "bottle-necks."

(iii) *Expert buying and selling.* Expert knowledge of the commodities bought and sold is required, and so the employment of specialists is essential, particularly where goods are bought and sold in those organised produce markets where it is necessary for the buyer to examine, test and assess the value of samples, as in the case of wool and tea.

(iv) *Marketing the product.* Manufacturers have to produce in anticipation of demand, but the wholesaler can often assist them by passing on to them information regarding consumers' demand which he has obtained from the retailers with whom he is in touch. This service is of greatest importance to the manufacturers. The wholesaler can also assist the manufacturer in developing the market for his products.

(v) *Financing production and distribution.* In addition to financing the holding of stocks, the wholesaler often helps to finance both the manufacturer and the retailer more directly. Manufacturers expect to be paid for their products as soon as possible, while many retailers have insufficient capital to carry large stocks of unsold goods. By prompt payment to the manufacturers and by allowing credit to the retailer the wholesaler helps to finance the activities of both.

(vi) *Preparing the product for sale.* The wholesaler often processes or prepares for sale the goods he receives from the manufacturer before passing them on to the retailer. This may take the form of packing, grading or branding. Sugar refining and the blending of tea are often carried out by the wholesalers of those commodities.

This brief survey of the functions of a wholesaler clearly shows the essential nature of his work. Indeed, all distributors are really engaged upon the final stage in the process of production. Division of labour requires specialisation of production in a limited number of places, but only a small percentage of the goods produced are required where they are made. Most of the goods, therefore, are of little economic value until they have been transferred to places where there is a demand for them. The greater the extent of specialisation, the greater will be the amount of distribution required, and therefore the greater is likely to be its cost. The increasing cost of distribution is thus the result of increasing specialisation and division of labour. Exchange is the logical corollary of specialisation, and similar commodities in different places are in the strict economic sense really different commodities. The middleman who assists distribution and exchange makes possible this greater volume of production. His work can therefore be considered to be productive.

(7) TYPES OF MIDDLEMEN

Only those wholesalers who carry stocks have warehouses, such as dealers in manufactured goods and some dealers in foodstuffs and raw materials. In Canada and the United States wholesalers store wheat in elevators until it is required. In some trades this type of wholesaler is known as a factor, as for example in boots and shoes and tobacco. Some wholesalers, however, merely organise the distribution of the commodity from the producer to the retailer, and so do not carry large stocks themselves, as for example, coal merchants and motor-car distributors, while others specialise in financing the holding of stocks.

The main functions of import and export merchants are indicated by their names. The importer may have an entire ship's cargo consigned to him, and he will be responsible for its warehousing after it has been disembarked, after which he will make arrangements for its sale, generally to other wholesalers, on one of the produce exchanges. This work is carried out by another group of middlemen who are experts in their own particular trades. Unlike the middlemen previously mentioned, they rarely own the commodities in which they deal, but are merely agents who are employed by other wholesalers, usually being paid on a commission basis. These are the brokers and the del credere agents, the latter guaranteeing payment for the goods they sell, and so receiving a higher rate of commission.

A smaller-scale wholesaler is often to be found in provincial towns. Sometimes these people buy from large regional wholesalers, as in the grocery and provision trades, the large number of retailers making it impossible for the large wholesalers to deal directly with them all. The local wholesalers, being in closer contact with the retailers in their area, are able to grant credit with less risk. Small-town wholesalers are also found in the tobacco trade, in which the numbers of retailers is very large, though most of them have only a small turnover. Their needs can best be served by a wholesaler in the same town, for the large tobacco retailers usually buy direct from the manufacturers. Thus the number of middlemen engaged in the distribution of a product depends on the particular character of the trade concerned.

(8) THE OMISSION OF THE WHOLESALER

There are some cases where the wholesaler has been cut out, goods being sent direct from manufacturer to retailer, or even direct from manufacturer to consumer. Since, as already shown, wholesaling is a vital link in distribution, the elimination of the wholesaler merely means that either the manufacturer or the retailer must take over his work. For a manufacturer this will involve the establishment of a warehouse, so that he can undertake the function of storing and the setting up of a selling department, and engaging a staff of commercial travellers. Instead of dealing with comparatively few bulk orders to wholesalers, he will now have to deal with a huge number of small orders to suit the requirements of his retail customers, and this will necessitate his having to employ a large additional staff in his administrative and packing and forwarding departments. In other words, such a manufacturer will have to incur the expenses of the wholesaler, and in relation to the extra capital involved it is unlikely that his profit, as a percentage of his capital, will be any greater than it was when he confined himself to manufacturing. If he decides to sell direct to consumers this requires the opening of retail shops or the setting up of a mail-order department, so incurring also the expenses of retailing.

Clearly, therefore, advertisements of sale direct from producer to consumer are often misleading and aim at influencing the ignorant and more gullible type of consumer. The manufacturer, however, may wish to ensure that his product is put on the market, and may think that a general wholesaler will not push its sale sufficiently. In such a case he may think the trouble and expense of doing his own wholesaling worth while, and either open his own retail shops, if his turnover justifies it, or appoint a limited number of retailers as his sole agents. Or, if he is a manufacturer of branded goods—that is, goods bearing registered trade names—he may prefer to advertise and himself market his product as far as the retailer.

The marketing of most boots and shoes is now done through manufacturers' own shops, and in recent times the number of wholesalers in this trade has declined. Even where there is insufficient demand for the product to make it economic for the manufacturer to open his own shops, he may prefer to appoint a limited number of "sole" agents for his goods in each town—a common practice with manufacturers of radio and television sets—and again act as his own wholesaler. The increasing tendency in many trades to brand goods, together with the consequent expansion of advertising, has brought about the disappearance of many small provincial wholesalers. The development of large-scale retail trade, through multiple-shop organisations and department stores, has led these businesses also to set up their own wholesaling departments.

III. HIGHLY ORGANISED MARKETS

(9) THE DEVELOPMENT OF ORGANISED MARKETS

The wholesaling of many commodities is carried on in highly organised markets, buyers and sellers meeting in a particular place in order to transact business. Such markets tend towards a high degree of "perfection," for, since buyers and sellers are in close touch, one price for the same commodity rules throughout the market. There is a tendency for an organised market to develop when the following conditions are fulfilled:

(i) The commodity should be fairly durable, in order that stocks can be held.

(ii) The annual production of the commodity must be sufficiently large to make it possible to deal in large consignments.

(iii) It is an advantage, too, if the commodity can be graded, but if not, it should be possible to test the quality easily by means of samples.

(iv) If the price of the commodity is apt to fluctuate widely, owing to the difficulty in the short period of increasing or curtailing the supply, this will act as an incentive to establish an organised market. It will also encourage the emergence of merchants specialising in carrying risks, with the probability of the development of some method of eliminating or reducing the risk of loss due to price fluctuation.

The commodities that fulfil these conditions are foodstuffs and raw materials, particularly those imported from abroad. Thus organised markets have been established for wheat, tea, coffee, sugar, cotton, wool, rubber, timber, lead, tin, copper, etc. The main markets for all these commodities are found in London, though there are cotton exchanges at both Liverpool and Manchester, a sugar exchange in Liverpool and a number of provincial corn exchanges.

(10) PRODUCE EXCHANGES

Highly organised markets exist, then, for many commodities, buying and selling being concentrated in some specific place or building. Usually business is carried on according to a definite set of rules, though the actual method of conducting business on a produce exchange depends primarily on whether the commodity is capable of being graded. The main advantages to be derived from grading are:

(i) the commodity need not be actually on view in the market, and in fact business can be done by telephone;
(ii) it makes possible dealings in futures (*see* 11).

Both cotton and wheat can be accurately graded, the grading of the former being carried out by the Liverpool Cotton Association (consisting of merchants, brokers and spinners), and that of the latter by the London and Liverpool Corn Trade Associations. Unfortunately the grades adopted for cotton in Liverpool and the United States are not identical, and this often causes delay on the arrival of the cotton at Liverpool, where the quality has to be decided. Where grading is possible, business is usually conducted by private treaty—that is, individual bargaining between buyer and seller.

Where grading of the commodity is not possible, as in the case of wool and tea, it becomes necessary for prospective buyers to take samples of the lots to be offered for sale. These commodities are then sold by auction to the highest bidders. Selling brokers acting on behalf of overseas producers are responsible for the warehousing of the wool after its arrival in port until arrangements have been made for its sale at the London auctions, which for fine wool take place six times each year. Buying brokers, acting on behalf of wool merchants, topmakers, spinners and merchants engaged in the entrepôt trade, inspect the wool, take samples and make their estimate of the quality before attending the auction.

At the London Commercial Sales Rooms such commodities as tea, coffee, cocoa, sugar, etc., are sold by auction, dutiable commodities, such as tea being imported on consignment and stored in bonded warehouses until auctioned. As with wool, expert buying brokers are employed to sample the commodities before bidding at the tea auctions.

(11) FORWARD MARKETING

It is because cotton can easily be graded that a market in "futures" developed. Ten distinct grades of cotton are recognised by the Liverpool Association, and thus it is possible to sell raw cotton before its arrival in Liverpool. The commodities dealt in on a futures market are "futures," these originally being contracts to deliver goods at a future date at an agreed price. Dealings in futures take place in both wheat and cotton. Prices for immediate delivery are known as "spot" prices. If a merchant thinks the spot price of cotton likely to rise in the next few months he will buy futures if they are quoted at a lower price than he expects to prevail in the future, as a hedge against a rise in the price of raw cotton. Speculators do not buy or sell the actual commodity, but instead buy or sell futures. The existence of such speculators makes it possible for those owning and holding the actual goods to "insure" against price fluctuations by themselves buying or selling futures. If the holder of a commodity which cannot be marketed for (say) six months fears a fall in price he can sell futures now, and so assure himself of receiving the present price. In this way he insures himself against a fall in price. Obviously, the buyer of the futures is speculating against such a fall in price, for he hopes to be able to sell at a higher price six months later. The existence of a futures market is particularly advantageous in the case of commodities subject to wide fluctuations of price.

The difficulty of satisfactorily grading wool prevented for a long time the development of a market in futures for that commodity, although such markets were operated with some measure of success at both Antwerp and New York. The wide fluctuations in the price of wool during 1950–52 led to demands for the establishment of a futures market for wool in Great Britain, and in 1953 a wool futures market was opened in London. This now makes it possible for wool merchants also to insure against price fluctuations through the medium of futures. Futures markets have also been established for coffee and cocoa.

The activities of the speculators are often condemned. Speculators, however, on commodity markets require to possess expert knowledge of the markets in which they deal. Their activities iron out price fluctuations, and they tend to make markets more nearly perfect. If a commodity is in plentiful supply immediately after harvest its price then will be low; but as the supply shrinks the price would tend to rise until the next harvest. If speculators enter such a market and buy while the price is low immediately after the harvest they will tend to force up the price at such times. Then, by holding stocks and releasing them later, they prevent the price from rising later as high as it otherwise would have done. Such speculation steadies prices. Speculation on the financial markets is considered below.[1]

[1] See pp. 438–9.

RECOMMENDATIONS FOR FURTHER READING

A. Marshall: *Principles of Economics*, Book V, Chapter 1.
J. G. Smith: *Organised Produce Markets*.

QUESTIONS

1. Why does the wholesaler play a very important part in the distribution of certain classes of goods, while in other classes he plays a small part or is entirely absent? (R.S.A. Adv. Com.)

2. Discuss the functions of the middleman with particular reference to recent criticisms that he is unnecessary and receives too high a remuneration for his services. (L.C. Com. C. & F.)

3. Write a note on economic markets. (C.I.S. Inter.)

4. The middleman is sometimes described as an unnecessary feature of the economic organisation. Discuss this view. (Exp.)

5. What are the essential features of a centralised and organised market? Illustrate by reference to any such market with which you are familiar. (Exp.)

6. What functions are performed by middlemen and what determines their regard? What happens when an industry is nationalised? (R.S.A. Adv.)

7. What is meant by "hedging"? How far is hedging possible in the absence of organised markets? (R.S.A. Adv. Com.)

8. Why is it that some commodities have a restricted market and others a very wide one? (A.I.A.)

9. It has been suggested that all wholesale dealing should be in the hands of the State. On what grounds do you think that such a statement could be made? Give your own views on the subject. (A.C.C.A. Inter.)

10. Write a short account of market speculation as an economic function and show its effect upon prices. (I.B.)

11. Does speculation on the organised commodity markets increase or diminish the range and frequency of price fluctuations? (Final Degree.)

12. What are the advantages of having markets where one can buy and sell what has not yet been produced? (Final Degree).

CHAPTER X

DEMAND CURVES AND SUPPLY CURVES

In Chapter I it was seen that all goods are scarce relative to the demand for them, for there is not a sufficient amount of anything to allow everyone to have as much of it as he would like. The central problem of economics is how to distribute these limited supplies among the people wanting them. One method is for the State to issue to each person a ration card, and to require the surrender of a coupon when a supply of the commodity is bought. Another method by which limited supplies can be distributed among those desiring them is through the price mechanism. It is the purpose of this chapter to show how the price mechanism works. People will generally buy less of a thing if its price rises, so that if supplies of a commodity are reduced a rise in its price will reduce the amount of it demanded; if supplies increase, price falls and more will be demanded. Thus, it becomes the function of price to equate demand with supply.

I. PRICE DETERMINATION

(1) HAGGLING

If there are few sellers and few buyers in the market the prices at which the commodities will be sold will probably be determined by a process known as haggling. In a sale by private treaty this method obtains, and the prices at which houses are sold are often arrived at by this means. A prospective buyer may approach a prospective seller, and after finding that the seller was asking £3,400 the buyer might offer him £3,000. If the seller prefers to keep the house himself rather than accept £3,000, and if this sum is the maximum the buyer is prepared to pay, there is no basis for further bargaining. However, it is more likely that there is a range of prices that would satisfy the seller, and he may, for example, be willing to accept £3,100, though he may be hopeful of obtaining more than that. Similarly, the buyer may be willing to pay up to £3,250, though he hopes to obtain the house for less. The actual price agreed upon will therefore lie somewhere between £3,100 and £3,250. If the buyer is keener to buy than the seller is to sell the price will be nearer £3,250. If, on the other hand, the seller is keener to sell than the buyer is to buy the price will be nearer £3,100. This range of prices over which bargaining is possible can be represented diagrammatically as follows:

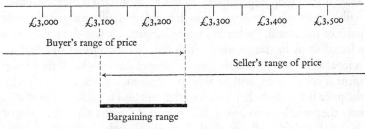

FIG. 6. THE RANGE OF BARGAINING.

(2) SALES BY AUCTION

Another method of determining the price at which a commodity shall be sold is to put it up for auction. In such a case there is one seller and a number of prospective buyers. The auctioneer offers an article for sale and asks for bids for it. Anyone desirous of purchasing it is then at liberty to make an offer, and the article will eventually be sold to the highest bidder—that is, to the keenest buyer: the one prepared to pay the highest price. The actual price he will pay depends on how much the second keenest buyer is prepared to pay. If four people—A, B, C and D—are bidding against one another for a house they may be willing to pay £3,400, £3,200, £3,100 and £2,800 respectively. The house may be sold to A for £3,225, because at that price B, C and D have all dropped out of the bidding. Sometimes rivalry between two bidders forces up the price to a level that neither of them would have paid had each not been carried away by a desire to score a victory over his rival. The important thing to notice, whether the sale is by auction or private treaty, is that the cost of building the house does not enter into the determination of the price at which it can be sold, since once it has come into the market, its price depends not on its cost, but on the relation between the keenness of buyers to buy and the keenness of sellers to sell.

(3) OFFERS AT FIXED PRICES

These two methods of determining price—haggling or private treaty and selling by auction—are still in operation at highly organised wholesale markets. It was seen in the preceding chapter that raw wool is sold by auction and raw cotton by private treaty. Both methods of sale are occasionally adopted for consumer goods, more particularly where the sales are infrequent. Works of art are often sold by auction. For consumer goods where there is a regular demand both these methods of sale are too cumbersome and would take up an unnecessary amount of time. For things such as foodstuffs, clothing, household goods, etc., it is customary for the sellers to mark their goods at definite prices. Most British shopkeepers today would be astonished if their customers wished to haggle over prices, though haggling is still customary in some parts of the world. What has really happened is that the sellers have selected from the range over which they were prepared to sell, some price at which they think they can dispose of their stocks. If their judgment is correct they will be able to sell all their stock at this price; if the price is too high they will find that business is slack, and sooner or later they will have to lower their prices; if they fix the price too low they will quickly sell out all their stock, though they will probably raise their price when they find demand stronger than they anticipated. Evidently then there is some price at which the whole of the stock, neither more nor less, could be sold. What this price will be depends on the strength of the demand for the commodity relative to the supply.

II. DEMAND

(4) THE MEANING OF DEMAND

By demand is meant the quantity demanded at a particular price, for it is impossible to conceive of demand not related to price. To want or need a thing is not the same as to demand it. To distinguish demand from need it is sometimes called effective demand. Most housewives would probably like to have a constant supply of hot water, and they might say that they needed water-heaters for the purpose. The demand for such heaters, however, may be fairly small if their price is high. It is quite certain that if the price were lowered more of them would be sold and installed, whereas if the price were doubled fewer would be demanded. Similarly, most housewives probably buy a smaller quantity of strawberries at the beginning of the season, when the price is high, than they buy later, when the price is lower. Generally at a high price less will be sold than at a low price, assuming, of course, that no change takes place in the intensity of demand.

(5) INDIVIDUAL DEMAND SCHEDULES

It thus becomes possible to compile an individual's hypothetical demand schedule for a commodity. Demand schedules are difficult to estimate, for statistics cannot be compiled to show demand at prices different from those ruling at a given time. For example, if the price of cocoa were 1s. 8d. per tin Mrs Gamp, a housewife, might buy (say) six tins per month; if the price were 1s. 10d. per tin she might buy only four tins per month, but at a price of 1s. 6d. per tin eight per month.

Mrs Gamp's demand schedule for cocoa might therefore run as follows:

TABLE XVI
An Individual Demand Schedule (1)

Price per tin	Demand per month (number of tins)
2s.	3
1s. 11d.	3½
1s. 10d.	4
1s. 9d.	5
1s. 8d.	6
1s. 7d.	7
1s. 6d.	8
1s. 5d.	9

It is necessary to emphasise again that this does not indicate any change in demand on the part of Mrs Gamp, but merely expresses what her *present* behaviour with regard to the purchase of this commodity would be at a series of different prices. With no change in the intensity of her demand for cocoa, she will buy only three tins per month if the price is 2s., or eight tins per month if the price is 1s. 6d. Such a demand schedule is purely hypothetical, but it serves to illustrate the principle that more of a commodity will be bought at a low than at a high price.

Other housewives will have different demand schedules for cocoa, because the intensity of their demand for this commodity is either stronger or weaker than Mrs Gamp's. For example, at all possible prices Mrs Prig may purchase a smaller quantity than Mrs Gamp, and Mrs Prig's demand schedule for cocoa might be as follows:

TABLE XVII
An Individual Demand Schedule (2)

Price per tin	Demand per month (number of tins)
2s.	0
1s. 11d.	1
1s. 10d.	1½
1s. 9d.	2
1s. 8d.	2½
1s. 7d.	3
1s. 6d.	4
1s. 5d.	6

On the other hand, the demand of Mrs Bardell may vary little over this range of prices, and her demand schedule might read:

TABLE XVIII

An Individual Demand Schedule (3)

Price per tin	Demand per month (number of tins)
2s.	3½
1s. 11d.	3½
1s. 10d.	4
1s. 9d.	4
1s. 8d.	4
1s. 7d.	4
1s. 6d.	4½
1s. 5d.	4½

(6) COMPOSITE DEMAND SCHEDULE

Theoretically, the demand schedules of all consumers of cocoa can be combined to form a composite demand schedule, representing the total demand for cocoa at various prices. This might be called the market demand schedule.

TABLE XIX

A Market Demand Schedule

Price per tin	Quantity demanded per month
2s.	100,000
1s. 11d.	120,000
1s. 10d.	135,000
1s. 9d.	150,000
1s. 8d.	165,000
1s. 7d.	180,000
1s. 6d.	200,000
1s. 5d.	240,000
1s. 4d.	300,000
1s. 3d.	350,000

These prices are called *demand prices*. Thus, the demand price for 200,000 tins of cocoa per month is 1s. 6d. per tin.

(7) DEMAND CURVES

The above demand schedule can be represented graphically (Fig. 7). The vertical scale *OY* represents the price per tin, and the horizontal scale *OX* represents the number of tins purchased. By convention the vertical axis is marked *OY*, and the horizontal axis *OX*, and it is usual

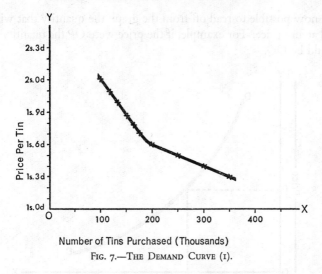

FIG. 7.—THE DEMAND CURVE (1).

also to show price along the vertical scale and the quantity along the horizontal. From this demand schedule it is possible to plot a demand curve (see Fig. 8). The curve *DD* then represents the state of demand for this commodity at a particular time and under particular conditions. Such a graph is merely a convenient way of showing at a glance the relationship between price and the quantity bought, and so it is not necessary to have the price and quantity scales marked off mathematically. It is sufficient to know that prices increase evenly from O towards Y and quantity from O towards X. The graph then becomes:

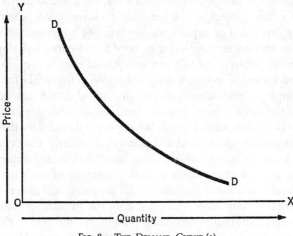

FIG. 8.—THE DEMAND CURVE (2)

It is now possible to read off from the graph the quantity that will be sold at any price. For example, if the price were *OP* the quantity sold would be *OQ*.

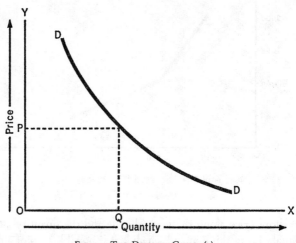

FIG. 9.—THE DEMAND CURVE (3).

The First Law of Supply and Demand—*the lower the price, the greater the quantity that will be demanded*—can be seen at a glance.

(8) EXCEPTIONAL DEMAND CURVES

The typical demand curve slopes downwards from left to right. An exceptional demand curve, therefore, will be one that slopes upwards from left to right, which means that the demand for the commodity will be greater at a higher than at a lower price. Clearly, the quantity demanded of any commodity will not be greater with every successive increase in price—that is, no demand curve will slope upwards in its entirety, but in a few exceptional cases it may slope upwards over a part of its length at a given period of time. The following are examples of cases where exceptional demand curves may occur:

(i) *Inferior goods.* Cheap necessary foodstuffs provide one of the best examples of exceptional demand. Most people do not vary their purchases of such things as bread and potatoes over fairly wide ranges of prices. Both are comparatively cheap commodities, and expenditure on them generally forms only a small percentage of one's total outlay on food. Even a very considerable fall in price would not encourage most people to buy more, though a steep rise in price, if continued, would eventually lead to less being bought. In the case of the very poor, however, it may be that, at the low price, they are able to buy a certain amount of these cheaper foodstuffs and still be able to afford in addition a small amount of more expensive foods, such as cakes and green vegetables. A rise in the prices of bread and potatoes, however, might mean that less of the more expensive commodities, cake and green vegetables, would be bought, even though their prices remained unchanged, their place being taken by increased amounts of bread and potatoes. The effect therefore of the rise in the price of bread and potatoes might be to increase the quantities of these commodities demanded, although the amount bought of the more expensive foods was reduced. Commodities of this type are sometimes known as *Giffen Goods*.

(ii) *Fear of a future rise in price.* If it is believed that the price of a commodity is likely to be higher in the future than at present, then, even though the price has already risen, more of the commodity may be bought at the higher price. This often happens with Stock Exchange securities, especially in the case of speculative buying. If the price of a security has been low for a long time a slight rise in price may be taken to indicate that the price is going to rise still further in the future.

On the outbreak of war in 1939 the prices of many commodities rose slightly, but there was a big increase in the quantity of goods bought, because many people remembered that during the First World War prices of most goods rose steeply. Demand similarly increased in the United States and some countries at the outbreak of the Korean War in 1950 and during the Cuban crisis of 1962. Fear of higher prices in the future, therefore, will often cause more to be bought at a higher than at a lower price.

(iii) *Articles of ostentation, etc.* There are some commodities that appear desirable only if they are expensive. Some articles of jewellery fall within this category. At a comparatively low price a smaller quantity might be sold than at a higher price, merely because the higher price gives the article greater exclusiveness in the eyes of purchasers. A fashionable dressmaker or milliner might often increase her sales by raising her prices. A luxury car might sell more readily at £7,500 than at £2,500. Since we cannot be expert buyers of everything, we tend to judge the quality of many things largely by the prices at which they are sold.

III. SUPPLY

(9) SUPPLY SCHEDULES AND CURVES

The second factor that affects prices is supply. By the supply of a commodity is meant the quantity that is called forth into the market over a particular period of time by a certain price. Just as demand is not the same as need, and means effective demand or demand at a price, so with supply. It does not necessarily comprise the entire stock of any commodity in existence, but only that amount drawn into the market by the price ruling at the time. The supply of oil is not the estimated resources of all the world's oil-fields, but only that amount which particular prices will bring onto the market. As one would expect, sellers will generally put a greater quantity onto the market the higher the price. As with demand, it is possible to construct a supply schedule showing the amounts that will be offered for sale at different prices by individual firms, these then being combined to form a supply curve for the industry. Such a supply schedule for tins of cocoa might run as follows:

TABLE XX

A Supply Schedule

Price per tin	Quantity offered for sale per month
2s.	400,000
1s. 11d.	370,000
1s. 10d.	350,000
1s. 9d.	320,000
1s. 8d.	285,000
1s. 7d.	240,000
1s. 6d.	200,000
1s. 5d.	160,000
1s. 4d.	120,000
1s. 3d.	80,000

These prices are *supply prices*. At a supply price of 1s. 9d. for example, 320,000 tins of cocoa per month will be supplied. From this supply schedule a supply curve can be plotted (Fig. 10). Or it will be again sufficient to express the curve generally (Fig. 11). Since usually more is supplied the higher the price, the typical supply curve slopes upwards from left to right. This illustrates the second Law of Supply and Demand—*the higher the price, the greater the quantity which will be supplied.* From this diagram it can be seen that at the higher price, OP^2, a greater quantity, OQ^2, will be put on to the market than at the lower price, OP^1, the amount offered for sale at this price being only OQ^1.

(10) EXCEPTIONAL SUPPLY CURVES

It is possible to conceive of the demand for a commodity being fixed over a narrow range of prices, especially if its cost forms only a small part of one's total expenditure, but there is no commodity the demand for which will be fixed whatever the price—that is, the demand curve will never be a vertical straight line at right angles to the base line OX.

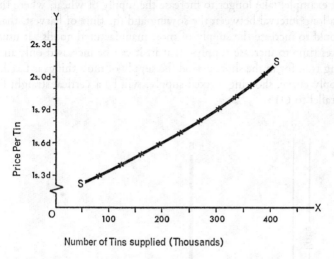

FIG. 10.—THE SUPPLY CURVE (1).

It is possible, however, for supply to be physically fixed, so that whatever the price, whether high or low, the same quantity of the commodity will be offered to the market. In the case of some rare things, each is unique (there is only one Mona Lisa, for example), and it is therefore

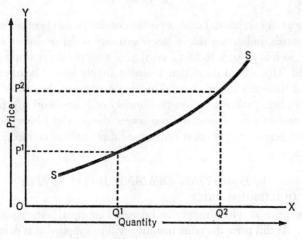

FIG. 11.—THE SUPPLY CURVE (2).

impossible to increase the supply. In fact, some time must usually elapse before the supply of any commodity can be increased, though to increase the supply of some things takes longer than others. It would, for example, take longer to increase the supply of wheat, where there is a long interval between the sowing and the time of harvest, than it would to increase the supply of most manufactured goods. It usually takes time to increase supply—that is, it can be increased only in the long run, for in the short period the supply of most things is fixed. A supply curve, showing a fixed supply, will be a vertical straight line, parallel to OY:

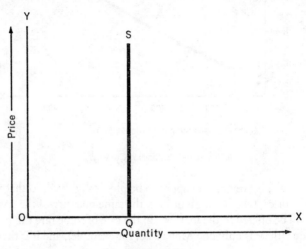

FIG. 12.—FIXED SUPPLY.

Just as in exceptional cases a portion of the demand curve can slope backwards, indicating that a larger quantity is demanded at a higher price, so it is possible to find a portion of a supply curve sloping backwards. This would mean that a smaller supply would be offered at a higher than at a lower price. This might occur in the case of labour (supply being taken to mean the number of hours worked), for men may wish to work shorter hours if wages (the price of labour) are high. This regressive supply curve is discussed more fully in connection with wages.[1]

IV. EQUATING DEMAND WITH SUPPLY

(11) EQUILIBRIUM PRICE

The price at which supply and demand are equal is the equilibrium price. At this price the same quantity will be supplied as is demanded.

1 See p. 301.

Returning to the example of the demand for and supply of cocoa and combining the market demand schedule (page 158) with the supply schedule (page 162) for the industry, the following table can be compiled:

TABLE XXI

A Combined Demand and Supply Schedule (1)

Price	Quantity demanded (number of tins)	Quantity supplied (number of tins)
2s.	100,000	400,000
1s. 11d.	120,000	370,000
1s. 10d.	135,000	350,000
1s. 9d,	150,000	320,000
1s. 8d.	165,000	285,000
1s. 7d.	180,000	240,000
1s. 6d.	200,000	200,000
1s. 5d.	240,000	160,000
1s. 4d.	300,000	120,000
1s. 3d.	350,000	80,000

From this table it will be seen that if the price of cocoa is 1s. 6d. per tin the quantity demanded will be 200,000 tins, this price also calling forth a supply of 200,000 tins. Under these conditions of demand and supply, then, 1s. 6d. will be the equilibrium price. This can also be represented graphically by superimposing the demand curve upon the

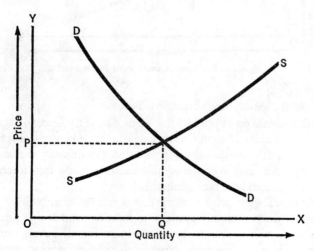

Fig. 13.—The Equilibrium Price.

supply curve (Fig. 13). At the point of intersection of the two curves demand and supply are equal. The *equilibrium price*, therefore, *OP*, at which price the quantity *OQ* will be supplied, *equates supply and demand.* This is the third Law of Supply and Demand. Price in a perfect market is thus determined by the interaction of the two forces of supply and demand, the intensity of demand in relation to the conditions of supply. At one time it was thought that the price of a commodity was determined solely by cost of production, but cost of production only influences supply, and this is only one of the two forces that affect prices. If, however, supply were fixed, price would depend principally on demand. Since supply often tends to be fixed in the short period, the shorter the period, the more important is demand (Fig. 14). At all prices the quantity available is *OQ*; the price *OP* equates demand with this supply.

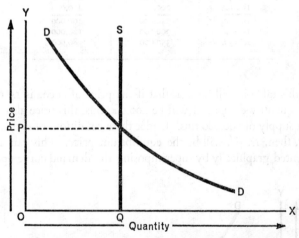

FIG. 14.—THE EQUILIBRIUM PRICE WITH FIXED SUPPLY.

(12) MARKET PRICE AND NORMAL PRICE

The determination of price by the interaction of the forces of supply and demand occurs through the working of what is known as the *price mechanism*. Both the quantity supplied and the quantity demanded vary with price, and so at the equilibrium price these two forces of supply and demand are brought into balance.

If the equilibrium price is charged in a market there will be just sufficient of the commodity available to meet demand at that price— that is, there will appear to be no shortage, for all buyers can be supplied at the prevailing price. Nor will there be any surplus, since the sellers will just be able to dispose of their entire stocks, for at the equilibrium price the market will be cleared. At any price higher than the equilibrium price the sellers will find some of the commodity left on their hands unsold; at a lower price than the equilibrium price demand will exceed supply and there will be said to be a shortage of the commodity.

The actual price charged in the market may be only the short-term equilibrium price, for in the short period the forces of supply and demand may be subject to temporary influences. The short-period equilibrium price is the *Market Price*. However, when conditions of supply and demand have settled down so that the rate at which the commodity is consumed is equal to the rate at which it is produced, then a long-period equilibrium price will become established. This is known as the *Normal Price*.

RECOMMENDATIONS FOR FURTHER READING

K. E. Boulding: *Economic Analysis*, Chapters 4 and 5.
H. Henderson: *Supply and Demand*, Chapter 2.

QUESTIONS

1. What exactly do you understand by the laws of demand and supply? Is it always true to say that a fall in price is followed by an increase in demand? (R.S.A. Inter.)

2. Explain briefly how the price-system works. (A.C.C.A. Inter.)

3. How are prices settled in a competitive market? (I.T.)

4. Within what limits may the prices of goods move in a free market? (A.I.A.)

5. Illustrate in diagrammatic form the equilibrium between demand and supply under conditions of perfect competition and decreasing cost. Explain the various parts and the meaning of the diagram. (C.I.S. Inter.)

6. Estimate the significance of demand curves in practical business as distinct from theoretical economics. (S.I.A.A.)

7. "In the short run price is determined by demand, and in the long run by the cost of production." Discuss this statement. (C.C.S. Final)

8. In what circumstances would a fall in the price of a commodity lead to a reduction in the quantity bought? (Final Degree.)

9. What determines equilibrium in a single market and what forces tend to establish it? (Final Degree.)

CHAPTER XI

SUPPLY AND DEMAND RELATIONSHIPS

I. CHANGES IN SUPPLY AND DEMAND AND THEIR EFFECTS

(1) CHANGES IN DEMAND

The next thing to consider is the effect of changes in demand, but first it is necessary to be perfectly clear what is meant by a change in demand. It might be thought that because a fall in price from 1s. 9d. to 1s. 6d. results in 50,000 more tins of cocoa being demanded, this indicates a change in demand. This, however, is not so, for it is merely a movement along the *same* demand curve, and the *entire curve* represents the state of demand at a particular time. A change in demand means that the new state of demand necessitates a new demand curve. The typical demand curve shows that at a higher price a smaller quantity is demanded than at a lower price. A change of demand results in *a different quantity being demanded at each of the old prices.* This can be more readily understood from a diagram:

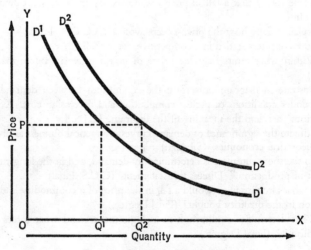

FIG. 15.—CHANGE IN DEMAND (1).

The state of demand before the change is represented by the curve D^1D^1. In these conditions at the price OP, the quantity demanded was OQ^1. It is now assumed that for some reason, to be considered shortly, the state of demand has changed, and is now represented by the new curve D^2D^2. At the old price, OP, the quantity now demanded is OQ^2, which is obviously greater than the former quantity, OQ^1. In fact, under the new conditions of demand a larger quantity is now demanded at each of the old prices. The new curve therefore illustrates an increase in demand. If the new curve had been entirely to the left of the original curve this would have shown a decrease in demand. Confusion frequently arises because sometimes movement along the same demand curve is spoken of as an increase or a decrease in demand. Strictly, an increase or a decrease in demand is the result of a change in demand, and therefore requires a new demand curve. To avoid ambiguity, it is better to speak of an increase or a decrease in the quantity demanded when this is merely the result of a change of price, and therefore refers to the same demand curve.

A change in demand need not, as in the above diagram, affect the whole of the demand curve. The new curve may partly overlap the old:

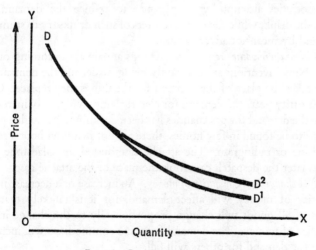

FIG. 16.—CHANGE IN DEMAND (2).

In this case the change in demand has brought about an increase in demand only over the lower ranges of prices.

(2) CAUSES OF CHANGES IN DEMAND

There are a number of reasons why demand may change:

(i) *Changes of taste or fashion.* The intensity of demand for a thing depends on the keenness of people to buy it, but it is often difficult to discover on what this keenness depends. Taste may depend on a number of factors, though education and training are often important influences, but taste probably varies more between one period and another than between different groups of people at the same period, and it generally changes fairly slowly. There is probably a greater appreciation of good music today than there was twenty-five years ago, and so during that period the demand for symphony concerts and opera has increased.

Fashion is apt to change more arbitrarily, and often apparently without reason. Few men in 1965 wore bowler hats, whereas in 1910 this was the most popular hat for men. In 1910 few men went hatless, whereas fifty years later many men rarely wore a hat. This change of fashion has decreased the demand for men's hats, and especially for bowler hats. Some fashions may be related to the weather, and a fine summer may increase the demand for panama hats. Some children's toys seem to have a brief period of popularity and then are seen no more, demand vanishing almost overnight. Advertisers and propagandists try, and often succeed in changing tastes or fashions. Temperance societies attempt by propaganda to reduce the demand for alcoholic drink, while the manufacturers of such drinks try to stimulate demand by means of advertising.

(ii) *New commodities replace old.* Things are always becoming out of date. New inventions are constantly being made, and the demand for these takes the place of the demand for the things they replace. Over the past fifty years the demand for electric lamps has greatly increased, while the demand for gas-mantles has been declining. Though a piano is now to be found in few homes, there are not many without a radio, television or radiogram. The attaché case ousted the Gladstone bag, just as later the despatch case took the place of the attaché case.

(iii) *A change in the quantity of money.* An increase or a decrease in the quantity of money will affect demand, for it is unlikely that the prices of all goods will change proportionately to the change in the quantity of money. The demand for some commodities will increase, while the demand for others will fall.

(iv) *A change in real incomes.* The distinction between money income and real income will be considered more fully later.[1] A change in real income means a change in the quantity of goods the money income will buy. A person's money income may rise, while his real income falls, if prices rise more than wages. On the other hand, his real income may rise, though his money income falls, if his wages fall more slowly than prices. An increase in people's real income may have little effect

[1] See p. 300.

on the demand for the cheaper foodstuffs, or on food at all after a certain point, but it may have considerable effect on the demand for luxuries and semi-luxuries.

(v) *Changes in the distribution of incomes.* Inequality of incomes between different groups of people may be lessened by taxing the rich more heavily than the poor, by subsidising foodstuffs and by the State providing free social services of which the poor may avail themselves more than the rich. This may result in an increase in demand for those things mostly bought by the poor—with a consequent rise in their prices.

(vi) *Changes in population.* Two kinds of change may be noted, (a) an increase or decrease in the total population or (b) a change in the proportion between the different age-groups, though if the first of these changes takes place it is almost certain to bring about the second change also. The effect of population changes has already been considered, and it was pointed out that if an increase occurred in the proportion of old people in the population and a reduction in the proportion of children, it would tend to increase the demand for the assortment of goods old people wanted and reduce the demand for goods primarily required for children.

(vii) *Changes in the prices of other goods.* The demand for one commodity may change as a result of a change in the price of some other commodity. To some extent all prices are affected in this way. A general increase in the prices of foodstuffs will reduce the demand for food to a less extent than a rise in the price of other goods, but its effect will be to reduce the demand for other things, if incomes remain unchanged. These are cases, however, where the demand for two or more commodities is more closely related. Where things are fairly close substitutes for one another, a fall in the price of one will reduce the demand for the other. A rise in the price of patent cocoa drinks might increase the demand for cocoa; a rise in railway fares might increase the demand for bus travel. Sometimes commodities are used together, and then a change in the price of one will affect the demand for both, even though the price of the second commodity remains unchanged. A rise in the price of motor cars, for example, might reduce the demand for petrol.

(viii) *Expectation of the trend of future trade.* The demand of business men for factors of production depends on their expectation whether business activity is likely to be maintained in the future, since they have to produce in anticipation of demand. This particularly affects the demand for new capital. If a slump is feared the demand for new machinery or plant will probably fall off.

(ix) *Expectation of future changes in prices.* This generally affects business men more than consumers. Expectation of a rise in the price of a raw material will stimulate the demand of merchants and manufacturers for it, whereas fear of a fall in prices will make them more cautious, and so check demand. Exceptional demand (that is, where more is bought at a higher than a lower price), resulting from a fear of a further rise in price, really falls within this category. This was considered in the previous chapter.

(x) *Taxation.* Taxes may be imposed either to lessen inequality of income or deliberately to reduce the demand for a commodity. Some alcoholic drinks are heavily taxed in order to reduce their consumption rather than to raise revenue. Duties are often imposed on imported goods in order to reduce the demand for them.

(3) CHANGES IN SUPPLY

Just as a change in demand requires a new demand curve, so it is with a change in supply. The fact that more will generally be supplied at a high than a low price does not indicate a change of supply, but merely shows the effect of a change of price on supply. As with demand, this ambiguity can be avoided if one speaks of changes in the quantity supplied when different positions on the same supply curve are being considered. A change in supply therefore requires a new supply curve:

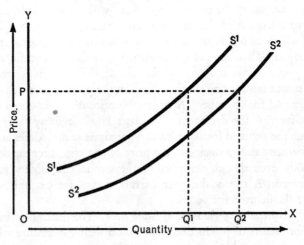

FIG. 17.—CHANGE IN SUPPLY.

In this case the change is an increase in supply, showing that at the old price OP the quantity OQ² will now be supplied, instead of the smaller quantity OQ^1. At all prices a larger quantity than before will be supplied.

(4) CAUSES OF CHANGES IN SUPPLY

The following are some of the reasons why conditions of supply may change:

(i) *Where the producer consumes more of his own product.* An improvement in people's standard of living may result in their consuming more of their own output of a commodity. For this reason the exports of meat from Argentina have been less in recent years than formerly. Similarly, Russia exports less wheat today than it did before 1914.

(ii) *Changes in the cost of production.* If the entrepreneur has to pay more to secure the services of the factors of production he employs, his costs of production will rise. Since no producer could remain in business for long if he failed to cover his costs of production, a rise in costs will generally, other things being equal, tend to reduce the supply coming on to the market. A fall in his costs will have the opposite effect.

(iii) *Changes in the technique of production.* This is probably the most important factor affecting supply. The development of a new method of production or the invention of a new machine may make possible a big expansion of output at lower cost and so increase supply.

(iv) *Effects of the weather.* In the case of agricultural products the actual output cannot be precisely estimated in advance, owing to vagaries of the weather. Even if the same area is devoted to wheat over a series of years, the variation in output between one year and another may be very considerable. Because of the long interval between seed-time and harvest, the response of supply to changes in the price of farming products is slow.

(v) *Effect of taxation.* Taxation of commodities is likely to raise their prices. The imposition of a tax on a commodity is equivalent to an increase in its cost of production and so will generally result in a decrease in supply. A reduction of taxation will have the opposite effect.

(5) EFFECTS OF CHANGES IN DEMAND

(i) *An increase of demand.* Consider first the effect of a change in demand, assuming the conditions of supply to remain unchanged. As previously emphasised, this requires the drawing of a new demand curve. SS represents the condition of supply for the commodity, D^1D^1 is the old demand curve and D^2D^2 the new demand curve after the change (in this case, increase) of demand. Before this change the equilibrium price was OP^1, at which the quantity OQ^1 was supplied. Supply adjusts itself slowly to changes of price, and in the short period supply may appear to be fixed. The immediate effect, therefore, of the

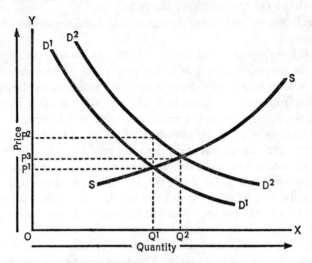

FIG. 18.—THE EFFECT OF INCREASE IN DEMAND.

increase in demand is for price to rise from OP^1 to OP^2 because supply remains for a time at OQ^1 as before. Sooner or later the effect of the rise in price will be to evoke the supply of a larger quantity of the com-

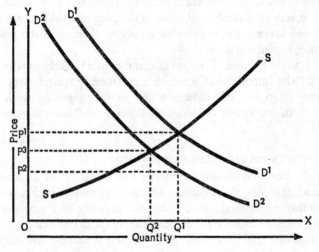

FIG. 19.—THE EFFECT OF DECREASE IN DEMAND.

modity. The point of intersection of the supply curve and the new demand curve indicates the new equilibrium position, the quantity supplied being OQ^2 and the price settling down at OP^3. The effect of the increase in demand has been both to raise price and increase the quantity supplied. The fourth Law of Supply and Demand therefore states that *an increase in demand tends both to increase price and to call forth a larger supply.*

(ii) *A decrease in demand.* A fall in demand will bring about a fall both in price and in the quantity supplied (Fig. 19).

Again there is an immediate effect, for a reduction in the quantity supplied does not take place at once. The immediate effect is for price to fall from OP^1 to OP^2, equilibrium ultimately being achieved at a price of OP^3 with the quantity OQ^2 supplied.

(6) EFFECTS OF CHANGES IN SUPPLY

(i) *An increase in supply.* Immediate and ultimate effects are possible in the case of changes in supply, but generally demand responds more

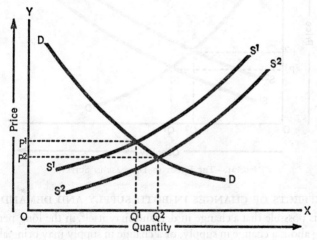

FIG. 20.—THE EFFECT OF INCREASE IN SUPPLY.

readily to changes in price than does supply (Fig. 20). *DD* represents the state of demand, S^1S^1 the conditions of supply at first, and S^2S^2 the conditions of supply after an increase of supply. Such a change might occur as a result of technical improvements. As a result of the change a larger quantity than before will be supplied at each price. The old equilibrium price was OP^1, at which the quantity OQ^1 was supplied. The new equilibrium price is OP^2, at which OQ^2 is supplied. The effect of the increase in supply has been to increase the quantity supplied and to lower the price. The fifth Law of Supply and Demand states that *an increase in supply tends to lower price and to increase quantity demanded*.

(ii) *A decrease in supply*. A decrease in supply will pull the supply curve to the left of its original position, and the effect will be to raise price and reduce the quantity demanded.

The new price, OP^2, is higher than the old, OP^1; the new quantity supplied is OQ^2, and this is smaller than the old, OQ^1. Such a change in the conditions of supply might be brought about by increased costs of production, just as the increase in supply in the previous example might have been the result of a fall in costs. Costs of production therefore affect price indirectly through an increase or decrease in supply.

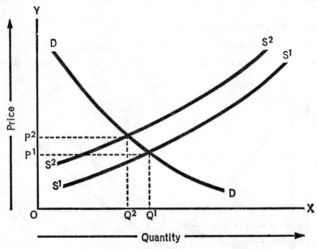

Fig. 21.—The Effect of Decrease in Supply.

(7) EFFECTS OF CHANGES IN BOTH SUPPLY AND DEMAND

It is possible that a change in demand may itself, in the long period, bring about a change in supply, or a change in supply may bring about a change in demand. Consider the example given in 5 (i). The effect of the increase in demand was to raise price and increase the quantity supplied under the existing conditions of supply—that is, without any change in supply. To put this increased quantity on the market may, however, make it possible for the firms in the industry to take advantage of economies of large-scale production. If so, this will bring about a more than proportionate increase in supply, and the ultimate effect therefore may be to lower price and increase the quantity supplied. In the reverse case of the falling off in the demand for a

commodity the decrease in the quantity demanded may increase the
average cost of production and so lead to a rise in price, as is the case
with the manufacture of motor cars.

For clarity, the immediate effect, considered in 5 (i), is omitted.
The original equilibrium position indicated by the intersection of the
original supply and demand curves S^1S^1 and D^1D^1 shows that the
quantity OQ^1 would be supplied at a price of OP^1. Demand then
increased from D^1D^1 to D^2D^2. Before any change took place in supply
a new equilibrium position was established after price had risen from
OP^1 to OP^2, and after the quantity supplied had increased from OQ^1 to

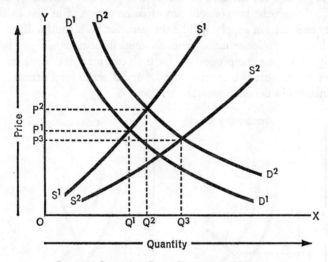

FIG. 22.—CHANGE IN BOTH SUPPLY AND DEMAND.

OQ^2. Finally, after the change in supply the ultimate effect was to
bring about equilibrium at a price of OP^3, at which quantity OQ^3
was supplied. Thus the ultimate effect of this change in demand was
to reduce price and increase output. The reader may find it of interest
to work out graphically the following further cases:

(i) The ultimate effect of an increase in demand where the increase
in the quantity supplied can be obtained only at increased costs of
production (that is, where expansion of an industry is under conditions of increasing costs).

(ii) The ultimate effect of a decrease in demand where the decrease
in the quantity supplied raises costs of production.

(iii) The ultimate effect of a decrease in demand where the decrease
in the quantity supplied lowers costs of production.

II. INTER-RELATIONSHIP OF SUPPLY AND DEMAND

(8) INTER-RELATED DEMANDS

(i) *Joint or complementary demand.* One commodity may be complementary to another, and so the two commodities may be jointly demanded, as for example bread and butter, tea and sugar, strawberries and cream, lamb and mint sauce, pens and ink, motor cars and petrol. In such cases changes in demand are generally in the same proportion for each of the linked commodities; if the demand for bread increases by 10%, then the demand for butter will probably increase by about 10%, though the proportions can often be varied. But it is unlikely that conditions of supply will be the same for both commodities, and so changes in price resulting from a change in demand will not necessarily be in the same proportion for both commodities. For example, let us assume that two commodities, A and B, are in joint demand, and an increase in demand occurs:

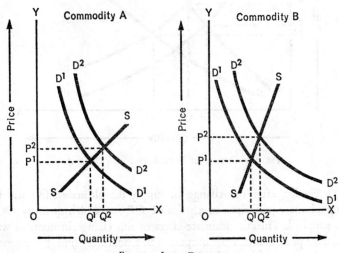

FIG. 23.—JOINT DEMAND.

OQ^2 represents a similar proportionate increase over OQ^1 in each case, but because the conditions of supply are not the same for each commodity (the supply of A being more responsive than B to changes of price), the price of commodity A will rise by only approximately $33\frac{1}{3}\%$, whereas the price of commodity B almost doubles.

If a change should occur in the conditions of supply bringing about an increase in supply of commodity A, the state of demand in this case remaining the same, the price of commodity A will fall and the quantity demanded will increase. Since *A* and *B* are complementary the increased demand for *A* means an increased demand also for *B*, and the conditions of supply for *B* being unchanged, its price will rise.

(ii) *Derived demand.* The term *derived* demand is frequently used where demand for one commodity is the direct result of the demand for another, as, for example, in the case of the demand for factors of production. The demand for land, labour and capital is derived from the demand for the commodities produced by these factors. The demand of entrepreneurs is for a number of factors jointly—for example, the woollen manufacturer has a joint demand for land, labour, factory buildings, machinery, raw wool, coal or other source of power, and transport. The demand for every one of these things can be said to be derived from the demand for woollen cloth, carpets or other woollen goods.

Joint, complementary or derived demand are similar to one another, in that an increase in the demand for one commodity brings about an increase in the demand for the other.

(iii) *Composite demand.* Sometimes a commodity can be used for two or more purposes, and the demand for it may vary as a result of a change in the demand for any one of these purposes. Steel may be used for making motor cars, or in shipbuilding; bricks may be used for building either houses or schools; wool may be demanded for making either into cloth or into carpets. This is known as composite demand, and it applies to most raw materials. An increase in the demand for carpets will raise the price of wool, and increase the amount of wool going to carpet manufacturers, but in the short period the supply available to cloth manufacturers will be reduced and they also will have to pay a higher price for wool.

(iv) *Competitive demand.* If two commodities are fairly close substitutes for one another an increase in the quantity demanded of one of them will reduce the demand for the other. To some extent all commodities are in competitive demand with one another, because the purchase of more of one thing necessitates the purchase of less of others, so that any change in demand for one thing to some extent affects the demand for all others. Where two things serve more or less the same purpose, to have more of one means that less of the other will be wanted. An increase in the quantity of butter demanded would probably reduce the demand for margarine; an increased demand for mutton might reduce the demand for beef; a change in the demand for fish might conversely affect the demand for meat.

Suppose that two commodities *A* and *B* are in competitive demand and that an increased demand for commodity *A* occurs (Fig. 24).

The increased demand for commodity A raises the price from OP^1 to OP^2 and increases the quantity supplied from OQ^1 to OQ^2. As a consequence of this increased demand for a commodity A there is a fall in the demand for commodity B from D^1D^1 to D^2D^2, as a result of which its price falls from OP^1 to OP^2 and the quantity supplied falls from OQ^1 to OQ^2.

In the case of competitive demand an increased demand for one commodity reduces the demand for the other.

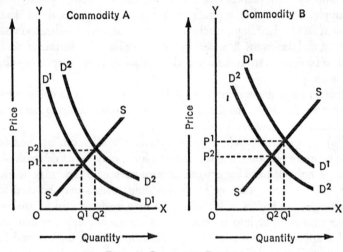

FIG. 24.—COMPETITIVE DEMAND.

The demand for factors of production is competitive to the extent that factors are capable of being substituted for one another. The employment of more capital by an entrepreneur may mean a decreased demand for labour.

(9) INTER-RELATED SUPPLY

(i) *Joint supply.* Some commodities are produced together, so that change in the supply of one can be brought about only by similarly changing the supply of the other. Wool and mutton, beef and hides, gas and coke and the various types of oil are examples of such joint supply. The seriousness of the problem of supply in these cases depends on the extent to which the proportion between the joint products can be varied. It is said that inability to vary the proportions is rare, although in many cases the extent of such variation may not be very great. It is true, for example, that Australian sheep produce better wool than mutton, whereas New Zealand sheep produce better mutton than wool. In response to an increase in demand, the supply of wool can therefore be increased without proportionately increasing the supply of mutton. Nevertheless, the supply of mutton will be increased to some extent. The increased demand for commodity *A* (wool) will cause a fall in the price of commodity *B* (mutton):

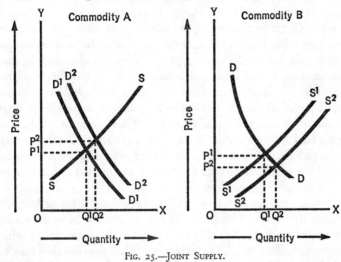

FIG. 25.—JOINT SUPPLY.

The increased demand for wool raises the price of wool from OP^1 to OP^2 and increases the quantity supplied from OQ^1 to OQ^2. This increases the supply of mutton from S^1S^1 to S^2S^2, increases the quantity supplied from OQ^1 to OQ^2, and lowers the price from OP^1 to OP^2.

(ii) *Competitive supply.* To expand the production of one commodity generally requires a reduction in the output of another. This is particularly true of farming products in a country such as Great Britain. To increase the supply of an agricultural product such as wheat means ploughing up more grassland and rearing fewer grazing animals. More meat may be produced, but only at the cost of less milk, or vice versa. There is a wider application, for every country's supply of factors of production is limited, so that if factors are used for one form of production, obviously they cannot be used for another. It is equally true, therefore, to say that an expansion of manufacturing means less farming. During the nineteenth century Great Britain neglected its farming, but this made possible the vast industrial expansion of the country during that period. When, during the two World Wars of the twentieth century, it was desired to increase the output of food, without at the same time curtailing industrial production, it is not surprising that shortage of labour became a serious problem.

(10) DO THE SUPPLY AND DEMAND CURVES REPRESENT INDEPENDENT FORCES?

It has already been seen that a change in the demand can bring about a change in supply, and that a change in supply may cause a change in demand. Can it be that the supply and demand curves are even more intimately related and, indeed, are responsive to the same influences? Is the supply curve really only a part of the demand curve? In some cases this may be so. If the seller has a reserve price—that is, a price below which he is not prepared to sell, a price at which the commodity is more preferred than money—then in reality the seller himself enters the market at that price, and when he refuses to sell he is in a sense buying back his own goods. It is common at auctions for the sellers to have such reserve prices. Even the farmer who takes eggs to market may decide to take them back for home consumption rather than sell them if the price is very low.

In certain markets some people may be either buyers or sellers, as opportunity occurs. This would be true of speculators in the various commodity markets. Not only have they a reserve price below which they are unwilling to sell, but if the price falls below this they may become buyers. The higher the price, the more they are willing to sell; the lower the price, the more they are prepared to buy. It is thus possible to compile for such a person a combined supply and demand schedule. Assume that the speculator is operating on the Stock Exchange, and, for the sake of simplicity, assume further that he is interested only in the ordinary shares of the Alpha-Beta Manufacturing Co., Ltd., his combined supply and demand schedule might run as follows:

TABLE XXII

A Combined Demand and Supply Schedule (2)

Price	Quantity bought or sold + = Bought — = Sold
16s.	+ 1,000
17s.	+ 450
18s.	+ 250
19s.	+ 100
20s.	—
21s.	— 50
22s.	— 200
23s.	— 400
24s.	— 700

It is possible now to represent this schedule graphically:

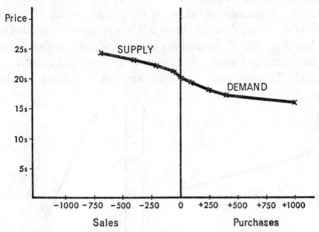

FIG. 26.—A COMBINED DEMAND AND SUPPLY CURVE.

Thus it becomes possible to represent both supply and demand by a single curve. The supply curve then becomes merely a part of the demand curve reversed.

III. THE CONCEPT OF ELASTICITY

(11) ELASTICITY OF DEMAND

By elasticity of demand or supply is meant the degree of responsiveness of demand or supply respectively to changes of price. If a slight change in price causes a big change in the quantity demanded, then demand is said to be elastic. If, however, a fairly considerable change in price makes little difference to the quantity demanded, then demand is

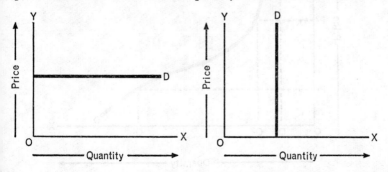

FIG. 27.—PERFECTLY ELASTIC DEMAND.   FIG. 28.—PERFECTLY INELASTIC DEMAND.

said to be inelastic. Demand is perfectly inelastic if the same quantity is demanded whatever the price.

Elasticity determines the shape of the demand curve. If demand is perfectly elastic the demand curve will be a straight line parallel to the base line (Fig. 27). If demand is perfectly inelastic the demand curve will be a straight line at right angles to the base and parallel to *OY* (Fig. 28). Between these two extremes are an infinite number of

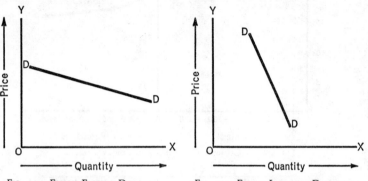

FIG. 29.—FAIRLY ELASTIC DEMAND.   FIG. 30.—FAIRLY INELASTIC DEMAND.

possibilities. A fairly elastic demand will be represented by a gradually sloping demand curve (Fig. 29). A fairly inelastic demand will be represented by a steeply sloping demand curve (Fig. 30). The less steep the curve, the more elastic is the demand, provided, of course, the

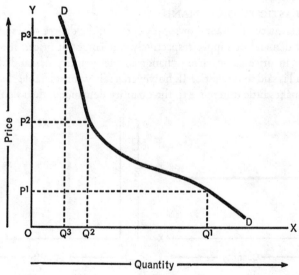

FIG. 31.—A DEMAND CURVE WITH VARYING ELASTICITY.

curves to be compared are drawn on graphs with identical price and quantity scales. Probably there is no commodity for which the elasticity of demand is the same at all prices, and most demand curves

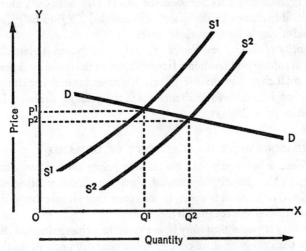

FIG. 32.—ELASTICITY OF DEMAND AND CHANGE OF SUPPLY (1).

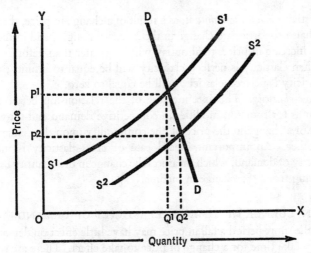

FIG. 33.—ELASTICITY OF DEMAND AND CHANGE OF SUPPLY (2).

will show different elasticities over different parts of their lengths (Fig. 31). This demand curve shows that at low prices up to OP^1 demand is inelastic, but between prices OP^1 and OP^2 demand is elastic, becoming inelastic again at high prices over OP^2. Reading from the

graph, it can be seen that when the curve is steep, as between prices
OP^2 and OP^3, there is little change (OQ^2 to OQ^3) in the amount
demanded, and so demand is inelastic: whereas when the curve has a
more gradual slope, as between the prices OP^1 and OP^2, there is a
considerable change in the quantity demanded (OQ^1 to OQ^2), and so
demand is elastic between these prices.[1]

Elasticity of demand and change of supply. If demand is elastic an increase in supply will result in a large increase in the quantity demanded,
but a small change in price (Fig. 32). If demand is inelastic an increase
in supply will result in a small increase in the quantity demanded, but a
big fall in price (Fig. 33).

(12) MEASUREMENT OF ELASTICITY OF DEMAND

If a change in the price of a commodity brings about a proportionate
change in the quantity demanded, then the elasticity of demand is
considered to be *equal to unity*. In such cases there is no change in total
expenditure on the commodity.

Elasticity is *greater than unity* if, as a result of a change in price, there is
a more than proportionate change in the quantity bought. In the case
of an increase in price, total outlay on the commodity will be less than
before.

Elasticity is *less than unity* if, as a result of a change in price, there is a
less than proportionate change in the quantity bought, and in the case
of an increase in price, total outlay will be greater than before.

When elasticity is perfect, elasticity will be equal to infinity; when
inelasticity is perfect, elasticity will be equal to zero.

Cross-elasticity. This is a measure of the relationship between the
demands for two commodities in competitive demand and shows the
effect of a change in the price of one commodity upon the demand for
the other. An important special case of cross-elasticity is income
elasticity of demand, which measures the change in the quantity bought
resulting from 1% change in income.

(13) INFLUENCE OF TIME ON ELASTICITY OF DEMAND

In the short period a fall in price may have little effect on demand, as
it may take time for a change of price to take effect. There are several
reasons why this may be so:

(i) it may be some time before all consumers become aware of the
change in price.

---

[1] The reader must beware of assuming from these illustrations that the *degree of elasticity*
is the same for any point on a straight line "curve."

(ii) If it is thought that price is likely to fall further, consumers will not increase their purchases at once.

(iii) From habit people may have become accustomed to buying a certain assortment of goods and so may be reluctant to change. This may be more important in the case of an increase in price. During a period of inflation those people whose incomes have risen proportionately less than prices may be unwilling to accept a lower standard of living 'and so, hoping the inflationary condition is only temporary, they may draw upon past savings in order to be able to obtain the same quantity of goods as before the rise in prices took place.

(iv) Some goods are durable, and consumers will obviously not replace them until they are worn out, even if their price has fallen.

(v) In the case of complementary commodities, jointly demanded, a fall in price of one of them will have little effect if the price of the other rises by a greater amount. Sometimes, in order to take advantage of a fall in price, it is necessary to purchase other commodities. For example, to benefit from a fall in the price of electricity, a householder would have to instal more electrical appliances.

(14) THE BASIS OF ELASTICITY OF DEMAND

A number of factors influence the responsiveness of demand to changes of price:

(i) *The possibility of substitution.* The most important influence on elasticity of demand is whether there are close substitutes for the commodity. The closer the substitutes, the more elastic is likely to be the demand for the commodity, but the substitute must be within the same price range. From the point of view of use, a Rolls-Royce may be a perfect substitute for a small car, but economically it is no substitute at all, for even a very large change in the price of the small car will have no effect on the demand for large expensive cars. The demand for cocoa is elastic because fairly close substitutes for it exist at approximately the same price. If there are no close substitutes within the same price range the demand for a commodity is more likely to be inelastic.

(ii) *The degree of necessity.* Whether goods are luxuries or necessaries is not therefore the chief determinant of elasticity of demand. Indeed, the demand for some expensive luxury goods may be very inelastic, not because they are luxuries but rather because they lack close substitutes. Similarly, the demand for bread and potatoes is inelastic because there are no close substitutes within the same price range and not merely because they are necessaries. If there are close substitutes it matters little whether the commodity is a necessary or a luxury, but if there are no good substitutes the extent to which the commodity is a necessary may then affect the elasticity of demand for it.

(iii) *Consumers' incomes.* Generally, the higher a person's income, the more inelastic will be his demand for commodities. The demand of a millionaire for all commodities may be quite unaffected by any changes of price. For the majority of people, however, a choice has to be made, and choice becomes more exacting the lower the income. Any re-distribution of income in favour of people in the lower-income groups will tend to make demand for some commodities more inelastic (that is, those things more particularly demanded by such people) and for other things more elastic (that is, those things desired by people in the higher income groups).

(iv) *Cheap commodities.* The smaller the proportion of total income expended on a commodity, the more inelastic will be the demand for it. For example, the price of a box of matches might rise considerably before it had much effect on the demand for it.

(v) *Habit.* It has already been noticed that once certain habits of expenditure have been formed, they may be sufficiently strong for a time to offset the effect of changes in price over a certain range. This has been particularly noticeable in the case of tobacco, for though the price has been enormously increased by taxation, the demand for it has remained almost unchanged. The demand for tobacco, obviously a luxury, has proved to be fairly inelastic, partly because the smoking habit is strong, and partly also because there is no close substitute for tobacco.

(15) ELASTICITY OF DEMAND AND TOTAL INCOME

If a small quantity of a commodity is supplied its price will be higher than if a larger quantity were supplied. How much the price of a com-modity rises as its quantity is reduced depends, as already seen, on the elasticity of demand for it. It is of interest to notice how the total in-come of suppliers will be affected by changes in the quantity supplied. This income will be shown by the area of the rectangle formed by the length representing quantity and the breadth representing price, since total income = price × quantity (Fig. 34).

For example, if *DAD* represents the demand curve for a commodity and *A* the point at which the supply curve cuts the demand curve, then *OQ* is the quantity supplied, and *OP* will be the price at which this quantity can be sold. Total income of suppliers will then be *OQ* (quantity) × *OP* (price)—that is, the rectangle *QOPA*.

Consider now the effect of a change in the quantity supplied. Suppose that the supply is increased from the quantity OQ^1 to the quantity OQ^2, and that demand is elastic (Fig. 35). It is clear that the expansion of output more than balances the fall in price, for the rectangle Q^2OP^2B is greater in area than the rectangle Q^1OP^1A.

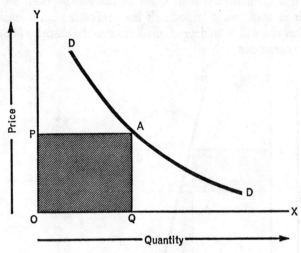

FIG. 34.—TOTAL INCOME.

When demand is elastic an increase in the quantity supplied will increase the total income of suppliers. If, however, demand is inelastic the greater quantity can be sold only after a large fall in price, and so the

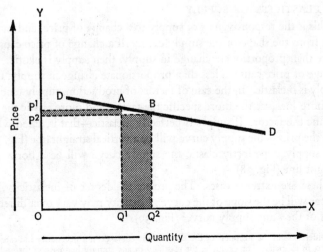

FIG. 35.—TOTAL INCOME WITH ELASTIC DEMAND.

total incomes of suppliers is less than before, as a comparison of the two rectangles Q^1OP^1A and Q^2OP^2B shows (Fig. 36). This is probably true of many farming products, the farmers having a smaller income when there is a good harvest than when the harvest is poor. Similarly, fishermen may find a large catch less profitable than a small one. Whether this will be so depends in all cases on the elasticity of demand for the commodity.

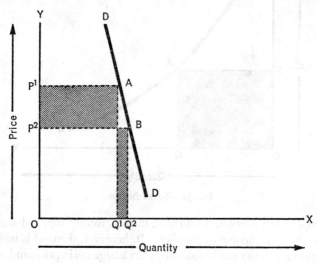

FIG. 36.—TOTAL INCOME WITH INELASTIC DEMAND.

(16) ELASTICITY OF SUPPLY

This is the responsiveness of supply to a change of price, and can be seen from the shape of the supply curve. If a change of price causes a more than proportionate change in supply, then supply is elastic. If a change of price causes a less than proportionate change in supply, then supply is inelastic. In the case of factors of production, supply tends to be more inelastic the more specific the factor, and more elastic the less specific the factor. If supply is perfectly inelastic—that is, fixed whatever the price—the supply curve will be a vertical straight line (Fig. 37).

If supply is perfectly elastic the supply curve will be a horizontal straight line (Fig. 38).

These are extreme cases. The greater the degree of inelasticity, the steeper will be the slope of the curve. Elasticity may vary over different parts of the same supply curve[1] (Fig. 39).

---

[1] Differences in the steepness of the slope of the curve do not necessarily indicate differences in elasticity. For example, the elasticity of any straight line passing through O, whatever may be its slope, is the same—unity.

Elasticity of supply determines the effect of change of demand on prices. If supply is fairly elastic an increase of demand will bring about

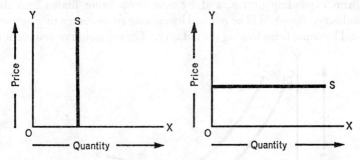

FIG. 37.—PERFECTLY INELASTIC SUPPLY.   FIG. 38.—PERFECTLY ELASTIC SUPPLY.

a big increase in the quantity supplied, but only a small increase in price (Fig. 40).

If supply is fairly inelastic an increase in demand will bring about only a small increase in the quantity supplied, but will cause a big rise in price (Fig. 41).

The more elastic the supply, the less variable will be the price.

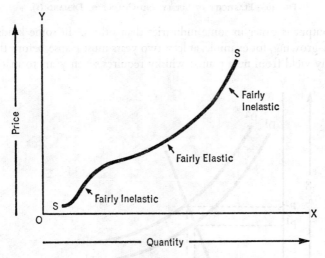

FIG. 39.—A SUPPLY CURVE WITH VARYING ELASTICITY.

Time has a greater influence on elasticity of supply than on elasticity of demand. In the short period, supply may be fixed, and it may take some time for an industry to adjust itself to a change of output.

Elasticity of supply will therefore depend on the time it takes an industry to make this adjustment. Supply will be increased by existing firms expanding output, and by new firms being drawn into the industry. Supply will be reduced by existing firms contracting output, and by some firms leaving the industry. The expansion or contraction

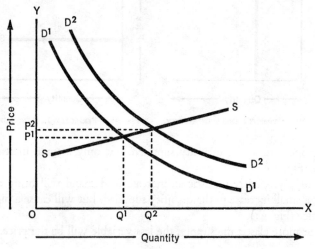

FIG. 40.—ELASTICITY OF SUPPLY AND CHANGE OF DEMAND (1).

of output is easier in some industries than others. In some kinds of fruit-growing, for example, at least two years must elapse before there is any yield from new plants; whisky requires seven years to mature,

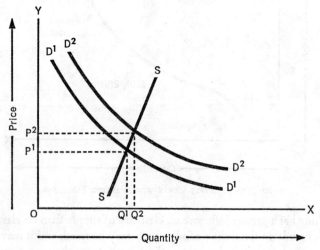

FIG. 41.—ELASTICITY OF SUPPLY AND CHANGE OF DEMAND (2).

and vintage wines much longer than that. Elasticity of supply depends on the ease with which changes in output can be accomplished.

IV. PRICE CONTROL

(17) THE PRICE MECHANISM

Demand, supply and price, then, depend on one another, and the equilibrium price equates demand with supply. It has already been seen that all goods are scarce relative to the demand for them, and the price mechanism is one method which enables goods to be distributed among the people who want them. Changes in either supply or demand will be reflected by changes in price, an increase in supply or a falling off in demand bringing about a fall in price, and a decrease in supply or an increase in demand causing price to rise. An increase in demand tends to make entrepreneurs increase supply, just as a fall in demand will make them reduce supply. The price mechanism not only distributes "scarce" goods among consumers but also distributes "scarce" factors of production among entrepreneurs.

The demand of consumers encourages entrepreneurs to expand supply, and this stimulates the demand of entrepreneurs for factors of production. The demand of consumers, therefore, through the price mechanism, determines what assortment of goods shall be produced, how much of this and how much of that. Under perfect competition the sovereignty of consumers is complete, and goods and resources go where they are most in demand. Furthermore, no elaborate administrative machinery is required to operate the price mechanism, and yet by means of it a vast assortment of goods and services can be produced and distributed in a way which people as a whole prefer. Adjustments to changes in conditions of supply or in intensity of demand can also be made without administrative action. These are its main advantages. On the other hand, it is pointed out that in actual conditions the market is imperfect, and in any case the demand of consumers is not the best way of determining what shall be produced, for it may result in the production of large quantities of (say) tobacco and only small quantities of (say) butter. The alternative is for a State planning committee to decide what shall be produced, but this requires a system of controls to ensure that industries obtain the share of resources apportioned to them. If it is felt, as in war-time, that the price mechanism will not distribute goods "fairly" control of prices and rationing may be introduced.

(18) PRICE CONTROL AND RATIONING

In conclusion, it will be useful briefly to consider some aspects of price control. The State may fix prices for any one of a number of reasons.

It may be considered desirable to protect buyers in general or the poorer section of the community, and in this case maximum prices will be fixed. It may be that the aim is to protect agricultural producers against a fall in income due to bumper harvests (*see* **15**), and in this case maximum prices will be fixed. Other weapons of price control are taxation (to raise prices) and subsidies (to reduce prices). The purpose of raising prices by taxation may be to check the consumption of certain commodities, either for "moral" reasons, as in the case of whisky and other spirits, or in order to check imports in the case of balance-of-payments difficulties. Subsidies may be imposed on certain foodstuffs in an attempt to keep down the cost of living or to encourage output. The effect of taxes and subsidies will be considered later.[1]

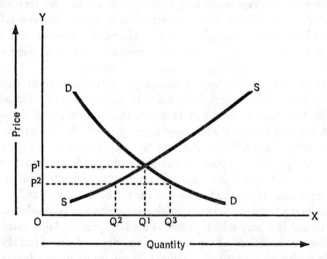

FIG. 42.—PRICE CONTROL AND RATIONING.

Consider now the effect of the fixing by the State of maximum prices for consumer goods. Such action will be necessary only if the equilibrium price, as determined by supply and demand, is considered to be too high. Let *DD* and *SS* be the appropriate supply and demand curves for the commodity (Fig. 42). The equilibrium price will be OP^1, and the quantity supplied will be OQ^1. Assume that the State now fixes OP^2 as the maximum price. At this price the quantity demanded will be OQ^3, but suppliers will now be willing to put on the market only the quantity OQ^2. The quantity demanded at this controlled price will be OQ^3, and this will exceed the quantity supplied by Q^2Q^3. Even if

[1] See Chapter XXX.

the State subsidised suppliers in order to call forth as large a supply as was forthcoming under equilibrium conditions, the quantity demanded will still exceed, by Q^1Q^3, the quantity supplied. If no further action is taken by the State retailers will now find that they have insufficient supplies to meet the demand of their customers. There will be a shortage of the commodity, with the result that customers will be dependent on the favour of retailers, goods not being offered for sale to everyone who wishes to buy. If prices are controlled below the equilibrium, either the State or retailers will have to introduce some form of rationing. In that case the fairest method of distribution would seem to be by some organised system of rationing.

RECOMMENDATIONS FOR FURTHER READING

K. E. Boulding: *Economic Analysis*, Chapter 7.
A. Marshall: *Principles of Economics*, Book V, Chapters 5, 6.
H. Henderson: *Supply and Demand*
G. J. Stigler: *Theory of Price*, Chapters 5–8.

QUESTIONS

1. Consider the different factors which may influence the effective demand for a commodity. When is the elasticity of demand greater than unity? (R.S.A. Adv.)

2. Show with examples, the practical importance of a large and of a small elasticity of demand. (C.I.S. Inter.)

3. (*a*) State briefly what is meant by "joint" and "composite" demand.
(*b*) What is elasticity of demand?
(*c*) What does an economist mean when he says that over short periods demand may be more elastic than supply, while over long periods supply may be more elastic than demand? (A.C.C.A. Inter.)

4. "Price control is impossible without rationing." Discuss. (B.S. Inter.)

5. What is meant by elasticity as applied to demand and to supply? What determines elasticity in each case? (C.C.S. Final.)

6. Define and explain the following economic terms: (*a*) elasticity of demand; (*b*) joint supply. (I.M.T.A.)

7. It has been said that the keynote of economic analysis is attention to the nature and working of the price mechanism. Explain this point of view, indicating carefully what is meant by the term "price-mechanism" in this context. (I.H.A.)

8. What determines the extent of the price change that follows any given change in supply? (D.P.A.)

9. Explain the concept "elasticity of supply with respect to price." Why might supply elasticities be lower in the short run than in the long run? (G.C.E. Adv.)

10. Define "elasticity of supply." Why might one expect the elasticity of supply of a commodity to be greater in the long run than in the short run? (G.C.E. Adv.)

11. What determines the elasticity of supply of wheat: (a) in the short run, and (b) in the long run? (G.C.E. Adv.)

12. "The demand for bread is inelastic." Explain what you understand by this statement, and give reasons why it is probably true. (G.C.E. Adv.)

13. Illustrate some of the defects in the price system which in your view should be remedied by State action. (Final Degree.)

14. "The so-called supply curve is simply a part of the total demand curve." (Wicksteed.) Explain and examine this contention. (Final Degree.)

THE TOOLS OF ECONOMIC ANALYSIS
(continued)

(ii) *The Concept of the Margin*

CHAPTER XII

THE BASIS OF DEMAND

I. MARGINAL UTILITY

Chapters X and XI were devoted to a consideration of supply and demand and the determination of price. An understanding of the technique of supply and demand provides the key to the solution of many problems in economics, but it is not a master key, and it requires to be supplemented by a second tool—the marginal analysis. By means of this it becomes possible to understand the basis upon which demand and supply curves are drawn. It is the purpose of this chapter to investigate the basis of demand: the following chapters will deal with the basis of supply.

(1) THE MARGIN

What, then, is meant in economics by the margin? The marginal unit of anything is the last to be added to or the first to be taken away from a supply. If a student already possesses three books on economics and is contemplating buying a fourth, this fourth book might be considered to be his "marginal" volume. Whether he buys it or not will depend on whether he thinks that the additional benefit to be derived from this fourth book is worth the price he will have to pay for it—that is, he considers its *marginal* worth to him. If a farmer has fifty acres of land under wheat a rise in the price of wheat may tempt him to devote another acre to wheat. This additional acre is the *marginal* unit. Alternatively, if he had decided to withdraw one acre from wheat cultivation the acre that ceased to grow wheat would be the *marginal* unit.

Marginal considerations concern the smallest possible increase or decrease in the stock or supply of anything. For this reason this branch of economics is sometimes called *microeconomics*. It is always marginal considerations that determine whether a person will add to his existing stock of a commodity. The marginal significance of any commodity, therefore, depends on how much of it is already possessed. If a student already possesses a number of books on economics the marginal significance to him of books on economics is likely to be low; if he has only one book on economics the marginal significance of such books may be high—unless he is a student of chemistry and has no interest whatever in economics! The margin is obviously not fixed, for an increase in one's supply will simply push the margin farther away, just as a decrease in one's supply will bring the margin nearer. A change in price will have a similar effect, a fall in price pushing the margin farther away and a rise in price bringing it nearer. It is therefore possible to speak of the marginal unit of a supply. Similarly, the term, margin, can be used in connection with cost, income, production, so that we can speak of marginal cost, marginal income and the marginal product.

The marginal unit is thus not a particular unit or any particular type or quality of unit. Some ambiguity arises from the use of the word in such phrases as "the margin of cultivation." Official use of the term "marginal land" has tended to make some people apply it to land of a particular grade of fertility, as a result of farmers being urged to expand production by cultivating marginal land. But what is marginal at one time is not necessarily marginal at another, and if present marginal land is cultivated this does not get rid of the margin, but merely pushes it farther away. The development of the United States in the nineteenth century gradually pushed the frontier farther to the west, but the frontier still remained, although its geographical position kept changing.

(2) UTILITY

As used in economics, the term utility may be defined as the amount of satisfaction to be derived from a commodity or service *at a particular time*. The utility of bread is the satisfaction to be obtained from consuming bread at a particular moment of time. There are two points to note. In the first place, the utility of a commodity has nothing to do with its usefulness; it may or may not be useful, though it must yield satisfaction. Nor has utility any ethical connotation. If we want something, whether it is good or bad for us, it possesses utility for us. The ordinary meaning of the word must therefore be put aside. It would perhaps have been better if Wicksteed's term, "significance," had been adopted instead of "utility."

The second point to be emphasised is its applicability to something *at a particular time*. A commodity does not possess a specific amount of utility. To a starving man bread will have great utility, whereas for a man who has just dined well, bread for the moment may possess no utility at all. If the starving man is given a good meal bread will also cease for a time to have utility for him. Utility therefore depends on the individual's own *subjective* estimate of the amount of satisfaction to be obtained from something. Thus there is *no such thing as intrinsic value*, for the same commodity has at the same time different utilities for different people, and even for the same person the utility of a thing is not constant, but differs at different times and in different circumstances.

(3) DIMINISHING MARGINAL UTILITY

The marginal utility of a good will thus be the amount of satisfaction to be obtained from the possession of a little bit more of it, or, alternatively, the loss of satisfaction due to giving up the smallest possible amount of it. Two demands of two different people for a commodity may differ for two reasons: (*i*) they may differ in their estimate of its desirability; (*ii*) they may already possess different quantities of it. Assuming that no change takes place in the strength of an individual's desire for it, its marginal utility to him will vary with the quantity possessed. The student with only one book on his subject has a high marginal utility for such books. When he acquires a second book marginal utility falls, and after acquiring a third, marginal utility falls again. With each additional book he obtains, the marginal utility of such books for him successively declines. Eventually a time will arrive when their marginal utility will be so low that an additional volume will have no utility at all for him. The marginal utility of a commodity therefore declines as one's supply of it increases until satiety is reached. It would be exactly the same with an homogeneous commodity like tea, each unit being identical, for marginal utility depends on the amount possessed. As a hungry man consumes more and more food, the marginal utility of food gradually declines for him. It is therefore the *marginal* utility of a thing, and not its *total* utility, that is important economically, for a person's demand for anything depends on the marginal utility of the commodity to him. Marginal utility can be applied to money, its marginal utility being the satisfaction to be obtained from the expenditure of one more unit of it. The Law of Diminishing Marginal Utility is a general law of life, as it applies to everything.

Since utility is the strength of the satisfaction to be derived from a thing, it cannot be measured. Assume, however, for the moment that the utility of tea for Mrs Gamp can be measured in units of utility:

TABLE XXIII
Marginal Utility

$\frac{1}{4}$ lb of tea	Total utility (units of utility)	Marginal utility (units of utility)
I	60	60
2	102	42
3	132	30
4	156	24
5	176	20
6	191	15
7	201	10
8	208	7

This table shows that for Mrs Gamp the marginal utility of a first $\frac{1}{4}$ lb. of tea stands at "60 units of utility." After purchasing $\frac{1}{4}$ lb. of tea its marginal utility falls to 42, and with each successive $\frac{1}{4}$ lb. purchased the marginal utility of the commodity falls, until for her eighth $\frac{1}{4}$ lb. of tea at 2 lb. its marginal utility has declined to four units of utility. Each additional $\frac{1}{4}$ lb. has less utility than the preceding one, showing that as one's stock increases marginal utility declines. Another method of illustrating the Law of Diminishing Marginal Utility is to consider how much Mrs Gamp would be willing to pay for each successive $\frac{1}{4}$ lb. of tea. For example, for the first $\frac{1}{4}$ lb. she might be willing to pay 5s., for the second 3s. 6d., third 2s. 6d., fourth 2s., fifth 1s. 8d., sixth 1s. 3d., seventh 10d., eighth 7d., ninth 4d.

The concept of diminishing marginal utility was developed about the same time (1871) by William Stanley Jevons in England and by Karl Menger in Austria, each working independently of the other. It is usual to couple with these two names that of Leon Walras, the Swiss economist, although his work was not published until 1874.[1] Jevons, however, used the rather misleading term "final utility" for marginal utility.

(4) THE ORIGIN

In the above example concerning tea the minimum unit taken was $\frac{1}{4}$ lb. Smaller units might have been taken—ounces, or even grains, but a very small amount may be of little use. Clearly, if the quantity possessed is too small to be of effective use it cannot have much utility, and an additional amount may then have greater utility than the first unit. In fact, the Law of Diminishing Marginal Utility begins to operate only after a certain point, called the *Origin*. Until the origin is reached—that is, until the minimum amount of the commodity that can be used effectively has been obtained—successive increments will show increasing utility.

(5) DIMINISHING MARGINAL UTILITY IS THE BASIS OF DEMAND SCHEDULES

In **3** the diminishing marginal utility of tea to a housewife, Mrs Gamp, was considered. She was willing, it will be remembered, to pay 5s. for her first $\frac{1}{4}$ lb., but for a ninth $\frac{1}{4}$ lb. she would only pay 4d. It can be assumed that if she is willing to pay 5s. for one $\frac{1}{4}$ lb. and 3s. 6d. for a second $\frac{1}{4}$ lb., then if the price is 3s. 6d. she will purchase

---

[1] See Sir A. Gray: *The Development of Economic Doctrine*, p. 341 n. The author also shows that Gossen, in a work published in 1854, was the first to propound a marginalist theory.

two ¼ lb. Similarly, if she is prepared to pay 2s. 6d for a third ¼ lb. she will buy three ¼ lb. if the price is 2s. 6d. These facts can be expressed in the form of a table:

TABLE XXIV

Diminishing Marginal Utility

Price	Amount purchased (number of ¼ lb.)
5s.	1
3s. 6d.	2
2s. 6d.	3
2s.	4
1s. 8d.	5
1s. 3d.	6
10d.	7
7d.	8
4d.	9

It is clear that this table is, in fact, Mrs Gamp's demand schedule for tea. If she estimates the marginal utility of tea at 5s. that is the price she is prepared to pay for it; if she considers the marginal utility of tea to be worth only 4d. she will pay no more than that amount. For example, if the price is 2s., and assuming she has no tea in stock, she will purchase (for 2s.) ¼ lb., because she assesses its marginal utility at 5s.; she will purchase a second ¼ lb. because she now assesses the marginal utility of tea at 3s. 6d., and a third ¼ lb. because she assesses its marginal utility at 2s. 6d., and a fourth because the price she pays (2s.) is still equal to what she considers its marginal utility to be worth. If the price is 2s. she will not, however, increase her purchase of tea beyond four ¼ lb., because the marginal utility of a fifth ¼ lb. is less than the price of tea. No rational person will pay a price higher than his estimate of the money value of the marginal utility of the commodity.

(6) CONSUMER'S SURPLUS

Consider once more Mrs Gamp's purchase of four ¼ lb. of tea at 2s. per ¼ lb. She was willing to pay 5s. for the first ¼ lb., whereas in fact she paid only 2s. for it. Similarly, she was willing to pay 3s. 6d. for the second ¼ lb., but actually paid only 2s. Again she obtained the third ¼ lb. for 2s., and would have been willing to pay 2s. 6d. Her actual expenditure on tea was 8s., but she obtained four ¼ lb. of tea which she considered to be worth 5s., 3s. 6d., 2s. 6d. and 2s. respectively—a total of 13s. Therefore she obtained 13s. worth of satisfaction for 8s.—a surplus of 5s. This is known as Consumer's Surplus.

Let us assume that a new book is published at 21s. Those people who consider that the amount of satisfaction they will derive from it not to be worth this price will obviously not buy it. Of those who buy a copy some would have been willing to pay more than 21s. Thus a person who would have been prepared to pay 30s. for the book can be considered to have obtained a consumer's surplus of 9s worth of satisfaction.

(7) EQUILIBRIUM DISTRIBUTION OF EXPENDITURE

In Chapter I it was seen that all things are relatively scarce, and that more of one thing can be enjoyed only by having less of another. A choice has therefore to be made, and this implies that each individual has a scale of preferences, a sort of list of his wants arranged in the order in which they press upon him. Though utility is not measurable, wants can, however, be arranged in order of preference. We can say that we prefer one thing to another, though we cannot calculate exactly the extent of this preference. It is clear now that the order in which commodities and services are arranged on such a scale is determined by their *marginal* utilities, and not by their *total* utilities. Bread and water, being necessaries of life, have a high total utility, and yet may occupy low positions on a person's scale of preferences because their marginal utility is low. For a consumer has not to decide between (say) bread and water, on the one hand, and (say) cake and milk, on the other, but instead his choice lies between a little more bread and a little less cake, or a little less bread and a little more cake.

Assume that a housewife goes to the market to purchase three commodities, A, B and C, and obtains the following quantities of each:

A	B	C
10 units	7 units	4 units

To maximise her total satisfaction she must buy so much of each commodity that its price in each case is exactly equal to her estimate of the money-value of its marginal utility. This must be so, because she has decided that the tenth unit of A stands higher on her scale of preferences than an eighth unit of B or a fifth unit of C; that a seventh unit of B is to be preferred to an eleventh unit of A or a fifth unit of C; that a fourth unit of C is preferable to an eleventh unit of A or an eighth unit of B. If the marginal utilities of these three commodities were not equal she could increase her total satisfaction by buying more of one and less of another. When deciding how much of each to buy it was their respective marginal utilities in relation to their prices that she considered —whether she should buy a little more of A and a little less of B or C, or a little more of B and a little less of A or C, etc. If she has no motive for changing the quantities that she has bought of these three commodities she will have achieved an equilibrium distribution of her expenditure. Perfect equilibrium can, however, be obtained only if all three commodities are capable of being divided into the smallest possible units.

Where there are many competing demands for a commodity, the more urgent will be fulfilled first. An increase in supply and a lower price not only allow more of the commodity to be used for existing purposes but also enable new uses for it to be developed. If electricity is dear its use may be restricted to lighting; if it becomes cheaper its use may be extended to cooking; if it becomes cheaper still it may come to be used for all kinds of other appliances—radiators, vacuum cleaners, washing machines, etc.

(8) SOME CRITICISMS OF THE LAW OF DIMINISHING MARGINAL UTILITY

The following are some of the main criticisms that have been levelled against the concept of diminishing marginal utility:

(i) *"The more one has the more one wants."* There are some things the marginal utility of which increases as one's supply increases. (This is, of course, quite apart from the fact that marginal utility in all cases increases until the origin is reached.) Supporters of the theory of diminishing marginal utility say that such cases are rare, but their opponents believe that they are common enough to make diminishing marginal utility far from being a general law. Instead of becoming satiated as more of something is enjoyed, the desire for more grows, so that the more one has of some things the more of them one wants. This may often be true of money, its accumulation merely increasing the desire to accumulate more. It is also true of anything for which a taste has to be cultivated, whether it be for fine wines or fine art, travel or sport. If acquisition stimulates the collecting instinct marginal utility increases even more strongly, whether the objects collected be postage stamps, gramophone records or pictures. Strictly, however, as a taste for something is being developed, a change of taste is taking place, and this creates a new condition of demand. In other words, the person who at one time did not care for Beethoven is not really the same person (economically, at least) as the one who has later developed a taste for Beethoven's music.

(ii) *Habit and impulse.* Much expenditure tends to become habitual, for people do not trouble to weigh carefully the marginal utilities of all the things that they buy, especially where the purchase of cheap, trivial articles is concerned. Few people, too, at some time or another have failed to resist an impulse to buy something which at a more rational moment they would have refused. Economists, however, assume that consumers always behave rationally.

(iii) *Large indivisible commodities.* The Law of Diminishing Marginal Utility assumes that all goods can be divided into small units, so that one's supply can be increased or reduced by the tiniest amount, whereas many durable goods are large and indivisible, as for example houses, furniture, motor cars. There are, however, many people who buy such things on hire purchase and so pay by instalments. In a sense, therefore, if payment for a piano is spread over (say) one hundred weeks each weekly instalment represents the purchase of one-hundredth of a piano.[1]

II. VALUE

(9) THE PROBLEM OF VALUE

At one time writers on economics devoted a great deal of attention to the question of value. Why, they asked, should the price of one thing be 5s. and that of another only 2s. 6d.? We have already seen that price depends on the interaction of the forces of supply and demand. The early economists, however, generally ignored the influence of demand and related price solely to cost of production. In the short period, once an article is offered for sale in the market its cost of production has no direct bearing on its price. Whatever it may have cost to produce, no consumer will be willing to buy it unless its marginal utility to him coincides with its price. If a speculative builder has erected a house at a cost of £3,000 he will not be able to sell it for that sum unless he can find someone whose marginal utility for such houses is £3,000. How much he sells the house for will, of course, determine his future building activity. If he finds he can sell it for £3,400 he may immediately set about building another similar house, but if he can sell it for no more than £2,600 he will cease building such houses. Costs of production, therefore, affect price indirectly through supply—high cost curtailing supply, and low cost tending to expand supply. In the short period, however, value depends entirely on marginal utility, which is the basis of demand.

(10) EARLY THEORIES OF VALUE

It will be useful to glance briefly at some of the early theories of value. They are essentially similar, and are merely different forms of the Labour Theory of Value. To Adam Smith there were two kinds of value, which he named "value in use" (this depending on the utility of the commodity), and "value in exchange" (determining the price at

[1] See P. Wicksteed: *Common-sense of Political Economy*, Book I, Chapter III.

which it could be sold). This distinction appeared to him to be necessary in order to explain the so-called "paradox of value," which greatly troubled early writers on economics. Water had great value in use, but generally a low exchange value, whereas diamonds had much less value in use, but had a high exchange value. It is clear, after considering marginal utility, that this paradox arose because these writers did not distinguish between *total* and *marginal* utility. In countries such as Great Britain, where water is plentiful and can be used for purposes low on the scale of preferences, the total utility of water is great, though its marginal utility is often low. In the case of diamonds the supply is relatively small, and so marginal utility tends to be high, though the total utility of diamonds is small. After noting this paradox, Adam Smith explained value in terms of "value in use." Therefore, the value of a thing depended on the amount of labour expended upon its production, for he said that it was "natural" that an article the making of which required two days' labour should have double the value of another article that was the result of only one day's labour. "Labour is the real measure of the exchange value of all commodities," he said.

Ricardo also recognised two forms of value, and agreed with his predecessor that the value of most things depended on the amount of labour required to produce them, but that there was another group of things, such as works of art and other rare articles, the exchange value of which depended on their scarcity. The supply of goods in the first category, he thought, could be increased "almost without any assignable limit," whereas the supply of goods in the second category could not be increased. It is not surprising that the Labour Theory of Value was eagerly seized upon by writers seeking support for preconceived political views. Karl Marx and his followers reiterated the view that the value of a commodity depended on the amount of labour required for its production, in order to be able to assert that the worker was entitled to the entire fruit of his labour. According to Marx, a thing can have value only if it is a product of human labour.

The Cost of Production Theory of Value as enunciated by J. S. Mill is really a refinement of the Labour Theory of Value. According to this theory, the value of any commodity is determined by its cost of production, including, of course, labour costs, but also including the profit of the entrepreneur.

(11) SOME CRITICISMS OF THE EARLY THEORIES OF VALUE

The following are some of the main criticisms of the early theories of value:

(i) *The difficulty of measuring labour or cost of production.* How is the amount of labour required in the production of a commodity to be measured? Adam Smith used time as his measuring rod, but workmen are not all of equal efficiency, and the less skilled may take longer than the skilled over a particular piece of work, and so put more labour into it. Labour, too, may be misdirected, and an article incapable of fulfilling the purpose for which it was intended can have no value, however much labour has gone to its manufacture, for even Marx admits that "nothing can have value without being an object of utility." Marx was aware of both these objections to the labour theory, and so he defined the amount of labour required as "socially necessary labour," for, he said, "mis-directed labour does not count as labour."

The term "cost of production" is no more precise than "quantity of labour." It is ambiguous, for the cost of producing a commodity depends on a number of factors, differing between one firm and another, and in any case can be considered only in relation to output.

(ii) *The early theories are not of universal application.* Apart from the special category of scarce goods mentioned by Ricardo, these early theories all fail to explain the value of rare things, such as works of art or antiques. It is a serious weakness of any theory of value if it does not explain the value of all things. The Law of Diminishing Marginal Utility, however, can be applied equally well to rare things as to articles in common use, for all goods are scarce relative to the demand for them, whether they are rare or not.

(iii) *The influence of demand is neglected.* The principal reason for the weakness of the early theories of value is that they ignore the influence of demand, while at the same time they explain very inadequately the influence of supply, the scarcity aspect of it being insufficiently stressed. Labour itself is limited in supply, and that explains to some extent why goods are scarce.

III. INDIFFERENCE CURVES

(12) THE MARGINAL RATE OF SUBSTITUTION

The problem of what determines value is still far from settled, and unlike J. S. Mill, who thought nothing further was to be said on the subject, there are some economists who doubt whether the problem ever will be settled. At one time the adherents of the Marginal Utility Theory believed that they had found the solution, but diminishing marginal utility is no longer generally accepted as an explanation of demand. More recently it has given way to the concept of the *marginal rate of substitution* and analysis by means of indifference curves.

Because all goods are relatively scarce, everyone has to make a choice between alternatives; therefore it can be assumed that everyone has a scale of preferences. This, it has been seen, is really a scale of marginal utilities. A little more of one thing is preferred to a little more of another. As Marshall said more than half a century ago: "The term, value, is relative and expresses the relation between two things at a particular place and time." Thus, the value of a thing can be regarded as the relation between preferences, for the value of one thing can be measured only in terms of another.

The valuation of one commodity in terms of another (one of which may be money) is known as the Marginal Rate of Substitution. Just so much of a commodity will be purchased in the market as will equate the Marginal Rate of Substitution of that commodity with the price that has to be paid for it.

Changes in price produce two effects:

(i) *A substitution effect.* If there are two commodities that are fairly close substitutes for one another, and there is a fall in the price of one of them, the one that has fallen in price will tend to be substituted for the other.

(ii) *An income effect.* A fall in the price of a commodity means that it is possible to buy the same quantity as before for a smaller outlay, and this may lead either to the purchase of more of that particular commodity or a quantity of some other commodity. This is similar, therefore, in its effect to an increase in the consumer's income.

(13) THE CONSTRUCTION OF INDIFFERENCE CURVES

Suppose that there are only two commodities available to the consumer—(say) x and y. If two commodities are considered these can be represented on a two-dimensional diagram. The Scales of Preference of individuals will differ. However, a consumer, Quilp, having the combination $9x + 14y$, may be willing to give up without any loss of satisfaction one x for two more of y, and the following table shows other combinations assumed to yield him equal satisfaction:

$23x + 7y$	$9x + 14y$
$20x + 8y$	$8x + 16y$
$17x + 9y$	$7x + 18y$
$15x + 10y$	$6x + 21y$
$13x + 11y$	$5x + 24y$
$11x + 12y$	$4x + 27y$
$10x + 13y$	$3x + 31y$

It will be noticed that as Quilp's supply of either commodity declines, its marginal utility increases, and so he is prepared to give up further units of it only in exchange for more of the other commodity. Thus, when he possesses $20x + 8y$ he will give up a unit of y only for $3x$, but when he has $6x + 21y$ he is prepared to exchange $3y$ for an extra unit of x. Quilp is indifferent between any of these combinations. If graphed they will form an indifference Curve, AA, any point on which shows a combination of x and y equally agreeable to him (Fig. 43).

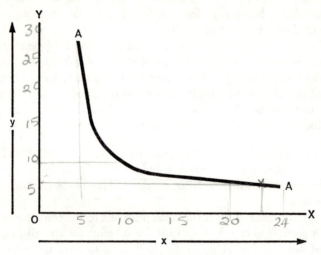

FIG. 43.—AN INDIFFERENCE CURVE.

Clearly, Quilp will prefer the combination $10x + 15y$ to any of those given in the above table, because this is obviously better than $9x + 14y$. Thus a second table of indifference can now be compiled showing all combinations of x and y that Quilp considers to yield him equal satisfaction to $10x + 15y$. This might run as follows:

$24x + 8y$	$10x + 15y$
$21x + 9y$	$9x + 17y$
$18x + 10y$	$8x + 19y$
$16x + 11y$	$7x + 22y$
$14x + 12y$	$6x + 25y$
$12x + 13y$	$5x + 28y$
$11x + 14y$	$4x + 32y$

A second indifference curve, BB, can now be constructed, and since any point in the curve BB is superior to any point on the curve AA, the second curve will fall slightly to the right of the first (Fig. 44).

In similar fashion further indifference curves can be added until a whole series of indifference curves has been drawn (Fig. 45).

Quilp will always prefer a position on a curve farther from O than a curve nearer to O, because the farther a curve is from O, the greater will be the satisfaction he will obtain. Since, however, he has only a limited amount of money to spend, this will limit his choice and prevent his selecting a curve very far to the right of O. Assume that if he spent the

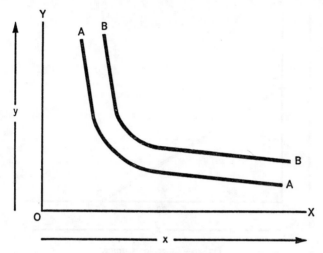

FIG. 44.—INDIFFERENCE CURVES.

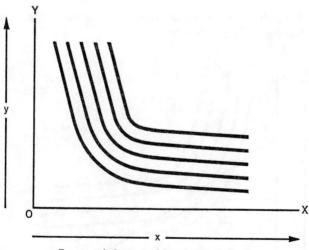

FIG. 45.—A SERIES OF INDIFFERENCE CURVES.

whole of his money on x this would give him 30x, or if he spent it entirely on y it would give him 20y, then because of his limited resources his actual choice must lie somewhere along the line *RS* that connects these two extreme choices:

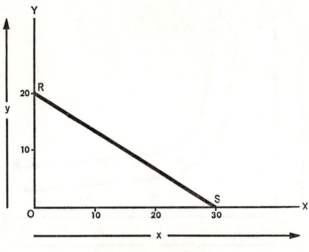

FIG. 46.—LIMITS OF CHOICE.

If Quilp's indifference curves are now superimposed on this diagram the following will be the result:

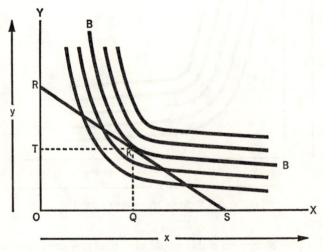

FIG. 47.—CHOICE AND MAXIMUM SATISFACTION.

Quilp's choice must be at some point on the line RS, and to obtain the maximum satisfaction, his choice must also be on the indifference curve farthest from O, and this must be the curve BB, which just touches RS at K—that is, the curve to which RS is a tangent. Quilp's actual combination of x and y will therefore be the quantity OT of y, together with the quantity OQ of x. If Quilp's demand changes as a result of his receiving an increase in income, or for some other reason, this will move the line RS farther away from O, and so enable him to move to a higher indifference curve. If the price of y rose, this would bring R nearer to O, reduce the slope of RS and bring K down to a lower indifference curve.

Indifference curves are therefore useful to illustrate choice between two alternatives. If choice lies between more than two, then x can be taken to represent one, and y the combined amount of the others. In favour of indifference curves it is claimed that they merely imply that the consumer is capable of balancing against one another different possible combinations of two commodities, so that it is no longer necessary to make the unreal assumption that he can measure in terms of money the utility of each additional increment of a commodity. Whether demand is analysed with the aid of the marginal utility concept or by means of indifference curves some assumption of human behaviour, however, is required. The main point is: is it more realistic to assume that the individual values a commodity in terms of a little bit more or a little bit less of it, or does he compare the satisfaction to be derived from different combinations of two commodities?

(14) SOME APPLICATIONS OF INDIFFERENCE CURVES

It will be useful to give a few simple illustrations of the application of indifference curves.

(i) *To show the effect of a rise in price* (Fig. 48). The amount of money possessed is OM. If this is entirely spent on the commodity before the rise in price takes place the quantity OQ can be bought. After the rise in price only the quantity OQ^1 can be bought.

Before the rise in price, the maximum satisfaction was obtained by purchasing OQ^2 of the commodity and retaining OM^1 of money, because this was the combination of the commodity and money indicated by the point on MQ at which the indifference curve I^1 was a tangent.

After the rise in price, maximum satisfaction is obtained by purchasing the quantity OQ^3 and retaining OM^2 of money. This combination is on indifference curve I^2, which is nearer the origin, O, than

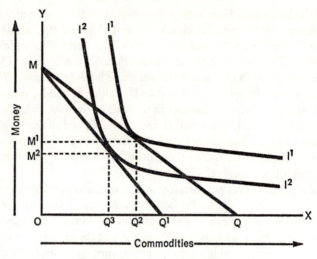

FIG. 48.—EFFECT OF A RISE IN PRICE.

the indifference curve I^1, showing that total satisfaction has been reduced.

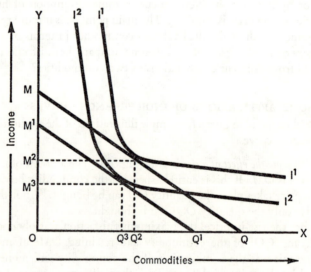

FIG. 49.—EFFECT OF A FALL IN INCOME.

(ii) *To show the effect of a fall in income.* The income at first is *OM*, and if this is completely spent, the quantity *OQ* of commodities could be bought. Maximum satisfaction is obtained when *OM²* of income is retained after purchasing OQ^2 of commodities, for this combination is on the consumer's highest indifference curve.

Income falls to OM^1, and total purchases cannot now exceed OQ^1. As a result, the highest indifference curve available to this consumer is now I^2. The curve I^2 is lower than the curve I^1, and so the consumer has suffered, as one would expect, a loss of satisfaction.

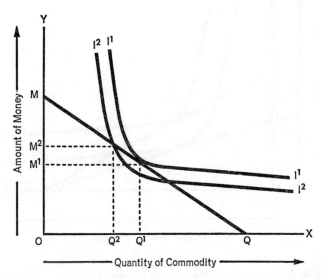

FIG. 50.—THE EFFECT OF RATIONING.

(iii) *To show the effect of rationing on consumer's satisfaction.* Before rationing was introduced, this consumer purchased OQ^1 of the commodity and retained OM^1 of his money. (If he had spent the whole of his money he would have been able to purchase the quantity OQ.)

As a result of rationing he can buy only the quantity OQ^2, but this leaves him with a larger amount of money unspent—namely, OM^2. This combination of money and the commodity is on a lower indifference curve (I^2 instead of I^1) and so, although he has more money to spend on other things, his total satisfaction is less than before. The closer the rationed quantity OQ^2 is to the previous quantity bought, OQ^1, the nearer the new indifference curve to the old, and the less the loss of satisfaction.

(iv) *To show the effect of inflation.* Assume that the prices of goods and services increase proportionately to income, so that if the entire income is spent, the same quantity of goods, etc., as before can be bought. Will, then, the satisfaction of the consumer also remain unchanged?

The consumer's income increases from OM^1 to OM^2, but this will still buy only the same quantity, OQ, of goods as before. If he purchases the same quantity of goods as before he will have more money left unspent than he had previously, although its value in terms of what it will

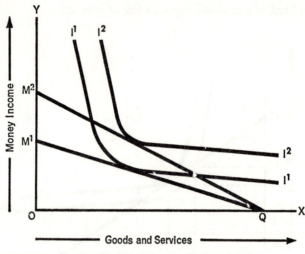

FIG. 51.—THE EFFECT OF INFLATION.

buy is the same. Nevertheless, this consumer is now on a higher indifference curve, and therefore appears to derive more satisfaction from the inflationary position than the earlier one. If he had spent his entire income his satisfaction would have remained unchanged, for the quantity of goods, etc., he purchased would also have remained exactly the same. However, he has more money left unspent, though this is of only the same real value as the smaller amount left unspent before, but evidently, according to the diagram, it yields him more satisfaction. Experience during the past twenty-five years of the falling value of money seems to indicate that it is probably true that many—perhaps most—people prefer to have a large money income rather than a smaller money income, even if real income in terms of the goods it will buy is the same in both cases.

It is necessary, however, to warn the reader that some economists object to money being employed as one of the two choices which indifference curves may be used to illustrate on the ground that, unlike other things, money is not wanted for its own sake but only as a medium of exchange.

RECOMMENDATIONS FOR FURTHER READING

A. Marshall: *Principles of Economics*, Book III, Chapter 6.
P. Wicksteed: *Common-sense of Political Economy*, Book I, Chapters 1–3.

For Indifference Curves:

K. E. Boulding: *Economic Analysis*, Chapters 33, 34.

QUESTIONS

1. Define and indicate clearly the relationship between *total utility, marginal utility* and *value*. (R.S.A. Inter.)

2. Explain the meaning of utility, and show what is meant by (*a*) total utility, (*b*) marginal utility. Give examples. (C.C.S. Inter.)

3. What relation has the amount of labour expended in the production of a commodity to the selling price of that commodity? (A.I.A.)

4. What is meant by consumer's surplus? (A.C.C.A. Inter.)

5. Explain and discuss the statement that the price actually paid for a commodity is a money measure of the marginal utility of that commodity. (I.B.)

6. "Where we talked of 'marginal utility,' we now talk of 'marginal preference'; and where we drew curves of 'marginal utility,' we now draw 'indifference curves.'" Explain with diagrams. (C.I.S. Final.)

7. Explain what is meant by consumer's surplus. What are the effects of (*a*) indirect taxes, and (*b*) rationing, on consumer's surplus? (I.M.T.A.)

8. Normally, more of a good will be demanded at a lower than at a higher price. Outline and comment on any theory which helps to explain why this is so. (G.C.E. Adv.)

9. What factors determine the demand for washing machines? (G.C.E. Adv.)

10. Taking an illustration from any part of the subject-matter of Economics, explain the importance of the margin in economic analysis. (C.C.S. Final.)

11. How does rationing of consumer goods affect the satisfaction that the consumer can obtain in the expenditure of his income? (Final Degree.)

12. In what ways has the use of indifference curves aided economic analysis? (Final Degree.)

CHAPTER XIII

THE BASIS OF SUPPLY:
(1) UNDER PERFECT COMPETITION

I. MEANING OF PERFECT COMPETITION

(1) THE APPLICATION OF THE MARGIN TO SUPPLY

In the previous chapter the concept of the margin was used to explain the basis of demand curves; in this and the next two chapters the marginal analysis will be used to explain the derivation of supply curves. It was shown that the demand for a good depends on the *marginal* utility—not on the *total* utility of the commodity. It is similar with the supply curve, which shows how much of a commodity will be put on the market over a range of prices. The amount of any commodity that will be produced at a given price will depend on its cost of production, but just as demand did not depend on total utility, so with supply it is marginal cost, and not total cost, that is the main determinant of how much will be supplied.

(2) PERFECT COMPETITION

Demand for most commodities comes from a large number of potential buyers, who act quite independently of one another, rarely making any concentrated effort to influence price by withholding their demand. Even when attempts have been made to persuade consumers to act together, they have rarely had much success, for it is difficult to get buyers to combine even for a limited period. In studying demand there is therefore no need to assume that there are many buyers, for such conditions are the normal experience of real life.

In the case of supply, however, for some commodities there are many producers, for others only a few. Thus the derivation of supply curves has to be considered under the influence of different environments, of which three may be recognised—perfect competition, imperfect competition and monopoly. The first and third of these—perfect competition and monopoly—exist only in the minds of economists, but it is necessary to consider supply under these unreal conditions before attempting a more realistic interpretation. First, the basis of supply will be explained in an environment of perfect competition; later supply under other conditions will be considered.

The assumptions of the perfect market were discussed in IX, 2. Though the existence of a perfect market does not necessarily ensure perfect competition, the two terms are on the whole very similar in meaning. Perfect competition relates more especially to the environment in which the production of a particular commodity is carried on. For a perfect market there must be a large number of buyers and sellers, and the commodity in which dealings take place must be homogeneous. Similarly, the primary assumptions of perfect competition are that there should be a large number of firms, each producing only a small fraction of the total output, so that no firm can influence the price of the commodity in the market by increasing or decreasing its output. Such firms must take the price of the commodity as fixed. At this price an individual firm can sell any quantity it pleases; to increase its sales it has no need to cut its price, for however great its own output, it still remains only a tiny fraction of the total output for the industry, and therefore it makes no material difference to the total supply of that commodity. In other words, the demand for the product of a *single* firm is perfectly elastic. Since, further, the commodity is homogeneous, there is no reason to prefer the product of one firm to that of another, and so, though a firm can sell any amount at the market price, its sales would be zero at any price above this. Under perfect competition, too, there is no restriction on the entry of new firms into an industry.

A certain ambiguity exists regarding the meaning of the term perfect competition. In addition to the assumptions just given, should one also assume perfect mobility of factors, their complete divisibility and an absence of all kinds of economic friction? If this were so, a change in demand from one commodity to another would immediately cause resources to be transferred from one form of production to the other, price moving to the new equilibrium without there being any intermediate effects. This difficulty would have been resolved if the suggestion made by an economist[1] many years ago had been followed. He suggested that the term be restricted to complete perfection in all respects, and the name "pure competition" be given to the less perfect conditions. Since this suggestion has not been generally followed, we are compelled to use the term perfect competition for a competitive state that is much less than completely perfect, and thus it is all the more necessary to make quite clear the assumptions on which it is based.

[1] E. H. Chamberlin: *The Theory of Monopolistic Competition* (1933).

II. COSTS

(3) COSTS OF PRODUCTION

The term "cost of production" also is ambiguous, for cost of production has meaning only when it is related to output. No answer can be given to the question: what is the cost of production of a fountain pen? for there is no such thing as *the* cost of production of any commodity. If only one pen is to be produced its cost of production will be very high: if 100 pens per week are to be produced it is fairly certain that the cost of production per pen will be much lower. If output is raised to 1,000 pens per week the cost of production per pen may be higher, lower or the same, depending on whether, between these two outputs, cost is increasing, decreasing or constant.

The word "cost" is ambiguous also because it has a variety of meanings; there are fixed and variable costs, prime and supplementary costs, average cost and marginal cost. It is best, therefore, to avoid the use of either the word "cost" or the phrase "cost of production," unless it is clearly stated what output is being considered.

(4) FIXED AND VARIABLE COSTS

Some costs vary with output, whereas others are said to be fixed because—at least over a fairly considerable range of output—they do not vary in this way. For example, once a firm has provided itself with a factory and installed the necessary machinery, these costs remain the same whether the firm is working at full or only half capacity. The same amount in rent and rates will have to be paid in either case. The number of clerks employed in the office does not vary with every change of output, and so the cost of administration is looked upon as a fixed cost in the short period. If, however, the firm is engaged in spinning wool the amount of raw material required will be directly related to output. If the machinery is driven by steam power less coal will be required if the firm is working below capacity. Whether the employees are on piece rates or paid by the hour, the wage bill will increase the larger the output. Rents, rates, interest on loans and any allowance for depreciation of machinery (machinery may depreciate even faster if idle) and administrative expenses are *fixed* costs; wages of labour, cost of power and raw materials are *variable* costs.

If, however, a firm is compelled by a falling off in the demand for its product to work short time for a lengthy period it is probable that administrative expenses also will have to be reduced. So another classification of cost groups the cost of administration with the variable costs, and calls these *prime* costs. The other fixed costs are then termed *supplementary* costs. The following diagram will help to make this clear.

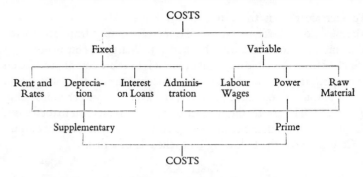

The importance of making a distinction between prime and supplementary costs is that in the short period a firm will generally continue in production if it covers only its prime costs. If it closes down temporarily it will still have to meet its supplementary costs, so it will suffer no greater loss by continuing in production if its revenue from the sale of its products covers only its prime costs. The loss of goodwill, and the difficulty of restarting production, consequent on the loss of its labour force and the depreciation of idle assets, all weigh against ceasing production if it is thought that a recession of trade is likely to be of short duration. In the long period, obviously, a firm must cover all its costs, supplementary as well as prime. Indeed, the distinction between fixed and variable costs is largely a short-period distinction. The so-called variable costs are merely those that are variable in the short period; administrative costs become variable in the medium period; and even the supplementary costs become variable in the long period; for when machinery wears out it need not necessarily be replaced and premises can be converted to other uses.

(5) AVERAGE AND MARGINAL COST

Marginal cost is the addition to total cost that results from increasing total output by one more unit. Average cost is the average cost of producing each unit of output. Consider the following example:

TABLE XXV
The Cost Schedule of a Firm (1)

Output	Fixed cost	Variable cost	Total cost	Average cost	Marginal cost
Units	£	£	£	£ s. d.	£
100	100	700	800	8 0 0	—
101	100	706	806	7 19 7	6
102	100	709	809	7 18 7	3
103	100	710	810	7 17 3	1

To increase output from 100 to 101 units adds £6 to total cost. Marginal cost, therefore, is £6. To increase output from 101 to 102 units increases total cost by a further £3. Marginal cost is now £3 It is clear from this table how important it is to relate cost of production to output. If only 100 units are manufactured their total cost is £800. At an output of 103 units, however, the average cost per unit is only £7 17s. 3d. The greater the proportion that fixed costs bear to total costs, the greater is the difference in average costs at different levels of output.

Consider now the following cost schedule of a firm:

TABLE XXVI
The Cost Schedule of a Firm (2)

Output	Total cost	Average cost	Marginal cost
Units	£	£	£
20	270	13·5	—
30	320	10·7	5
40	400	10·0	8
50	500	10·0	10
60	630	10·5	13
70	790	11·3	16

The table shows that if average cost is falling, marginal cost will be less than average cost; if, however, average cost is rising, then marginal

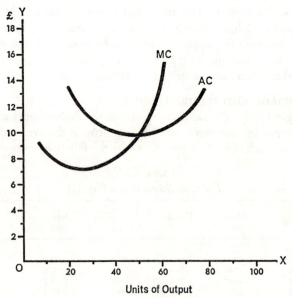

FIG. 52.—AVERAGE COST (AC) AND MARGINAL COST (MC).

cost will be greater than average cost. It also shows average cost and
marginal cost are equal when average cost is at a minimum. When,
therefore, average cost and marginal cost are represented graphically
the marginal cost curve should cut the average cost curve at the lowest
point on the average cost curve (*see* Fig. 52).

III. OUTPUT

(6) NORMAL PROFIT AND THE SIZE OF AN INDUSTRY

In economics cost is taken to include *normal profit*. By normal
profit is meant the payment necessary to keep an entrepreneur in a
particular line of production. Normal profit will vary between one
industry and another, being greater where uncertainty is greater. If a
firm persistently earns less than what is considered to be normal profit
for the industry the entrepreneur will leave that industry and seek
more profitable employment for its resources elsewhere. The *marginal
firm* will thus be the one just capable of earning normal profit. If profits
in the industry fall, the marginal firms will be the first to leave, and a
new margin, again comprising firms just earning normal profit, will be
created. If profits rise, all firms will earn more than normal profit, and
so new firms, whose costs previously were too high, will be drawn into
the industry. Thus, an industry expands or contracts according to
whether the firms comprising it earn more or less than normal profit.
Profit above normal is sometimes called *surplus profit* or *net revenue*. If
normal profit is reckoned as part of cost the marginal firm's profit—
that is, surplus profit or net revenue—will be zero.

(7) THE MOST PROFITABLE OUTPUT

It is an assumption of economics that all people, both consumers and
producers, at all times behave rationally. Thus it is assumed that the
aim of each entrepreneur is to try to maximise his profits, although
in actual conditions this is not always true, for it may necessitate an
expansion of his business that, for any one of several reasons, the entrepreneur may be unwilling to undertake. It is, however, essential to
make this assumption if a satisfactory theory of the firm is to be built up.

Profit will be at a maximum at an output where marginal cost is
equal to marginal revenue. By marginal revenue is meant the additional revenue accruing to a firm as a result of selling one more unit of its
output. Since to a firm working under conditions of perfect competition the price of its products is fixed, marginal revenue must be equal
to the price of one unit of the commodity, since the increase in revenue

from the sale of an extra unit is the price of that unit. Profit must therefore be at a maximum when marginal cost equals marginal revenue. So long as marginal revenue is greater than marginal cost, it will be to a firm's advantage to go on increasing its output, for in such circumstances each addition to its output will add to its profit. But if output is pushed beyond this point the addition to cost will be greater than the addition to revenue, and so total profit will be less. Marginal cost must therefore equal marginal revenue, and this is true of all forms of competition—perfect or imperfect.

It has already been shown that in perfect competition marginal revenue is equal to price; thus marginal cost also must be equal to price. It has been seen above that for the marginal firm average revenue is equal to average cost (since there is no profit other than normal profit), and since average revenue is the same thing as price, then in the case of the marginal firm operating under conditions of perfect competition the following conditions are fulfilled:

Marginal revenue = Marginal cost;
Marginal cost = Price;
Price = Average revenue = Average cost.

Therefore:

Price = Marginal cost = Marginal revenue = Average revenue = Average cost.

The main point to emphasise is that in perfect competition price is equal to marginal cost. This can be clearly seen from the following table:

TABLE XXVII

The Marginal Firm under Perfect Competition

Output	Average cost	Total cost	Marginal cost	Average revenue (price)	Total revenue	Marginal revenue	Surplus profit
Units	£	£	£	£	£	£	£
50	12	600	—	10	500	10	− 100
60	11	660	6	10	600	10	− 60
70	10·4	730	7	10	700	10	− 30
80	10·1	810	8	10	800	10	− 10
90	10	900	9	10	900	10	—
100	10	1,000	10	10	1,000	10	—
110	10·1	1,110	11	10	1,100	10	− 10
120	10·2	1,230	12	10	1,200	10	− 30

At an output of 100 units of the commodity marginal cost is £10, marginal revenue is £10, average revenue (price) is £10, and average cost is £10. Output will not be pushed beyond this point because surplus profit will be negative at any higher output—that is, there will be less than normal profit.

Under perfect competition firms always operate at an output where marginal cost is always rising (as in Tables XXVII and XXVIII), since under perfect competition no firm will restrict its output, and diminishing returns will set in sooner or later. Tables similar to the above can easily be constructed to show that if price is £6 the most profitable output will be sixty; if price is £8 the most profitable output will be eighty; and if price is raised to £12, then output will be increased to 120 units.

(8) HIGH-COST AND LOW-COST FIRMS

In any industry some firms are more efficient than others, and therefore make higher profits. This is not necessarily due to some firms being more efficiently managed than others; it may be due to the advantages of situation or some other influence outside the control of the entrepreneur. Whether a firm is a high-cost or a low-cost firm depends on the quality of the factors of production it employs, and the entrepreneur is only one of these factors. Nevertheless, the standard of efficiency of the management is of paramount importance, and the efficiency of the other factors may in no small measure be dependent on it, as for example the quality of its capital—whether it is up-to-date or old-fashioned. The firm's location may have been deliberately selected on account of its suitability for its particular line of production. In an area where an industry has been long established the local labour may be superior to that in other districts.

Consider now the cost schedule of a low-cost firm working under perfect competition:

TABLE XXVIII

Perfect Competition: a Low-cost Firm

Output	Average cost	Total cost	Marginal cost	Average revenue (price)	Total revenue	Marginal revenue	Surplus profit
Units	£	£	£	£	£	£	£
80	7·3	590	—	10	800	—	210
90	7·5	675	8·5	10	900	10	225
100	7·6	765	9·0	10	1,000	10	235
110	7·8	860	9·5	10	1,100	10	240
120	8·0	960	10·0	10	1,200	10	240
130	8·2	1,065	10·5	10	1,300	10	235
140	8·4	1,175	11·0	10	1,400	10	225

Again, it will not pay the firm to expand its output beyond 120 units, because that is the point where marginal cost is equal to marginal revenue, and this is clearly its most profitable output. The low-cost firm differs from the marginal firm in that total revenue exceeds total cost, so that surplus profit, additional to normal profit, is earned over a range of output.

It is sufficient for a firm to earn normal profit for it to continue in production, since surplus profit is really a type of economic rent, being a payment to factors over and above what is necessary to keep them in their present employment.

(9) THE FIRM AND INDUSTRY IN EQUILIBRIUM

(i) *Equilibrium of the firm.* Under perfect competition a firm will be in equilibrium when it is of no advantage to it to increase or decrease its output, or to change its method of production by altering the proportion in which its factors of production are combined. Its average cost will be at a minimum, for marginal cost is equal to average cost at minimum average cost (*see* 5). In such circumstances any change in output will result in a smaller total profit.

(ii) *Equilibrium of an industry.* Under perfect competition an industry will be in equilibrium when there is no tendency for the size of the industry to change—that is, when no firms wish to leave it and no new firms are being attracted into it. This means that the highest-cost or marginal firm will be making normal profit, neither more nor less, for if its profit were above normal new firms would wish to enter the industry, and if it had been making less than normal profit some firms would wish to leave. If every firm in the industry is making normal profit, and no more, the industry can be said to be in *perfect equilibrium.* Under perfect competition economic forces will generally pull an industry in the direction of this goal. Lack of complete divisibility of factors and differences in their quality may, however, result in the industry having a permanent cost structure of high- and low-cost firms. When its marginal firm is making more than normal profit an industry is said to be in imperfect equilibrium.

(10) THE RESPONSE OF SUPPLY TO CHANGES IN PRICE

A rise in the price of the commodity calls forth a bigger supply, and this is brought about partly by existing firms expanding their output and partly by new firms being attracted into the industry. The entire additional output is not provided by existing firms, because under perfect competition no firm will expand beyond the optimum size. A fall in price produces the reverse effect. It has been seen that some firms have high and others low costs, and that a fall in price drives out the high-cost (that is, marginal) firms, just as a high price makes it possible for new high-cost firms to come in. These high-cost firms found production unprofitable before the rise in price. The ease with which this adjustment of output to price takes place determines the elasticity of supply of a commodity. If expansion or contraction of an industry is easy supply will be elastic; if expansion or contraction is difficult supply will tend to be inelastic.

If marginal cost is rising very sharply—that is, if the marginal cost curve is steep—it will require a considerable rise in price to call forth an increase in supply. The shape of the supply curve therefore depends on the shape of the marginal-cost curve. If one is steep, so also is the other, and hence a steep marginal curve indicates that supply is inclined to be inelastic.

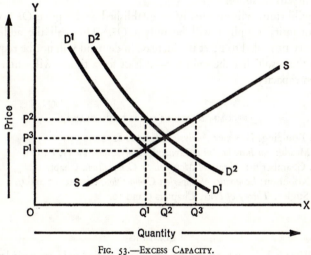

FIG. 53.—EXCESS CAPACITY.

If there are many firms enjoying more than normal profit it shows that the industry is too small. This may arise because special difficulties stand in the way of firms wishing to enter that particular industry, and these hold back newcomers, with the result that the price of the product is high. If there are many firms with less than normal profit it shows that the industry is too large, but that for some reason firms are unable or unwilling to leave it. In this case the price of the product will be low, and the industry may agitate for the fixing of a higher price. To accede to the industry's request, however, will provide no remedy, for it will merely perpetuate its excessive size. The ease or difficulty of contraction of an industry depends largely on its cost structure. If there is considerable difference between the costs of individual firms, with only a few firms at each level—that is, if the "cost ladder" of the industry is steep—contraction of the industry is easy, the few high-cost firms dropping out if there is a fall in price. If, however, there is little difference between the costs of one firm and those of another contraction is difficult and the industry will tend to remain over-large.

Where the response of supply to a fall in price is slow, producers may plan to produce more than the new equilibrium position justifies. For example, the impact effect of an increase in the demand for a commodity may be to raise its price to OP^2 (Fig. 53). At this price producers have an incentive to produce the quantity OQ^3, and so additional factors may be drawn into the industry to enable this quantity to be supplied (Fig. 53).

Equilibrium will eventually be established at the price OP^3, where the quantity supplied will be only OQ^2. Thus, all the additional capacity provided to meet the increase in demand will not be required, with the result that the industry—at least for a time—will suffer from excess capacity.

RECOMMENDATIONS FOR FURTHER READING

K. E. Boulding: *Economic Analysis*, Chapters 22–24.
J. E. Meade: *An Introduction to Economic Analysis and Policy*, Part II.
E. H. Chamberlin: *Theory of Monopolistic Competition*, Chapter 2.
Joan Robinson: *Economics of Imperfect Competition*, Chapters 7 and 9.
G. J. Stigler: *Theory of Price*, Chapters 9 and 10.

QUESTIONS

1. What is the meaning of market price, short-period and long-period normal price? Illustrate by referring to prices today. (R.S.A. Inter.)

2. Distinguish between prime and on-costs. How does this distinction affect the selling policy of a firm? (I.T.)

3. What do you understand by "normal profits"? Explain the relevance of this concept for the determination of the output of an individual firm. (B.S. Inter.)

4. Distinguish between prime and supplementary costs, and explain the importance of the distinction in the fixing of prices under conditions of imperfect competition. (I.T.)

5. "The fact that cost of production varies with output is constantly overlooked. People speak of *the* cost of production of an article as though there were only one cost, irrespective of the *amount* of the article produced. But it is well

known that in some industries (*e.g.* motor) costs fall when a substantial increase in output takes place, while in other industries (*e.g.* wheat farming) costs rise when output is increased." (Cairncross.) Why is this? (A.C.C.A. Inter.)

6. Distinguish between "short period" and "long period" in economic analysis and show the significance of the distinction in the theory of prices. (I.B.)

7. State exactly what you mean by prime and supplementary costs or overhead charges. Show by means of examples the importance of this classification in the fixing of prices. (I.B. Econ.)

8. Discuss the relationship of cost of production to both output and time. (C.I.S. Final.)

9. Bring out clearly the connection between Cost of Production and Price. (C.C.S. Final.)

10. Explain the problems raised in agriculture by the intervals which elapse between the producer's decisions and the consequent effects upon supplies reaching the market. (Final Degree.)

CHAPTER XIV

THE BASIS OF SUPPLY:
(2) UNDER MONOPOLY

I. OUTPUT UNDER MONOPOLY

(1) ABSOLUTE MONOPOLY

For a monopoly to be absolute two conditions must be fulfilled. Firstly, the production of the commodity or service must be in the hands of a single producer. (The monopolist could, of course, be a combine comprising all the producers of the commodity.) Secondly, there must also be no substitute for the commodity.

The second condition would be even more difficult to fulfil than the first, since there are few things for which there is not some sort of substitute. There may be no very close substitute for coffee, but if its price rose considerably the demand for it would be influenced by the existence of other beverages such as tea, cocoa, beer, wine, etc. A person's demand for any commodity is affected by his demand for all other commodities; the mere assumption that everyone has a scale of preferences implies that every purchase involves a choice between alternatives. A monopolist producer of motor cars is free from competition from other producers of motor cars, but he is still subject to competition from producers of other things, not merely other forms of transport but also quite different things, such as, for example, houses. Thus, absolute monopoly does not occur in real life.

Just as monopoly occurs when there is a single producer of a commodity, so monopsony means that there is only one buyer of a commodity or service. For example, there is only one "buyer" of the services of railway engine drivers, the industry now being nationalised.

(2) THE MONOPOLIST AND DEMAND

Even though a monopolist may have complete control over the supply of a commodity, he cannot control demand, though he may sometimes attempt to influence it by means of advertising. He has therefore to take account of the fact that more can be sold at a low than at a high price—that is, his power is limited by consumers' demand. He can increase his sales only by lowering price not only of his additional but of his entire output. Thus the monopolist can, if he wishes, fix his price, and then allow consumer-demand to decide what quantity he shall sell; or he himself can decide what output to produce, but in that case the price at which this output can be sold will depend on consumer-demand. This is what is meant by saying that even a monopolist is subject to the "sovereignty" of the consumer. For example, if DD represents the demand for a commodity the monopolist, if he wishes, can charge the price OP^a, but if he does he will sell only the quantity OQ^a. If he decides on an output of OQ^b, then he can sell this quantity only if he charges the price, OP^b. By reducing his output, therefore, from OQ^b to OQ^a the monopolist would be able to raise the price of the commodity from OP^b to OP^a. He can decide either his output or the price at which he will sell, but not both.

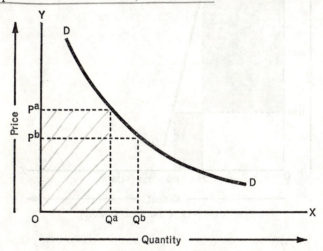

FIG. 54.—DEMAND AND THE MONOPOLIST.

Elasticity of demand and monopoly. Whether a monopolist can increase his revenue by restricting his output depends on the shape of the demand curve—that is, on the elasticity of demand for the commodity. The monopolist will increase his revenue only if a reduction in output brings about a more than proportionate increase in price. Thus the more inelastic the demand for the commodity, the greater is the opportunity to obtain monopoly profit. Consider the following cases, where A, B and C are commodities with different elasticities of demand —the demand for A being fairly inelastic, the elasticity of demand for B being equal to unity and C being in fairly elastic demand. In all cases it is assumed that production is in the hands of monopolists, and that at first the output was 100 units and the price 1s. per unit, so that the total revenue of each was 100s. Suppose now that each producer reduces his output to 75 units. The new price will then depend on the elasticity of demand for each commodity. The price of *A*, for which there is a fairly inelastic demand, will rise to 3*s*.; the price of *B*, for which the elasticity of demand is equal to unity, will rise to 1*s*. 4*d*.; and the price of *C*, for which demand is fairly elastic, will rise only to 1*s*. 2*d*. The following diagrams show the effect of curtailment of output in these three cases:

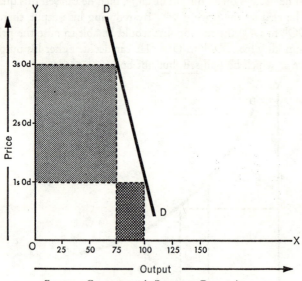

FIG. 55.—COMMODITY A (INELASTIC DEMAND).

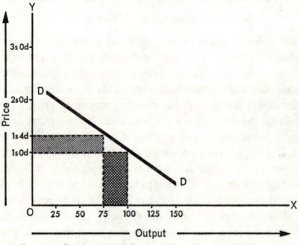

FIG. 56.—COMMODITY B (ELASTICITY OF DEMAND = UNITY).

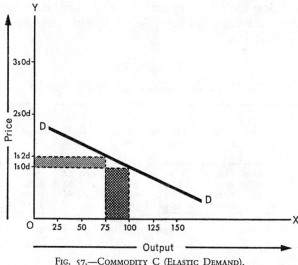

FIG. 57.—COMMODITY C (ELASTIC DEMAND).

It is clear therefore that the effect on total revenue of a reduction of output depends on the elasticity of demand for the commodity. In the case of *A*, where demand is inelastic, total revenue increases from 100*s*. to 225*s*.; for *B*, with unit elasticity of demand, total revenue remains the same; for *C*, where demand is elastic, total revenue falls from 100*s*. to 87*s*. 6*d*. Where demand is elastic the monopolist cannot increase his income by curtailing output, but he may try to increase demand through advertising. Demand, however, is not the sole determinant of monopoly output: the problem of cost also has to be considered.

(3) MONOPOLY OUTPUT

The essential feature of monopoly is that the monopolist can influence the price of the commodity by expanding or contracting supply. The monopolist's aim will be to produce that output which will yield him maximum profit. The monopolist's output is shown in the following tables, giving the cost and revenue schedules of three monopolists, the first working in conditions of increasing marginal cost, the second in conditions of decreasing marginal cost and the third in conditions of constant marginal cost. In perfect competition, it will be remembered, firms always expand their output to a point where marginal cost is increasing (see pp. 224–5).

(i) *Increasing marginal cost.* From Table XXIX it can be seen that if the monopolist has an output of 70 units (per week) he can sell them at 8*s*. 9*d*. each, his total revenue being 70 × 8*s*. 9*d*. (612*s*. 6*d*.), and his total cost (including normal profit) 432s. 6d. If the total cost is subtracted from the total revenue this leaves the monopolist a surplus (or mono- poly) profit of 180s.

TABLE XXIX

The Cost and Revenue Schedule of a Monopolist

Units of output	Average revenue (price per unit)	Total revenue	Marginal revenue	Average cost	Total cost	Marginal cost	Surplus profit
70	8s. 9d.	612s. 6d.	—	6s. 2d.	432s. 6d.	—	180s.
80	8s. 6d.	680s.	6s. 9d.	5s. 4d.	457s. 6d.	2s. 6d.	222s. 6d.
90	8s. 3d.	742s. 6d.	6s. 3d.	5s. 5d.	492s. 6d.	3s. 6d.	250s.
100	8s.	800s.	5s. 9d.	5s. 6d.	550s.	5s. 9d.	250s.
110	7s. 9d.	852s. 6d.	5s. 3d.	5s. 8d.	620s.	7s.	232s. 6d.
120	7s. 6d.	900s.	4s. 9d.	5s. 11d.	710s.	9s.	190s.

If he increases his output to 80 units he has to reduce the price to 8s. 6d. in order to sell his entire output. This increases his total revenue by 67s. 6d. to 680s., but since his total costs increase by only 25s., he achieves a higher surplus profit than before—namely, 222s. 6d. His marginal revenue is 6s. 9d. (67s. 6d. ÷ 10) and his marginal cost is 2s. 6d. (25s. ÷ 10). (It is necessary to divide the difference in total

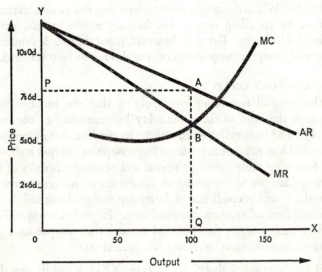

FIG. 58.—MONOPOLY OUTPUT WITH INCREASING MARGINAL COST. (MC = marginal cost. AR = average revenue (demand curve). MR = marginal revenue. AC = average cost.)

revenue and total cost shown in the table by 10, because the table shows outputs only at intervals of 10 units.) The monopolist will continue to expand his output so long as marginal cost does not exceed marginal revenue. In this case he will not exceed an output of 100 units, because at this point his surplus profit is at a maximum. This occurs where marginal revenue equals marginal cost. Under perfect competition marginal cost is equal to price, but under monopoly average revenue (price) is greater than marginal cost. In the above examples the monopolist's output is 100 units, the price is 8s. and his marginal cost only 5s. 9d. The graph (Fig. 58) shows the monopolist's output to occur when marginal revenue equals marginal cost, but also where average revenue (price) exceeds marginal cost by AB.

(ii) *Marginal cost decreasing.*

TABLE XXX

The Cost and Revenue Schedule of a Monopolist

Marginal Cost Decreasing

Output	Price	Total revenue	Marginal revenue	Average cost	Total cost	Marginal cost	Surplus profit
20	12s. 7½d.	252s. 6d.	—	7s. 10d.	156s. 3d.		96s. 3d.
30	9s. 4d.	280s.	2s. 9d.	6s. 0d.	180s.	2s. 4½d.	100s.
40	7s. 6d.	300s.	2s.	5s. 0d.	200s.	2s.	100s.
50	6s. 3d.	312s. 6d.	1s. 3d.	4s. 4d.	216s. 3d.	1s. 7½d.	95s. 9d.
60	5s. 3½d.	317s. 6d.	6d.	3s. 10d.	228s. 9d.	1s. 3d.	88s. 9d.

As before, the monopolist will not increase his output beyond the point where marginal cost equals marginal revenue, for at this point his surplus profit is at a maximum.

(iii) *Marginal cost constant.*

TABLE XXXI

The Cost and Revenue Schedule of a Monopolist

Constant Marginal Cost

Output	Price	Total revenue	Marginal revenue	Average cost	Total cost	Marginal cost	Surplus profit
50	11s. 6d.	575s.	—	9s. 0d.	450s.	—	125s.
60	10s. 8d.	640s.	6s. 6d.	8s. 4d.	500s.	5s.	140s.
70	10s.	700s.	6s.	7s. 10d.	550s.	5s.	150s.
80	9s. 4½d.	750s.	5s.	7s. 6d.	600s.	5s.	150s.
90	8s. 10d.	795s.	4s. 6d.	7s. 3d.	650s.	5s.	145s.
100	8s. 3d.	825s.	3s.	7s. 0d.	700s.	5s.	125s.

Again surplus profit is at a maximum when marginal revenue is equal to marginal cost. Cases (ii) and (iii) also can be shown graphically as follows:

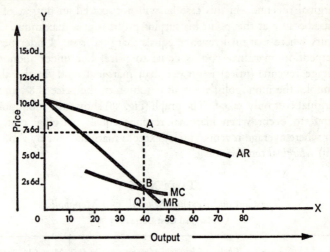

FIG. 59.—MONOPOLY OUTPUT (DECREASING MARGINAL COST).

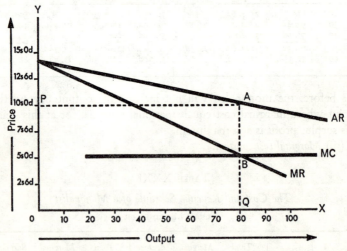

FIG. 60.—MONOPOLY OUTPUT (CONSTANT MARGINAL COST).

All three tables show that in the case of monopoly, average revenue (price) is greater than average cost or marginal cost or marginal revenue.

The following graph (Fig. 61) shows that a monopolist's output therefore will be that at which there is the greatest difference between his total revenue and his total costs, since this yields him his maximum profit. Total cost is, as usual, assumed to include normal profit. At the output OQ^1 the gap between the two curves is widest, and so surplus profit is at a maximum. OQ^1 is therefore the monopolist's output.

Under monopoly, therefore, marginal cost may be increasing, decreasing or constant, but in all cases maximum profit is achieved when marginal cost equals marginal revenue. Under perfect competition marginal cost is always increasing, but again the most profitable output is where marginal cost equals marginal revenue. Under perfect competition, however, marginal revenue is equal to price, whereas under monopoly and imperfect competition price is greater than marginal revenue.

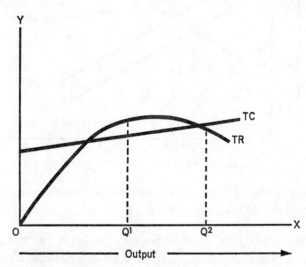

Fig. 61.—Monopoly Output. (TC = Total Cost. TR = Total Revenue).

(4) CHANGES IN DEMAND UNDER MONOPOLY

If the demand for a commodity increases its price also will rise and an expansion of its output will occur under monopoly, as under perfect competition (Fig. 62). D^1D^1 represents demand and MR^1 marginal revenue before a change in demand. D^2D^2 represents demand and MR^2 marginal revenue after the change in demand. MC is the marginal cost curve. If the expansion of output makes possible economies of scale the marginal cost curve will move farther to the right.

Before the change of demand output will be OQ^1, for at that output MR equals MC, and so price will be OP^1. After the change of demand output will increase to OQ^2 because MR^2 equals MC at this output, and the price will rise to OP^2. In this example marginal cost is increasing. If marginal cost is constant the effect of the increase in demand will be to increase output further, but with a smaller rise in price than when marginal cost is rising. If marginal cost is falling there will be an even greater increase in output and a still smaller increase in price.

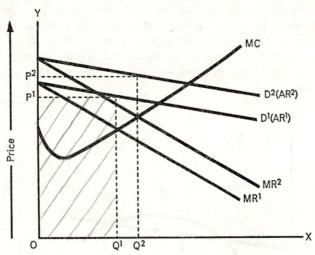

FIG. 62.—CHANGE OF DEMAND UNDER MONOPOLY.

A fall in demand will produce exactly reverse results, again assuming marginal cost to remain unchanged.

(5) THE EFFECT ON A MONOPOLIST OF A RISE IN COSTS

Consider now the effect of a rise in costs on a monopolist's output. In the diagram (Fig. 63) TC^1 represents total cost before the rise in costs takes place and TC^2 total cost after the rise.

Before the rise in costs output will be OQ, because at that output the difference between TC^1 and TR (total revenue) is at a maximum. It will be seen that if the increase in costs is the same whatever the output, as with TC^2, the monopolist will have no incentive to alter his output, since his profit is at a maximum at the same output as before, though of course reduced in amount.

The effect of a fixed lump-sum tax on a monopolist would be similar to an increase in his costs. Even if the tax was equal to his entire surplus profit, the monopolist would still have no motive for changing his output, (OQ).

A lump-sum tax equal to surplus profit at the monopoly output and

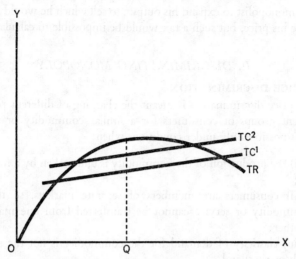

FIG. 63.—RISE IN COST UNDER MONOPOLY.

at all lower outputs, but decreasing with each output beyond monopoly output, would encourage the monopolist to increase his output. The heavily dotted line (Fig. 64) represents total cost after the imposition of such a tax. The monopolist will expand his output from OQ^1 to OQ^2 because his surplus profit is now greatest at this larger output. It has been suggested that the imposition of a tax of this kind would encour-

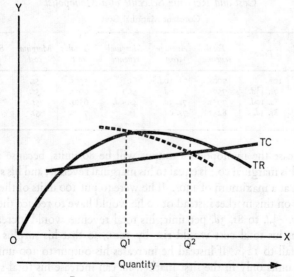

FIG. 64.—TAXATION OF A MONOPOLIST.

age a monopolist to expand his output, to sell which he would have to reduce his price, but such a tax would be impossible to calculate.

II. DISCRIMINATING MONOPOLY

(6) PRICE DISCRIMINATION

By price discrimination is meant the charging of different prices to different groups of consumers for a similar commodity or service. This is possible only under conditions when:

(i) the production of the commodity is undertaken by a monopolist;

(ii) consumers are members of separate markets, so that the commodity or service cannot be transferred from one market to another;

(iii) elasticity of demand for the commodity is not the same in each market; and

(iv) the cost of keeping the markets separate is not too great.

The monopolist can increase his total surplus profit if he sells his monopoly output in the first market and an additional amount in a second market.

Consider again the following portion of Table XXXI:

Cost and Revenue Schedule of a Monopolist
Constant Marginal Cost

Output	Price	Total revenue	Average cost	Marginal revenue	Total cost	Marginal cost	Surplus profit
70	10s	700s.	7s. 10d.	6s.	550s.	5s.	150s.
80	9s. 4½d.	750s.	7s. 6d.	5s.	600s.	5s.	150s.
90	8s. 10d.	795s.	7s. 3d.	4s. 6d.	650s.	5s.	145s.
100	8s. 3d.	825s.	7s. 0d.	3s.	700s.	5s.	125s.

In this case the monopolist's output will be 80 units, because at this output his marginal cost is equal to his marginal revenue, and his surplus profit is at a maximum of 150s. If he were to put 100 units of the commodity on this market instead of 80 he would have to reduce the price from 9s. 4½d. to 8s. 3d. per unit; his total revenue would increase by 75s., but his total cost would rise by 100s., so that his surplus profit would fall to 125s. If instead he increases his output to 100 units but sells 80 units only in the first market, he can increase his total surplus profit by disposing of the additional 20 units for any sum above their marginal cost of 100s. Assuming that his price in the second market is 5s. 6d., then:

Total cost of producing 100 = 700s.
Sale of 80 at 9s. 4½d. each = 750s. ⎫
Sale of 20 at 5s. 6d. each   = 110s. ⎬ 860s.
                                     ⎭

Surplus profit = 160s., an increase of 10s.

The reason why he is able to increase his total surplus profit in this way is that in order to increase sales in the first market he had to reduce the price of his *entire* output, whereas if the markets can be kept separate he can sell the additional output at a low price in the second market without having to reduce his price in the first market.

How much he will sell in each market will depend on the elasticity of demand for the commodity in each market. His total profit for the two markets will be at a maximum when he produces that output at which marginal cost is equal to marginal revenue in each market, for if this condition is not fulfilled it would be more profitable to transfer some of the output from one market to the other. In the above example (Table XXXI) this condition was fulfilled in the first market at an output of 80 with selling price at 9s. 4½d., marginal revenue and marginal cost both being 5s. To maximise his profit from the two markets together he will charge such a price in the second market that in that market also marginal cost equals marginal revenue at that output. If elasticity of demand is the same in each market there will be no incentive for the monopolist to charge different prices, for he cannot increase his profit by so doing. When a monopolist divides his output between two markets the price will be higher and the quantity sold less in the market where demand is more inelastic.

To make price discrimination possible markets may be kept separate by tariffs. In the above example the first market may be the home market, and the monopoly might be maintained by a high tariff on foreign imports. The extra output is then exported and sold much more cheaply abroad, the high tariff also serving the purpose of preventing a foreign purchaser making a profit by re-exporting the commodity back to the home market. This practice is generally known as dumping. Producers have often complained of foreign manufacturers dumping their goods at prices, which they said, were below "cost of production." This complaint shows again the ambiguity of the term "cost of production." Consider once more the above example. Assume the commodity to be produced under conditions of perfect competition in the second market at an average cost of 5s. If the price of the imported article is only 1s. 6d. this is obviously below the *average* cost of production of producers in either market, but is above the *marginal* cost of a monopolist selling in separate markets. A protective tariff is almost certain to be demanded by home producers as a protection against such dumping.

Sometimes markets are not so clearly separated. For example, a new novel may sell for 18s.; later a cheaper edition at 5s. may be published; later still there may be a cheap reprint at 2s. 6d. These markets may be completely separated from one another by time, but there is nothing to prevent a prospective purchaser waiting until the cheapest edition is brought out. If, however, most of the consumers who buy the 5s. edition are people who would not in any case have been willing to pay more, then the prospect of a cheaper edition will not seriously affect the sales of the more expensive first edition. Similarly, the 2s. 6d. edition may serve a third market. In order in such a case to assist price discrimination and make it less obvious there may be some attempt at differentiation of the commodity by means of different bindings.

Price discrimination and consumer's surplus. A bookseller may be able to sell ten copies of a particular book if its price were 5s., six copies if the price were 10s. 6d., but only two if the price were 18s. If actually the book is published at 5s. two people can obtain for 5s. a book for which they would have been willing to pay 18s., with the result that each of them enjoys 13s. worth of surplus satisfaction; three others who are willing to pay 10s. 6d. each have 5s 6d. worth of surplus satisfaction. When discriminatory prices can be charged consumer's surplus can be reduced to a minimum and the producer's surplus profit thereby increased. If everyone had to pay the maximum price he was willing to pay for everything he bought, consumer's surplus would completely disappear.

(7) FURTHER EXAMPLES OF PRICE DISCRIMINATION

Railway freight rates used to provide one of the most frequently quoted examples of discriminatory charges. Goods were arranged in twenty-one categories, the more expensive the commodity, the higher the charge for carrying it. The railway classification of goods was based on the principle of "charging what the traffic will bear," since if all goods had been charged at the same rate, some of the cheaper goods would never have been carried at all. This method of charging came into existence when the railways were monopolist carriers. Discriminatory charges were possible because the markets were quite separate—a high category commodity could not be transferred to a lower class in order to obtain the advantage of the cheaper rate (woollen cloth, for example, could not be passed off as coal!). In the case of discriminatory passenger fares the markets are not quite so easily kept separate. It will not pay to issue cheap return tickets, available for travel by ordinary trains, if this ruins the market for tickets at the full rate. To prevent this, restrictions are generally imposed on the use of cheap tickets—for example, the tickets may not be available until too late an hour for most ordinary travellers. If the issue of cheap tickets brings people to the railways who would not otherwise have travelled, then it is clear that the two markets are separate. Where special excursion trains are run the separation of markets becomes easier. The railways, too, have heavy fixed costs, and marginal cost is relatively low, for the additional cost of running an extra train is comparatively small, though the cost of maintaining the additional rolling stock is very high relative to its use.

Airlines similarly charge discriminatory fares, with lower rates for mid-week or night travel or at certain seasons. A lower fare is often charged to those travelling for pleasure than to those on business by linking fares to "packaged" holidays.

Before the introduction of the National Health Service in 1948 doctors were said to have different scales of charges for different groups of patients, the poor being charged at a lower rate than the rich. This was possible because the service was personal and could not be transferred from one person to another.

Gas and electricity undertakings, like railways, have very heavy fixed costs and relatively low variable costs. The two-part tariff—a fixed minimum charge and a further charge proportional to the amount consumed—is an attempt to apportion the charge over fixed and variable costs. Marginal cost, therefore, is low, and so sometimes lower charges are made where large quantities of the commodity are consumed. Again the markets are distinct, for the lower price can be obtained only after a stated amount of gas or electricity has been consumed. Sometimes price discrimination in the case of electricity can be applied also to the purpose for which it is used, a lower charge being made for its use as power than for lighting. Or discrimination may be in favour of a certain type of consumer, industrial concerns being charged at a different rate from householders. Since there must be sufficient plant to meet the heavy demand at peak periods, lower charges may be imposed at other times to encourage consumption at off-peak periods, as with storage heaters, which consume electricity only during off-peak periods but supply heat at other times, separate meters being required to keep the markets separate. For this reason long-distance telephone calls are cheaper in the evening than earlier in the day. In all cases the aim is to tap new markets, success depending

on the elasticity of demand for the commodity or service and the ease
and extent to which the markets can be kept separate.

RECOMMENDATIONS FOR FURTHER READING

K. E. Boulding: *Economic Analysis*, Chapter 25.
E. A. G. Robinson: *Monopoly*.
Joan Robinson: *Economics of Imperfect Competition*, Chapters 3 and 10–15.
E. H. Phelps Browne: *A Course in Applied Economics*, Part II.

QUESTIONS

1. What factors determine how much of a commodity a monopolist will
produce? (R.S.A. Inter.)

2. What do you understand by the phrase: "charging what the traffic will
bear"? (L.C. Com. C. & F.)

3. "The monopolist can sell his product at whatever price he likes." Comment on this statement and show how the monopolist reaches an equilibrium
position. (B.S. Inter.)

4. How, exactly, does a monopolist decide the price he will charge for his
product in order to maximise his profits? (I.T.)

5. Is it inevitable that the monopoly price of a commodity must be higher
than its competition price? In your answer, outline the major differences in the
determination of these two types of price. (I.H.A.)

6. What is the relevance of elasticity of demand to the fixing of prices under
monopolistic conditions? In what circumstances could a monopolist charge
differential prices? (Exp.)

7. "Given a certain elasticity of demand, the supply which the monopolist
will produce (and therefore the monopoly price) will depend upon the conditions of production." Discuss this statement. (I.B.)

8. Explain the term Monopoly in your own words; and discuss the effects of
monopoly (*a*) under private, (*b*) under public ownership. (A.C.C.A. Final.)

9. What do you understand by price discrimination? In what circumstances
is it (*a*) practicable, (*b*) profitable? (G.C.E. Adv.)

10. Discuss the view that charges for electricity should vary with the time of
day during which electricity is used. (Final Degree.)

CHAPTER XV

THE BASIS OF SUPPLY:
(3) UNDER IMPERFECT COMPETITION

I. IMPERFECT COMPETITION

(1) COMPETITION IS IMPERFECT

Until fairly recently economists considered that economic forces tended to pull market and competitive conditions towards an equilibrium position of perfection. Therefore, the working of the forces of supply and demand, they thought, tended to bring about a distribution of resources among those occupations where they could be most efficiently employed, and so produce that assortment of goods which would yield maximum satisfaction to consumers. Such hindrances to perfect competition as existed were considered to be exceptional. At the opposite extreme from perfect competition was monopoly. Under perfect competition there is a large number of firms producing a homogeneous commodity, so that buyers have no preference for the product of any particular seller; whereas under monopoly there is a single producer for whose product there is no close substitute. Under perfect competition sellers accept price as something beyond their control and have no incentive to restrict supply; the monopolist, on the other hand, can influence price by restricting his output.

Neither perfect competition nor monopoly, however, exist, and actual conditions lie between these two extremes. Unfortunately, in ordinary speech—and Acts of Parliament too—the term, monopoly, is loosely used to describe forms of very imperfect competition, including cases where producers are responsible for much less than half the total output of a commodity. Sellers are often driven by a community of interests to combine together; entry to an industry may be difficult if large capital is involved, or if there are considerable economies of scale, or new competitors may be kept out of the field by devices such as patent rights, or if similar products are differentiated by branding. In these and other ways competition has been rendered imperfect, and far from being exceptional, these conditions are now the rule. Under perfect competition there is a single price at which the entire supply can be sold. A feature of imperfect competition, however, is that there is no single selling price for the commodity.

The study of production under conditions of imperfect competition is more difficult than the study of either perfect competition or monopoly, for whereas these are two well-defined cases—just because they happen to be extremes—imperfect competition has many varieties, ranging from near perfection to near monopoly, so that generalisation becomes difficult.

(2) TYPES OF IMPERFECT COMPETITION

It is impossible to consider all forms of imperfect competition, but there are a few well-defined types that are worthy of notice. The two principal conditions for perfect competition, it has been seen, are (i) many producers, and (ii) a homogeneous commodity, so that buyers have no preference for the product of any particular producer. In one form of imperfect competition we find a large number of producers, but imperfection results from differentiation in the commodity produced or in the service provided. This is generally known as *monopolistic competition*. Another type of imperfect competition relates to cases where there are only a few producers, and to this the name oligopoly (Greek *oligoi* = few) has been given. Duopoly (two producers or sellers) is thus a special case of oligopoly. If the commodity is homogeneous we have perfect oligopoly; if there is differentiation between the products of different sellers we have imperfect oligopoly. The following table shows the distinguishing features of monopoly and the various kinds of competition:

TABLE XXXII

Features of Competition and Monopoly

Type	Producers	Commodity
Perfect competition ·	Many	Homogeneous
Imperfect competition:		
(i) Monopolistic competition . .	Many	Differentiation
(ii) Perfect oligopoly (or duopoly) .	Few (or Two)	Homogeneous
(iii) Imperfect oligopoly (or duopoly) .	Few (or Two)	Differentiation
Monopoly	Single	Single

II. MONOPOLISTIC COMPETITION AND OLIGOPOLY

(3) MONOPOLISTIC COMPETITION IN THE RETAIL TRADE

A feature of monopolistic competition, as of perfect competition, is that there are many producers or sellers, but unlike perfect competition, the commodity or service is not homogeneous. The retail trade provides an interesting example of monopolistic competition.

Differentiation takes many forms. Two shops may be selling similar goods, and yet there may be differentiation in the form of better service at one shop, or greater convenience of situation. In the case of shops in the suburbs of a town, it is unusual to find two shops in the same branch of trade very close together (though this is common enough in the town centre). Suppose A and B to be two grocers' shops. Each has a sort of hinterland in which its customers live, and

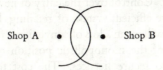

Shop A • • Shop B

within its own hinterland each shop has some measure of monopoly, owing to the greater convenience of its situation to people living in that area. Competition between A and B is therefore restricted to the small area between the two shops where the two hinterlands overlap. To people living well within the hinterland of A, Shop B is not a perfect substitute. If the two shops are close together some people may still prefer one to the other because they consider that they obtain better service there. The differentiation between them may consist of nothing more than the contrast between the pleasant smile of one shop-keeper and the surly nature of the other. As a result, if one retailer cuts his prices he will not attract all the customers away from the other retailer.

The reason why shops in one branch of trade tend to be found in the same street is that new entrants generally wish to reduce to a minimum any differences between those already in the trade and themselves. So in London tailors are concentrated in or near Savile Row, jewellers in Bond Street, newspaper offices in Fleet Street, doctors in Harley Street.

The typical retailing unit is the small shop. The retail trade is easy to enter because there is no need to have any special training before doing so, and the amount of initial capital required is relatively small. It now offers almost the sole remaining opportunity to the small man to set up in business for himself. Consequently, the effect of retailing being carried on under conditions of monopolistic competition is to produce *excess capacity* rather than surplus profit, for the high-cost firms are not driven out, as they would be if competition were perfect.[1] Other factors making for excess capacity in the retail trade are: (i) many small shops are family businesses, other members of the proprietor's family assisting him at peak periods for little or no wages; (ii) a very small

[1] The number of retail establishments in Great Britain, according to the latest census of distribution is 580,000.

shop may consist merely of a room of a dwelling-house converted into a shop, retailing being only a sideline to the proprietor's ordinary occupation. It has been suggested that by means of a system of licensing excess capacity in retailing could be avoided. In fact, some local authorities already restrict the number of certain kinds of shops—for example, those selling fish and chips. In some trades, for example, the sale of newspapers, wholesalers will supply only a limited number of retailers in a district. Control over the entry of new firms by licensing may provide a more efficient system of retailing, but if this results in fewer retail shops it will mean a loss of convenience for some consumers, and strengthening of the monopolistic position of retailers who are fortunate enough to secure licences. The cost to the consumer of greater efficiency in retailing is a curtailment of his choice of supplier. He may, of course, prefer greater freedom of choice to efficiency and the lower prices that should result from it.

(4) OLIGOPOLY

A common form of imperfect competition, known as oligopoly, occurs where there are only a few producers. Two forms of oligopoly can be distinguished—perfect and imperfect:

(i) *Perfect Oligopoly*. In the case of perfect oligopoly the commodity is homogeneous. This is true also of perfect competition, but in perfect competition there are many producers. Because the commodity is homogeneous there can be only one price under either perfect competition or perfect oligopoly. Under perfect competition, however, each firm must take price as being something outside its control, whereas under perfect oligopoly this is not so. Under either form of oligopoly a firm contemplating a cut in price must consider the possible effect of such action on the price policy of the other firms in the industry. Where the commodity is homogeneous, consumers have no preference for one producer as against another, and so if oligopoly is perfect a cut in price by one producer must lead to a similar cut by other producers. Generally, but not always, price leadership will be with the largest firm. In Great Britain the manufacture of cement and sugar refining provide examples of perfect oligopoly.

(ii) *Imperfect Oligopoly*. When production is in the hands of only a few firms and the commodity is not homogeneous—that is, where there is some differentiation between the product of one firm and that of another—imperfect oligopoly exists. If firm A cuts its price, there is then no certainty that Firms B, C, D and E will all follow suit immediately. Meanwhile Firm A will probably find that its sales have expanded sufficiently to increase its surplus profit. Any advantage in price-cutting goes to the first firm to indulge in it, but this can only yield a temporary advantage, for what A has done can also be done by B, C or D, and a price-cutting war may follow. The smaller the number of firms, the more severe will be the competition, so that duopoly tends to produce the most extreme example of cut-throat competition. In the end, the duopolists, in order to prevent each ruining the other, may decide to divide the market, each agreeing to allow the other a monopoly of its own area. The tobacco war resulted in such an agreement. Cut-throat competition takes the form of price-cutting or an advertising war. Price-cutting may be by an actual reduction in prices or through gifts of trading stamps; advertising may be supplemented by free samples.

(5) IMPERFECT OLIGOPOLY IN BRANDED GOODS

In imperfect oligopoly there are only a few producers, each one of whom tries to differentiate his product or service in some way from those of others. The extent of this differentiation may not always be very great, for all are producers of similar products, but because of some slight difference the product of one is not regarded as a perfect substitute for the product of another. For example, they may all be makers of strawberry jam, but Cheeryble's strawberry jam is not regarded as a perfect substitute for Boffin's strawberry jam, because some consumers believe Boffin's to be slightly superior in quality to Cheeryble's, while others believe Cheeryble's to be the better. Excelsior chocolates may differ only slightly from Superb chocolates, but some people may prefer Excelsior because they consider them to be more attractively packed, or there may be some who merely prefer the name. As a result, Superb chocolates are not considered to be a perfect substitute for Excelsior chocolates. In other words, the differentiation may be purely artificial and in no way adding to the quality of the commodity. Differentiation reduces the elasticity of demand for a commodity. Most branded goods are produced and sold under conditions of imperfect oligopoly.

As a result of this differentiation, Boffin may be able to charge a penny more for his jam. If competition were perfect this would result in all consumers buying Cheeryble's jam, and Boffin's sales would fall to zero. Under monopolistic competition some people will still prefer Boffin's jam, because they do not look upon Cheeryble's as being a perfect substitute for it. Again, if the makers of Superb chocolates cut their price they will not gain all those customers who previously preferred Excelsior chocolates, for many consumers do not consider Superb chocolates to be a perfect substitute for Excelsior.

Under conditions of imperfect competition there is always the opportunity for surplus profit to be made by any firm that is first in the field with something new. The possibility of surplus profits will attract a train of imitations (except so far as the idea is protected by patent rights) and profits will again fall. It will be necessary for the innovation to be an "improvement" on an existing commodity, for it is essential that its differentiation from the products of other firms should be slight; otherwise, if it is an entirely new article, a new market will have to be created. For example, suppose that Dorrit, a competitor of Boffin's and Cheeryble's in the market for strawberry jam, invents a new method of preserving the commodity, which makes it more convenient to use. Boffin and Cheeryble will not be driven out of the market, for some of their customers will remain loyal to them, but Dorrit may for a time capture a much larger share of the market, and increase his surplus profit until other firms imitate his invention.

This possibility of surplus profit, even for a temporary period, is the great stimulus to the invention of the new "gadgets" that are constantly coming on to the market. Because many consumers occasionally like to try something new, manufacturers of branded goods often add new brands to their range of products. It has been known for a manufacturer deliberately to market two brands, sold under different names, but otherwise identical, in order to obtain a larger share of the market.

(6) RESALE PRICE MAINTENANCE

Reference has already been made to the practice of differentiating similar varieties of products by branding. This may take the form of an invented name (often a misspelling of the name of a commodity, for example, the name "Sope" for a brand of soap), or the name of the firm may be used in a distinctive way. The invented name is the more popular, and some of these words have almost been accepted into the language. The Trade Marks Acts give protection to the manufacturer against the improper use of his trade name by unscrupulous rivals, provided the name has been legally registered. An important result of the branding of goods is that the manufacturer himself generally takes over the marketing of the commodity direct to the retailers, and such goods are usually extensively advertised.

To the retailer the branding of goods has both advantages and disadvantages. Since the goods are made up in packets or containers of uniform weight and quality, they are more conveniently handled, and there is no necessity for the retailer to inspect them before placing his order. On the other hand, retailers have to carry stocks of a large number of different varieties of similar goods in order to pander to the whims and fancies of their customers. If the manufacturer insisted on a fixed price this safeguarded a retailer against price cuts by his competitors. The more efficient retailer, however, was debarred by the fixed price from attempting to increase his turnover by selling at lower prices than his rivals; the maxim "small profits quick returns" ceased to operate. Resale price maintenance was thus a consequence of the sale of branded goods.

Resale price maintenance was first introduced in the 1890s after agitation by the smaller, independent retailers against price-cutting by multiple shops and department stores, which at that time were seeking to increase their turnover by this method. More recently, however, pressure for price maintenance has come chiefly from manufacturers. Insistence on resale at a fixed price was chiefly due to the manufacturer's desire to place goods with as many retailers as possible, in order to secure for himself the maximum number of selling points, and to do this he had to ensure that the more efficient retailers did not under-cut the others, since price-cutting might drive out the less efficient. Thus, the sale of fixed-price branded goods still further encourages excess capacity. Another effect of price maintenance is to substitute competition in service for price competition between retailers. Both the Lloyd Jacob Committee (1949) and the *Restrictive Trade Practices Act* (1956), however, condemned concerted action by manufacturers against retailers who had cut the prices of the products of any one of them. This was regarded as a restrictive practice. Most of the large multiple shops, supermarkets and self-service stores took advantage of this Act to sell goods below the fixed prices, thereby again introducing price competition into retailing. The *Resale Prices Act* (1964) made resale price maintenance illegal from 1965, except where manufacturers could satisfy the Restrictive Practices Courts, set up under the Act of 1956, that it was in the public interest for a fixed price to be retained.

(7) SELLING COSTS

Selling costs are costs incurred in order to stimulate sales, and thus advertising is the principal selling cost. Advertising can be undertaken for either of two purposes. Sometimes it is merely a way of making an announcement more widely known, this type being known as informative advertising, and to this there are no economic objections. Most advertising, however, is of the persuasive or competitive kind, and its purpose is to persuade the public that a certain manufacturer's brand of a particular commodity is different from, and superior to, all other manufacturers' brands. Under perfect competition, therefore, there could be no advertising of this second type, on account of the homogeneity of the commodity, although sometimes an industry as a whole might advertise in some such form as *Eat more bread* or *Eat more fruit*. Selling costs are therefore a consequence of imperfect competition, being associated with imperfect oligopoly and, to a lesser degree, with monopolistic competition. In the case of branded goods a fall in price is likely to increase sales only slightly, for people often prefer one brand to others. Advertising is essential, too, to keep constantly before consumers the names of the various brands. To some extent, therefore, all advertising is informative. In the production of some commodities selling costs form a very high proportion of total costs, being as high as 45%, for example, in the case of patent medicines. Selling costs are regarded as one of the greatest wastes of imperfect competition. Consequently, economists condemn competitive advertising, partly because of the wasteful employment of factors of production on advertising when they might have been used in some other form of production, and partly because this kind of advertising only increases costs of production. An advertising campaign may, of course, be advantageous to an individual producer, but competitive advertising cannot increase the *total* demand for all kinds of goods and services.

III. THE PROBLEM OF MONOPOLY POWER

(8) BASES OF MONOPOLY POWER

Although absolute monopoly does not exist in the real world, a large measure of monopoly power can nevertheless sometimes be obtained, as in the following circumstances:

(i) *Where one firm (or group of firms working together) controls a large proportion of the total supply* of a commodity. These are sometimes called natural monopolies. Most of the world's supply of rubber comes from Malaya; and Canada has almost a monopoly of the world's output of nickel. The few producers of tin have often combined to make price agreements. Brazil is the principal producer of coffee and it is distributed through a central agency, the Coffee Institute of Brazil. By the United Nations International Coffee Agreement of 1962 Brazil was allotted a quota of 40% of world export of coffee, Colombia 14%.

(ii) *Where large, specific plant is required,* as in some branches of the iron and steel industry. In such cases it is difficult for new firms to enter the industry, because of the considerable amount of capital required to do so. Even if capital is available, however, it will not be drawn into such industries immediately profits rise above normal, for where an industry consists of a small number of large firms the addition of one more firm may make the industry over-large and unprofitable. As a result, existing firms enjoy a certain degree of monopoly, but if profits rise much above the normal for a lengthy period rival firms will, of course, be tempted to enter the industry, and so in the long period surplus profit may disappear.

(iii) *Where duplication of a service would be wasteful.* Wherever fixed costs are very heavy proportionately to variable costs, as in the case of many public utilities, such as electricity, gas and water undertakings, an inferior service would result if rival suppliers each laid pipes or cables down every street. To the extent that gas and electricity undertakings compete against one another, wasteful duplication to some extent already exists in many places, and a more efficient service would result if it could be avoided. Similarly with railway transport, the desire of Parliament to ensure competition between different companies, in the days when the railways were being constructed, resulted in Great Britain in an unnecessary overlapping of routes and a less efficient railway system. Keen as was the desire of Parliament to maintain competition between railways, it had to allow them—until the coming of the motor vehicle—a monopoly over large portions of their systems. It may be that at the present time there is wasteful competition between road and rail services. Similarly, the early motor-bus operators were small firms, and often competed against one another over the same routes until 1931 when, in the interest of the safety of the general public rather than economic efficiency, road traffic was regulated, and competition in road passenger operation abolished. Competitive postal services, too, would obviously be wasteful, as is the practice of some nationalised industries of delivering their own bills to customers.

(iv) *Branded goods.* By the use of trade marks and trade names, manufacturers try to differentiate their products from those of other producers. The element of monopoly in such cases is restricted, but imperfection exists, as has been seen, in the form of imperfect oligopoly.

(v) *Patent rights.* A patent is a grant by the Crown to the inventor of a new machine or process, giving him a monopoly of its use, in the first instance, for a period of sixteen years, with the possibility of renewal for a further five years or in some cases ten years. Copyright is somewhat similar, and grants the owner the sole right to reproduce a literary or musical work for a period, in the case of an author of fifty years after his death, and for gramophone records of fifty years after the making of the matrix. Both patent right and copyright, therefore, give rise to forms of imperfect competition.

(vi) *Local monopolies.* These may arise in a number of ways. In the first place, where transport costs are very heavy and only one firm is near the market for the commodity, this firm may be able to raise its charges by an amount equal to the costs of transport of its nearest rival, and as a result obtain surplus profit. Suppose, for example, there is a coal-mine, A, near to a certain town, and no other mines nearer than B, C, D. Suppose, further, that the cost of raising a ton of coal is the same in all cases, but that it costs 5s. per ton to carry coal from mines B, C and D to the town. Then mine A will be able to charge nearly 5s. per ton more than the others and yet sell its coal more cheaply in the town, and so obtain monopoly profit. In the same way, local brick-works and stone quarries possess an element of local monopoly. Before the development of road passenger transport, village shops also often possessed local monopolies.

Another way in which a somewhat similar type of monopoly may arise occurs where an old-established firm has acquired a very high reputation, with the result that it may be able to continue to charge a little more than its rivals, even though its product is no better.

(vii) *Tariffs.* These can be used in order to maintain a home producer's monopoly in the home market or for the purpose of separating two markets in order to make price discrimination possible in a foreign market.

(viii) *Restrictions on entry to occupations.* In order to keep up wages in an occupation, a professional organisation may make entry more difficult by insisting upon a period of training or the passing of certain entrance examinations. In many cases the character of the occupation may require a high standard of knowledge and training, as in the medical and legal professions, but in some cases it is merely a device for restricting the number of people permitted to practise a particular calling. Similarly, trade unions, for example, may insist on an unnecessarily long period of apprenticeship.

(9) TYPES OF MONOPOLISTIC ASSOCIATION

In order to obtain the advantage of monopoly, firms may form themselves into voluntary associations, or they may combine together permanently.

Horizontal and vertical combines. Where the firms are all at the same stage of production (for example, if they are all engaged in dyeing), the association or amalgamation is said to be of the horizontal type;

where the firms are at different stages of production (for example, spinning, weaving, dyeing, etc.) the amalgamation is described as vertical. Voluntary associations of firms, price rings, pools and cartels are of the horizontal type, whereas trusts are generally of vertical structure.

The voluntary association aims either to fix a minimum price or to restrict output. Price agreements are easier to enforce among the members than agreements to limit output, and so quite loose associations, such as the price ring, can be formed for this purpose. The *Restrictive Trade Practices Act* (1956) made it illegal for a group of firms to agree not to sell below an agreed price.

Cartels. More complex organisation, such as that of the cartel (or Kartell), is required where the policy is to restrict output. In the cartel, which is of German origin, the member firms establish a central selling organisation. Thus the members retain their individuality and independence as producers, except in so far as they agree not to exceed a given output. Unless the members are loyal to the arrangement made for restricting output, the cartel will fail to make monopoly profit. In some of the German cartels a code of rules was drawn up, and member firms had to agree to abide by them. To enforce these rules the cartel appointed officials to visit individual firms, and, if necessary, inspect their books. A firm discovered to have exceeded the output assigned to it would be fined. There is a tendency, however, for all such voluntary agreements to break up. Changing conditions make the more progressive firms increasingly unwilling to maintain the *status quo*, until in the end they withdraw from the cartel in order to fight alone for a larger share of the market. No cartel is likely to include all the producers of a commodity, and those outside take advantage of the higher prices resulting from the cartel's restriction of output to expand their own output. For both these reasons voluntary monopoly agreements tend to be unstable, although where governments are responsible for the schemes success is more likely to be achieved. The setting up of a cartel or central selling agency can then be made compulsory, and the various Marketing Boards that have been set up in Great Britain for milk, hops, potatoes, eggs and a number of other farming products are of this type. In the case of some of these commodities restriction of output was not the aim, although this was so in the case of hops, but in all cases production for the market is restricted to producers holding the necessary licences. The extent to which a cartel can obtain monopoly profit depends on its powers (i) to restrict output, (ii) to restrict the entry of new firms into the industry.

Trusts. One of the chief weaknesses of the German type of cartel is that the members retain independence of management and, in many cases, the right to withdraw from the association after an agreed period. A complete amalgamation of firms overcomes this difficulty, for the old firms—at least, the weaker of them—completely lose their identity. The Trust is of American origin, though the *Sherman Act* of 1890 declared it to be an illegal form of business enterprise. The Trust is a large-scale amalgamation of firms, frequently of the vertical type, the shareholders in the constituent firms receiving Trust certificates in exchange for their shares.

The holding company. This is a more recent development for bringing a number of firms under a single control. It is a purely financial institution which uses its capital to acquire controlling interests in other firms—often in different industries to give greater diversification of product—generally by taking up 51% or more of their shares to form what is known as a "Group" of companies. The holding company has become the typical form of business organisation in both Great Britain and the United States. Although it has control over its subsidiaries, it can, however, retain their original names and the goodwill attached to them. A serious drawback to the holding company is that it makes possible what is known as "pyramiding"—that is, the control of a huge amount of capital by a person who may possess only a relatively small proportion of it. Suppose, for example, Z is a holding company with a capital of £100,003, in which Snodgrass holds shares to the value of £50,002. The holding company, Z, acquires controlling interest in companies A, B and C. Company A has two subsidiaries, D and E, while company C has one subsidiary, F. The following diagram shows the structure of the organisation:

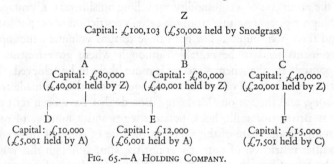

Z
Capital: £100,103 (£50,002 held by Snodgrass)

A
Capital: £80,000
(£40,001 held by Z)

B
Capital: £80,000
(£40,001 held by Z)

C
Capital: £40,000
(£20,001 held by Z)

D
Capital: £10,000
(£5,001 held by A)

E
Capital: £12,000
(£6,001 held by A)

F
Capital: £15,000
(£7,501 held by C)

Fig. 65.—A Holding Company.

There are six manufacturing companies—A, B, C, D, E and F—with a combined total of £237,000, entirely under the control of Snodgrass, whose total investment is only £50,002—that is, only a little over 21% of the total capital involved. Sometimes only a limited number of the ordinary shares issued by a limited company carry the right to vote at shareholders' meetings, most of the ordinary capital being in the form of non-voting "A" shares. The issue of non-voting shares makes pyramiding even easier. It has been suggested that no further issues of such shares should be permitted.

(10) ADVANTAGES AND DISADVANTAGES OF MONOPOLY AND IMPERFECT COMPETITION

(i) *Advantages.* In some cases production or distribution can be carried out more efficiently in the hands of a monopoly. Rationalisation of any industry—that is, reorganisation to secure greater efficiency—makes possible the elimination of excess capacity by closing down production centres where costs are high, and concentrating production in those where costs are lower; instead of all factories working below capacity, a smaller number will then work at full capacity. The Government recently assisted the Lancashire cotton industry to reorganise itself in this way. Similarly, at an earlier period Woolcombers Ltd. had purchased many wool-combing businesses in order to close them, and so reduce the total capacity of the industry.

It has already been seen that competition in the supply of gas, electricity and water would be wasteful and result in higher prices to consumers.

A reduction in the number of retail shops would probably make possible a reduction in the prices of many consumer goods. Under monopoly it becomes possible to reduce the number of varieties of products, whereas under competitive conditions each firm strives to offer as many designs as possible. A reduction, for example, in the number of models of motor cars would to some extent reduce consumers' choice, but the production of an excessive number of designs increases their average cost. Fewer models would mean "longer runs." The same applies to cloth and many other things. Standardisation is the basis of cheaper production. Restriction in the number of designs, however, may not always be a desirable policy. It would not, for example, be in the interests of British worsted manufacturers to put cheapness before variety of pattern, for it is chiefly in the market for high-quality goods that they can compete successfully against foreign manufacturers.

(ii) *Disadvantages.* Though the chief aim may often be to obtain economies of large-scale production, the creation of monopoly brings with it the danger of the misuse of monopoly power by exploitation of the consumer. For, under monopoly, prices are almost certain to be higher, and output lower, than they would be under perfect competition.

The principal disadvantage, however, of monopoly is that consumers lose some of their freedom of choice, and the assortment of goods produced is not that desired by them. Under perfect competition it is the demand of consumers that determines what goods and how much of each shall be produced. By restricting output the monopolist prevents as large an amount of resources going into the production of his commodity, as consumers would wish, and so resources are forced into other forms of production which consumers consider to be less desirable. Under monopoly, prices are likely to be more stable than under perfect competition, but output is liable to fluctuate more, and so, therefore, is the level of employment.

So long as a number of firms are competing against each other to supply the market with a certain commodity, each firm has a strong incentive to make itself as efficient as possible. Each firm will readily adopt improved methods of production in order to try to push ahead of its rivals. Under monopoly this incentive is weakened, and if new inventions are costly to introduce there may be reluctance to abandon the older methods. Perhaps one of the chief drawbacks to nationalisation is the loss of this spur to efficiency.

(11) CONTROL OF MONOPOLY POWER

One of the chief problems that confronts a State wishing to maintain a free economy is how to prevent the exploitation of consumers by producers who possess some element of monopoly power. Labour has been protected by factory legislation and by trade unions, and nowadays there is probably a greater danger of the trade unions exploiting the rest of the community than of labour itself being exploited. Company law has been tightened up to regulate more effectually the activities of limited companies. Consumers, however, have never succeeded for long in organising themselves to protect their particular interests. In general, however, monopolists are disinclined to exercise their power to the full for fear of attracting State action against them. The following are some of the ways by which it might be possible to control monopoly.

(i) *Legal action against monopolies.* The American policy of declaring monopolies to be illegal was not particularly successful before 1914, although under the anti-trust laws the Standard Oil Company was broken up into sixteen smaller companies in 1911. More recently, however, the courts of the United States have vigorously attacked many undesirable monopolistic practices, including some of those indulged in by oligopolists, and the firms concerned have been compelled to cease these activities.

In 1948 a Monopolies and Restrictive Practices Commission was set up to inquire into the conditions of manufacture in Great Britain of a number of commodities. Altogether the Commission reported on the manufacture and distribution of over twenty commodities, including matches, electric lamps, motor-car tyres, linoleum and cathode-ray tubes used in television sets. It is of interest to note that the Act setting up the Commission defined a monopolist as a producer of at least one-third of the total output of a commodity. The power of the Commission was limited to reporting its findings to Parliament. Under the *Restrictive Trade Practices Act* (1956), however, five Restrictive Practices Courts were established to decide whether existing agreements among producers or distributors, all of which had to be reported to a Registrar, were in the public interest, and these courts have power to enforce their decisions. Any agreement found to be undesirable must be immediately dissolved. Since the passing of the Act the members of some trade associations, however, have made "open price" arrangements, the price-leader informs its rivals of the price that it intends to charge, and these other firms can then of their own volition decide to charge the same price if they so wish. This practice is as yet outside the jurisdiction of the courts. The *Resale Prices Act* (1964) encouraged competition by abolishing resale price maintenance except in cases specifically exempted by the Restrictive Practices Courts. In 1965 the practice developed of putting before the Monopolies Commission proposals for mergers that would give producers 30% or more of the total output of a commodity, and since then the Commission has refused to sanction more than one proposed merger.

Thus in both Great Britain and the United States a more effective war is now being waged against monopolists and oligopolists.

(ii) *Legal control*. When it has been recognised that some degree of monopoly is unavoidable, if wasteful competition is to be obviated, charges and profits have often been legally restricted. Canal and railway rates in Great Britain were at an early date made subject to Parliament's control. In the case of some monopolies—gas, electricity and local transport undertakings, for example, where these were operated by joint-stock companies—no increase in dividend was permitted unless at the same time they reduced their charges. Since 1931, when road passenger traffic was regulated, no changes in either service or fares have been allowed without the sanction of the Traffic Commissioners for the area.

(iii) *State or municipal operation*. Monopolies of the public-utility type have for long been considered to be best administered by local authorities or the State, the presumption being that neither of these authorities would exploit consumers. Most municipalities in Great Britain operate passenger transport services, and formerly many of them also owned their own electricity and gas undertakings until these services were nationalised. The postal service from the seventeenth century has been looked upon as an appropriate activity of the State, and the Post Office took over telegraph and telephone[1] business in 1897. When it was decided in 1933 to co-ordinate the various types of passenger transport serving London—omnibuses, tramways, underground railways—a public corporation, the London Passenger Transport Board was set up. In this country it was considered desirable too that broadcasting should be a monopoly, and though at first it was under the control of the British Broadcasting Company, it was eventually taken over by the British Broadcasting Corporation. The public corporation gives the State a measure of control through the periodic review of its Charter by Parliament. For its television service, however, the B.B.C. since 1954 has had a rival in the Independent Television Authority (I.T.A.).

(iv) *Taxation.* Suggestions have been made that monopolists should be subjected to some special form of taxation in order to encourage them to increase their output. The most ingenious of these suggestions is that a tax, inversely proportional to his output, should be imposed on every monopolist. If such a tax could be imposed it would prevent a monopolist increasing his profit by curtailing output. In practice, a tax of this kind would be very difficult—if not impossible—to operate. The effects of different kinds of taxes on the monopolist have already been considered.[2]

RECOMMENDATIONS FOR FURTHER READING

K. B. Boulding: *Economic Analysis*, Chapters 27 and 28.
G. J. Stigler: *The Theory of Price*, Chapters 11–15.
E. H. Chamberlin: *The Theory of Monopolistic Competition,* Chapters 3–6.
Joan Robinson: *Economics of Imperfect Competition*, Chapters 25 and 26.
D. Braithwaite and S. P. Dobbs: *The Distribution of Consumable Goods.*
M. Hall: *Distributive Trading.*

QUESTIONS

1. "Combination does not necessarily imply monopoly, nor does monopoly involve combination." Illustrate this statement by examining the several types of combinations of business units with which you are familiar. (R.S.A. Adv. Com.)

---

[1] Except the Hull telephone service.
[2] See above pp. 238–9.

2. Write a short essay on the main features of cartels, combines and trusts in industry and their advantages and disadvantages to the consumer. (L.C. Com. Econ.)

3. Distinguish with examples, between horizontal and vertical combination. (A.I.A.)

4. How does a Trust differ from a Cartel in structure and policy? (I.T.)

5. It has been suggested that Combines operate at the expense of the consumer. What do you understand by this statement, and do you consider it necessary to modify it in any way? (L.C. Com. C. & F.)

6. Discuss the use and limitations of advertisement as an aid to trade. (Exp.)

7. What is meant by imperfect competition? Distinguish any types of imperfect competition which are known to you. (C.I.S. Inter.)

8. In what ways may competition be "imperfect"? Are the consequences necessarily undesirable? (C.I.S. Inter.)

9. Explain briefly the major points of difference between "perfect" and "imperfect" competition. (C.I.S. Final.)

10. Discuss the differences between monopoly and competition, and compare the results of these systems. (C.C.S. Final.)

11. In what circumstances, if any, can price discrimination be justified? (C.I.S. Final.)

12. Why do monopolies arise? Discuss the possible causes of the emergence of monopolistic organisations, with special reference to the conditions in the United Kingdom. (G.E.C. Adv.)

13. What are the advantages and disadvantages in the practice of putting branded consumable goods upon the market? (Final Degree.)

14. "Resale price maintenance only serves to shelter the inefficient retailer from the salutary pressure of competition." Discuss. (Final Degree.)

15. "Monopolistic competition involves a less economical use of resources than perfect competition." Do you agree? (Final Degree.)

16. Why are monopolies considered to be harmful? Can they ever be beneficial? (Final Degree.)

17. Implicit collusion always converts oligopoly into monopoly." Discuss. (Final Degree.)

PART FIVE

THE NATIONAL INCOME AND ITS DISTRIBUTION

CHAPTER XVI

THE NATIONAL INCOME

I. PERSONAL INCOME AND NATIONAL INCOME

(1) TYPES OF INCOME

As a result of the co-operation of the factors of production during a particular period of time, a certain output of goods and services is achieved. Factors of production are generally paid for their services in money, these payments being variously known as rent, wages, interest and profit. It is tempting to regard these four payments as the rewards accruing to the four factors of production for their share in the work of production—rent to land, wages to labour, interest to capital and profits to entrepreneur. Unfortunately, this is too simple an arrangement. Wages are easily recognised as the particular reward of labour, but it is not nearly so easy to assign the other payments to appropriate factors. Rent is paid for the use of land, but there are often elements of rent both in wages and in profit, and it is not always easy to distinguish between interest and profit. All these four types of payment are, however, income, and all income is received by someone. The total income of a community depends, then, on the total volume of production—in fact, as will be shown shortly, it *is* the total volume of production. The purpose of this chapter is to consider the national income and its importance, and then in the chapters that follow to discuss how this total income is distributed among different sections of the community. In other words, these later chapters will be devoted to that branch of economics known as distribution.

If production is regarded from the point of view of the entrepreneur all payments made to factors are expenses of production—that is, the costs of all the goods and services produced. To the factors of production, however, these payments are income. Some of the factors of production are persons; others are inanimate things, such as most forms of capital. Payments, however, can be made only to persons, and not to inanimate objects. Payment is made for the services of a factor, and these may be personal services, such as those of labour or the entrepreneur, or impersonal services, such as those of land and capital, and in the case of impersonal services payment is made to the owners of the factors.

Income therefore is derived from two sources:

(i) the performing of personal services—work or organisation;
(ii) the ownership of factors providing impersonal services.

The term "property" is used for any impersonal thing that yields an income. The following diagram shows the different sources of income:

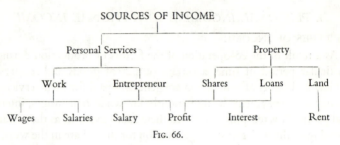

FIG. 66.

(2) INEQUALITY OF INCOME

Inequality of income can be attributed, then, to one of two causes: (i) differences in payments made for personal services; or (ii) differences in the amount of property possessed. A discussion of the causes of differences in wages in different occupations must be reserved for Chapter XVIII. Many people have only income of this kind; others derive considerable income from the ownership of different kinds of property. Incomes derived from the possession of property vary enormously, because property is very unequally distributed. Property of all kinds—land, buildings, shares in companies, Government Stock, etc.—can be acquired either by inheritance, or by saving, or in both these ways. It should be noted that it is not merely the possession of property that yields income; the owner receives payment because he allows someone else the use of his property, that is, he is paid for a service he renders. Large accumulations of property have been built up partly by inheritance and partly through saving, where successive generations of owners have aimed at adding to their possessions during their lifetime.

Before the growth of large-scale industry during the past hundred years the rate of accumulation was slow, for most property consisted of land and buildings, and openings for profitable investment were few. In England the system of inheritance, whereby all the landed property and most of the personalty were left to the eldest son, tended to increase inequality. The younger sons generally entered the professions or trade, and many of them—especially those who took up law or trade—saved enough in their lifetimes to purchase estates for themselves and found new landowning families. In countries where on the death of the father the property is shared among all the children there will be a more widespread ownership of property and less inequality. Industrial development has increased the possibility of building up a large accumulation of property in one's lifetime, and big fortunes have been made in many different types of production. In Great Britain some income from property is usual among even the lower-salaried grades of the middle classes and the better-paid artisans. Thrift, for long preached as a great virtue, is still practised by people within a wide range of income derived from work. Savings Certificates and balances in the Post Office and Trustee Savings Banks are widely held, and in the largest companies shareholders often number many thousands. The custom of home ownership has increased enormously in the last quarter of a century, and though much of such property is mortgaged with Building Societies for periods up to twenty years, the houses eventually become the property of the occupiers, and as such yield income—in this case notional—the rent that otherwise would have to be paid. The thrifty are not limited to any particular income group—just as spendthrifts are to be found among rich and poor alike—though, of course, the thrifty rich can save more than the thrifty poor. Inequality of income has, however, been reduced by steeply progressive income taxes, which make it difficult to accumulate large amounts of property by saving, and by heavy death duties which reduce the amount of property that can be acquired by inheritance.

(3) THE NATIONAL INCOME = THE VOLUME OF PRODUCTION

The terms "national income" and "volume of production" are simply alternative names for the same thing. For, as we shall see later (p. 521), the amount paid for a commodity really comprises a number of payments for the services undertaken in its production, and all payments become income to those who receive them. Consequently, the national income can be regarded either as the money value of all goods and services produced during a particular period—usually a year, or the sum of all personal incomes derived from economic activity during that time. A Census of Production records the quantity of ships, motor cars, sewing-machines, wireless sets, bedroom suites, carpets, worsted cloth, cotton goods, boots and shoes, wheat, oats, potatoes, jam, etc., produced in the country during a certain year; but it does not show how much medical and dental service, how much teaching, how many hours of entertainment and music have been provided. Even if it did show the total of services, as well as of goods, produced in the year, the total would still be a clumsy one, and not easily compared with that of other years.

A common denominator must therefore be found, and the money value of all these things provides an obvious unit of measurement, though by no means a perfect one, for money itself may change in value. Marshall defined national income as "the aggregate net product of, and the sole source of payment for, all the agents of production."[1] Sir John Hicks has given the following definition: "The national income consists of a collection of goods and services reduced to a common basis by being measured in terms of money,"[2]

The total volume of production is, then, expressed as a sum of money. For example, it was calculated in 1964 that the total volume of production of the United Kingdom was worth 26,452 million, that is to say, the total value of all the goods and services produced in this country in that year was £26,452 million. The total income of the producers of those goods and services, therefore, together must have been £26,452 million. The entrepreneurs received payment for the goods they were responsible for producing, out of these sums paid rent, wages and salaries, and interest on loans, keeping the balance of profits as their own reward. Those people who provided services were paid either in fees or salaries, and the value of their services was assessed at the amounts they received. For clarity, some complications have for the moment been omitted, but these will be considered shortly. It is evident, therefore, that the total volume of production and the total of all incomes are one and the same. In other words, the price paid for a commodity is equal to the sum of the payments to the factors of production that have assisted in its manufacture.

The calculation of the national income can consequently be approached either from the side of the output of goods or from the side of income. If full information were available, either method of calculation should yield the same result. A third approach is possible: from the side of consumption. Since income is either spent or saved, the total amount spent on consumers' goods, added to savings, should also be equal to the national income, provided there has been no hoarding.

(4) INCREASED INTEREST IN THE NATIONAL INCOME

Though economists from the time of Marshall onwards have given consideration to the national income, it is only comparatively recently that the study of its measurement and distribution has assumed a

---

[1] A. Marshall: *Principles of Economics*, VI, I, 10.
[2] J. R. Hicks: *The Social Framework*, Part IV.

prominent place in economics. This has been rendered possible because Governments have now begun to take more interest in the subject, for serious analysis and study were impossible until current statistics were available, the compilation of which was too vast a task for the resources of private institutions devoted to economic study. The British Government has established a permanent body known as the Central Statistical Office, which since 1941 has provided the material for the Government's annual White Paper on National Income and Expenditure. In the United States the National Bureau of Economic Research of the Department of Commerce fulfils a similar function. This matter has received most attention in the United States and in Great Britain, but many other countries are now interested in the subject, as also is the United Nations.

II. THE MEASUREMENT OF THE NATIONAL INCOME

(5) WHY MEASURE THE NATIONAL INCOME?

Why, then, is so much interest taken in the national income? In Chapter II we saw that the aim of production is to increase economic welfare. In the first place, economic welfare depends on the volume of production, for an increase in the volume of production will increase economic welfare, provided (i) that it does not increase inequality of income, and (ii) that it is not achieved at the cost of health. A reduction in inequality of income will generally increase economic welfare, unless it results in a fall in production. As an indication of economic progress, Marshall considered national income to be a more suitable measure than national wealth. "The money income, or inflow of wealth," he says, "gives a measure of a nation's prosperity, which, untrustworthy as it is, is yet in some respects better than that afforded by the money value of its stock of wealth."[1] An increase in the national income in real terms is an essential pre-requisite to a rise in the general standard of living of a people.

The fact that in this country the State began to measure the national income in 1941—at perhaps the greatest crisis in the nation's history—is some indication of the practical importance by that time attached to knowing the extent of the volume of production. It then became possible to see how much of production was being devoted to the war effort and how much to civilian needs. Since then it has become an important instrument of economic planning. Directly and indirectly

---

[1] A. Marshall: *Principles of Economics*, p. 80.

the public sector of the economy has been expanding, the State playing an ever more important rôle in the national economy. The acceptance by the State of responsibility for full employment has made it more than ever necessary for it to know the trend of business activity, and particularly the proportion of the national income devoted to investment. Nowadays one of the principal aims of economic policy of Governments throughout the world is to improve the standard of living of their people. In the first place, the standard of living of a people depends on the size of the national income, for clearly the greater the volume of production, the greater the quantity of goods and services available for distribution. An increase, therefore, in the national income makes possible a rise in a people's standard of living. A second influence on the standard of living is the way in which the national income is distributed, the less the inequality of individual incomes, the higher the general standard of living.

Governments, too, are concerned to promote economic growth. The rate at which total volume of production expands is generally taken as a measure of a country's economic progress. During the 1950s and 1960s the rate of economic growth in West Germany and Japan was very impressive, and there was a feeling in some quarters that Great Britain was lagging behind, as its rate of growth was much less.

(6) FACTORS DETERMINING THE NATIONAL INCOME

A number of influences determine whether a country shall have a large or small income. It is for the following reasons that one country has a larger national income than another.

(i) *The stock of factors of production.* The quantity and quality of a country's stock of the factors of production will be one of the most important influences on its national income. Land may be fertile or infertile, for reasons outside the control of the community. Climate and soil are the prime factors that determine what type of agriculture (if any) can be undertaken, for handicaps of climate can be overcome only to a limited extent. Irrigation can offset lack of rainfall; glasshouse production can mitigate a lack of heat; but the Sahara Desert is too vast to be treated in the one way, as the Canadian tundra is too vast for the other. Agricultural production may also vary quite considerably from one year to another, merely because of vagaries of the weather.

The quality of the labour will depend partly on the inborn intelligence of the people, though perhaps mainly on the quality of its education and training. The supply of labour must be large enough to make the best use of other factors, but too great a supply will mean smaller shares for all. In other words, the population should be near the optimum.

Capital can vary from simple, primitive tools to the most modern type of automated industrial plant. The extent of a country's stock of modern forms of capital is the most important influence on its total volume of production. The supply of factors in any country is limited, and whether or not the best use is made of them will depend on the entrepreneurial ability available, for only if the factors are combined in the optimum proportions will the maximum output be achieved.

The quantity and quality of factors of production vary enormously between one country and another.

(ii) *The state of technical knowledge.* A second influence on the national income is the state of technical knowledge in the country. Until the middle of the eighteenth century methods of production had remained substantially unchanged for many centuries, but since then technical progress has become ever more rapid, especially in the more economically advanced countries. In spite of the assistance given to the less-developed nations, there is a wide difference in the state of technical knowledge of the most advanced industrial countries as compared with the developing ones. The most recent development has been the introduction of automation, an important feature of which is the linking together of machines with automatic control. To speed up technical progress in Great Britain, the Government in 1964 established a Ministry of Technology to co-ordinate and encourage industrial research.

(iii) *Political stability.* If production is to be maintained at the highest level, political stability is essential. The development of many countries —for example, some of the South American Republics—has been hindered in the past by political instability. At some period of their history all countries have suffered setbacks to their economic progress on account of political instability resulting from wars and revolutions.

One country can be considered to be richer than another if its national income averaged per head of its population is greater. Such comparisons, however, are difficult, since each country calculates its national income in its own currency. Different peoples demand different assortments of goods, and in some countries people perform more services for themselves.

(7) SOME DIFFICULTIES OF MEASURING THE NATIONAL INCOME

Measurement of the national income is beset with difficulties:

(i) *Information is incomplete.* Although the Inland Revenue returns provide particulars of sources of income that is subject to Income Tax, and the Ministry of Labour has information on wages, there still remain some items that have to be estimated. Some income is not recorded, as for example when a joiner, electrician or plumber does a job in his spare time for a friend or neighbour.

(ii) *The danger of double counting.* The cost of raw materials and of finished goods must not both be counted, for that would mean that the cost of raw materials would be included twice. In reckoning the output of a firm the cost of materials purchased from other firms must be deducted. All services performed by one firm for another, including transport, insurance and banking, must therefore be excluded, as their cost is included in the price of the product.

(iii) *Unpaid services.* Only those goods and services for which payment is made are included. All those services that people do for themselves, or do gratuitously for others—a woman making her own clothes, or doing embroidery; a man painting his house or growing a few vegetables—have to be excluded. It is very difficult to know exactly where to draw the line between what to count and what to leave out, but the only practicable method is to exclude all unpaid employment. This method of surmounting the difficulty, however, produces some anomalies. The fewer services people do for themselves—that is, the greater the division of labour—the larger will be the national income, even if no increase in actual output results. If Jingle, a house-painter, attends to his own garden, and Trotter, a gardener, paints his own house, neither of these tasks will add anything to the national income. If, on the other hand, Jingle paints Trotter's house, and Trotter does some gardening for Jingle, the national income is increased by the charge each makes for the work he has done. Therefore, the greater the extent to which division of labour is carried—that is, the less people do for themselves—the greater will be the national income, even though the actual volume of production is the same in both cases. For this reason the national income of India—only about £27 per head in 1966—appears to be even lower than it actually is. If the Mersey Tunnel was freed from toll, or if a charge was made for using the Woolwich ferry, the national income would be affected, but clearly in neither case would there be any change in the volume of services provided.

(iv) *Depreciation.* If it is the *net* national income that is to be calculated, then the amount set aside for replacing worn-out or out-of-date fixed capital assets must be deducted from the total. If the national income is being considered in terms of volume of production the reasonableness of this is at once clear, for the production, for example, of motor lorries to replace vehicles that are no longer fit for service obviously does not increase the total stock of such vehicles. However, for the sake of uniformity with other countries the British White Paper on National Income and Expenditure shows the *Gross* National Product.

(v) *Housing.* If Cratchit lives in a house for which he pays his landlord a rent of £52 per annum this rent is clearly income to the landlord; it will not, of course, be net income, for out of it the cost of repairs to the property will have to be met. If Cratchit buys this house he will no longer pay rent—at least, not to some other person. This rent payable to himself is known as notional income. For purposes of calculating the national income it is justifiable, therefore, to credit Cratchit with an addition to his income equal to the rent of the house in which he lives as owner-occupier. In the British White Paper on National Income and Expenditure this item is included under the heading, Dwelling-houses; newly-built houses come under the heading, Building.

(vi) *Public income and expenditure.* Government expenditure falls into three main categories: (a) the maintenance of internal law and order and external defence; (b) the provision of social services—education, medical and dental services and social security payments; and (c) the payment of interest on the National Debt. Part of the expenditure in category (b) falls on local authorities, as also does some of the expenditure of an entirely local character, as, for example, street lighting and the upkeep of parks. Government income is principally derived from direct taxes, such as income tax, and indirect taxes, such as purchase tax; Local Authorities raise revenue by levying rates. State activity may also include the operation of nationalised industries, some of which may be a cost to the tax-payer. Much of Government expenditure presents no difficulty if it is considered as a collective payment by the Government on behalf of tax-payers for the various services provided, but from the tax-payers' point of view it becomes compulsory consumption. The National Debt payment, however, is interest on a debt created in the past, which tax-payers pay to holders of Government Stock. Since it is merely a transfer of income from one group of people to another, income from this source must not be included in addition to the full incomes of those who paid it, otherwise there will be double counting. Similarly, social-security payments for sickness, etc., are also merely transfers of income from one group of people to another. Such transfer income must not be counted twice.

Indirect taxes, such as purchase tax and duties on beer and tobacco, are generally deducted from the market prices of the commodities on which they are levied, in order to show output at factor cost, that is, the cost in terms of the payments to the factors of production used in their manufacture.

(vii) *Foreign payments.* There are people in this country who receive income from abroad in the form of dividends from shares in foreign enterprises, or interest payments on foreign Government Stocks; and also there are foreigners who receive dividends and interest from their investments in this country or who send gifts to relatives abroad or make use of this country's shipping, banking and insurance facilities, and therefore have to pay for them; or again, the Government may receive interest payments for loans made in the past to foreign countries, or foreign tourists may come to Great Britain and spend money on hotel accommodation and transport. From all these sources income may come from abroad, or for any one or all of these reasons payments may have to be made to foreign countries, but to some extent payments and receipts will offset one another. These items must therefore be added to (or subtracted from) internal income. In calculating the national income of a country, only its net income from abroad (total receipts less total payments) will be included.

(viii) *Inventory revaluation.* The term *inventory* is used in the British White Paper on National Income and Expenditure, but more generally used in the United States, denotes the value of stocks and work in progress at the end of the year, as shown in a firm's balance sheet. In the trading account compiled to enable the firm's profit to be calculated the opening and closing stocks are the inventories of the current and preceding years. If prices rise during the year gross profit on stocks held will increase, but the replacement cost of such stocks will also rise. Business profits include any such gains, but in the calculation of the gross national product, for national-income purposes, it is more useful to show this item separately and make the necessary adjustment for it.

(ix) *Changes in the value of money.* Money is a poor measuring rod, since its own value is liable to change, but it is, nevertheless, the only common denominator we possess for adding together the heterogeneous mass of goods and services that comprise the national income. Nevertheless, the total national income in terms of money has little meaning. Comparison between one year and another is impossible unless the relative value of money at the two dates is known. To say that for Great Britain the national income in 1913 was £1,968 million, that in 1938 it was £5,175 million and in 1964 £26,452 million gives no indication of whether the *real* income was greater in 1913 or 1938, or in 1938 or 1964. In order to compare real income in these two years it is necessary to know that £1 in 1913 would buy approximately what £5 would buy in 1964. Even so, the comparison may not be very accurate, for the construction of index-numbers of prices is a problem with its own peculiar difficulties, as will be seen later. Nevertheless, the *Blue Book on National Income and Expenditure*, published by H.M. Stationery Office, now includes a table showing total expenditure of consumers (i) at current prices, (ii) in terms of prices ruling in a selected base year, so that comparison between different years becomes possible (see Table XXXVII, p. 278).

III. THE DISTRIBUTION OF THE NATIONAL INCOME

(8) THE WHITE PAPER ON NATIONAL INCOME

Let us now take a closer look at the White Paper on National Income and Expenditure of the United Kingdom presented to Parliament annually since 1941, usually in March, and the more detailed Blue Book, published each year in September. The White Paper and the Blue Book give the money value of the total production of goods and services for the previous year at factor cost. This is known as the gross national product, which in 1964 was made up as follows:

TABLE XXXIII

Gross National Product

Product or service	1964	196–*
	£ million	£ million
Goods and services produced by		
Agriculture, forestry and fishing . . .	1,019	
Manufacturing	10,114	
Mining and quarrying	741	
Building and construction	1,966	
Transport	1,851	
Distribution	3,434	
Insurance, banking and finance . .	944	
Public utilities	936	
Dwelling houses	1,172	
Services provided by public authorities .	2,917	
Other services	1,592	
Net income from abroad . . .	−234	
NATIONAL INCOME	26,452	

* The reader is recommended to complete this column with the latest figures available.

The White Paper also shows the national income as the total of all forms of income derived from economic activity (Table XXXIV).

Employers' insurance contributions appear in the table because it is now general practice to regard them as part of employees' incomes deducted at source. Whether the national income is calculated as the total volume of production or the total of all incomes, it is clear now that it must yield the same total. The national income and the volume of production are indeed the same thing. It is clear that this may be so, since what is paid by a consumer for a commodity becomes income to all those who have had a share in its production. Every commodity, it is said, represents merely a collection of the services of those who have obtained the raw material, changed its form in some way, transported and marketed it at the wholesale and retail stages.

TABLE XXXIV

National Income

Type of income	1964	196–†
	£ million	£ million
Wages	10,700	
Salaries	6,965	
Pay in cash and kind of the Forces	455	
Employers' insurance contributions	1,457	
Professional earnings	405	
Income from farming	562	
Profits of other sole traders and partnerships* . .	1,370	
Profits of companies*	2,900	
Profits of public enterprises*	700	
Rent of land and buildings	1,172	
Net income from abroad	−234	
NATIONAL INCOME	26,452	

* Including depreciation.   † For the latest figures.

A third method of calculating the national income is to take the sum of all expenditure personal and public (Table XXXV).

Finally, it becomes possible to allocate the national income among the factors of production (Table XXXVI). From this it can be seen that in 1964 70% of the national income went to labour, 4% to land and 26% to capital and the entrepreneurial factor.

In 1964 the national income, expressed as an average per head of the population, was £533 for the United Kingdom, over £1080 for the United States and about £240 for Russia. The only possible basis on which such comparisons can be made is to average the national income per head of the population. But before that can be done the total income for one country has to be recalculated in terms of the currency of the other at the rate of exchange current at the time, and this may not necessarily give a very accurate indication of the relative internal value of the two currencies.

If national income figures are used as a basis for comparing standards of living in different countries—or even of the same country at differ-

TABLE XXXV

Expenditure

	1964	196–
	£ million	£ million
Personal consumption:		
Food	5,557	
Clothing	1,919	
Rent and rates; fuel and light.	3,234	
Alcoholic drink	1,317	
Tobacco	1,344	
Household goods	2,454	
Books, newspapers, etc.	312	
Cars and motor-cycles	771	
Travel	691	
Entertainment	338	
Other goods and services	3,447	
Total personal consumption	21,334	
Expenditure of public authorities	5,410	
Gross domestic capital formation	3,672	
Subsidies	520	
Net income from abroad	−234	
	30,702	
Deduction:		
Indirect taxes on goods and services	4,250	
Gross national expenditure at factor cost	26,452	

TABLE XXXVI

Allocation of the National Income to Factors

	1964	196–	Factor
	£ million	£ million	
Wages	17,665		Labour
Profit and interest	7,849		Capital and entrepreneur
Rent	1,172		Land
Net income from abroad	−234		
	26,452		

ent periods of time—allowance must be made for (i) price changes; (ii) differences in the size of the population; (iii) the rate of exchange between the different currencies; (iv) the amount of production for such things as armaments; (v) the amount of unpaid work undertaken by the people for themselves; (vi) how the national income is distributed among the people, that is, whether there is great inequality or not.

Table **XXXVII** shows the national income in recent years.

TABLE XXXVII

The National Income

(i) No allowance for changes of prices

Year	£ million	Date	£ million
1870	929	1958	18,584
1910	2,062	1960	20,835
1938	5,175	1961	22,270
1946	8,783	1962	23,211
1950	10,792	1963	24,680
1952	14,005	1964	26,450
1954	14,597	1965	
1956	16,837		

(ii) Calculated in terms of 1958 prices

Year	£ million
1958	18,584
1960	20,077
1962	21,271
1964	22,730
1966	

These tables show that between 1958 and 1964 the national income increased in real terms by 22½%, whereas in money terms the increase was 42½%.

(9) SOCIAL AND PRIVATE NET PRODUCT

A. C. Pigou[1] drew a distinction between what he called social and private net product. The national income shows the value of the goods and services produced during a certain year, but it takes no account of any harmful effects of production. There are some things the production of which adds to the national income, but which at the same time create a dis-service. The net social product might therefore be defined as the private net product *less* the value of any disservices entailed in its production.

In this category might be placed the manufacture of intoxicants, for if it can be shown that the consumption of intoxicants leads to an increase in crime, thereby creating additional expense to the State for the maintenance of prisons and larger police forces, social welfare would be increased if the production of such commodities were curtailed. The production of cheap gin in London in the early eighteenth century increased the private net product but not the social net product, one-

[1] A. C. Pigou, *Economics of Welfare*.

fifth of the deaths occurring in London at that time being attributed to excessive consumption of gin.[1]

All the so-called "wastes" of imperfect or monopolistic competition increase the private net product by amounts greater than the social net product. Especially is this true of competitive advertising, for its effect is merely to persuade people to buy one thing instead of another, nothing being added to the total volume of goods and services produced.

Profits from organised gambling, such as the running of football pools and bookmakers' business, add to the private but not to the social net product.

The expansion of the social net product owes a great deal to scientific research, but the application of research to new means of destruction adds nothing to the social net product.

All people who live in industrial towns have to suffer to a greater or lesser degree from the effects of an atmosphere heavily laden with smoke and other impurities. Laundry bills are heavier and the sickness rate is higher in such places than in more salubrious districts. If the atmosphere is also polluted with chemical impurities, as it is near chemical or tin-plate works, curtains and other household fabrics may deteriorate more rapidly than elsewhere. From the private net product a deduction to cover these disservices must be made in order to obtain the social net product.

Some people believe that the employment of married women in industry reduces the social net product, as it may lead to neglect of children, though this loss may be reduced by setting up day nurseries.

Similarly, the social net product will exceed the private net product wherever the production of a commodity or the provision of a service is conducive to healthier conditions. Examples of such things are the provision of parks and other open spaces in large towns, the substitution of electric power for coal, or the extension of "clean air" zones in the larger towns.

RECOMMENDATIONS FOR FURTHER READING

J. R. Hicks: *The Social Framework*, Part IV.
A. C. Pigou: *The Economics of Welfare*, Part II, Chapter 8.
White Paper on National Income (annual).
Blue Book on National Income (H.M.S.O.).

QUESTIONS

1. What do you understand by the National Income? How is it measured? (C.C.S. Final.)

[1] G. M. Trevelyan, *English Social History*, Chapter II.

2. How can economic growth be assisted? (C.I.S. Final.)

3. Compare any two ways of measuring the National Income. (C.I.S. Final.)

4. What do you understand by the income of (*a*) an individual and (*b*) a nation? (C.I.S. Final.)

5. What main economic factors affect the standard of living? (I.B.)

6. What is meant by the real national income? What are the main difficulties involved in a comparison of the real national income today with that of twenty-five years ago? (B.S. Final.)

7. Define the National Income, distinguishing between the different senses in which the term can be used. Indicate any recent improvement in National Income Statistics for the United Kingdom with which you are familiar. (C.I.S. Final.)

8. "The national income consists of a collection of goods and services reduced to a common basis by being measured in terms of money." Comment upon this statement and discuss the view that the national income provides the best single measure of a nation's economic progress. (I.B.)

9. Account for the rise in National Income since 1939. (G.C.E. Adv.)

10. Why is the National Income per head higher in the United Kingdom than it is in Italy or Greece? (G.C.E. Adv.)

11. Describe the methods of calculating the national income. How far can the national income be used as a measure of economic growth? (I.B.)

12. The National Income of the United Kingdom was £13,711 million in 1953 and £24,212 million in 1963. Does this mean that either the country as a whole or each individual in it was better off in 1963 than in 1953? What further information would you require to study this question fully? (C.C.S. Inter.)

13. Explain what is meant by: (*a*) money national income; (*b*) real national income. (G.C.E. Adv.)

14. How has real national income per head changed in the United Kingdom in the past thirty years? What do you consider to be the chief causes of this change? (G.C.E. Adv.)

15. "The standard of living in country A is twice as high as in country B." Discuss the conceptual and practical difficulties involved in this statement. (Final Degree.)

16. What factors will influence the possibility of doubling the standard of living in the United Kingdom during the next twenty-five years? (Final Degree.)

CHAPTER XVII

THE THEORY OF DISTRIBUTION

I. THE MARGINAL PRODUCTIVITY THEORY

(1) THE FACTOR MARKET

We have now to consider what determines the share of the national income received by labour and the owners of the other factors of production. In the markets for consumers' goods prices are determined by the interaction of the forces of supply and demand. This problem of pricing has already been considered. The marginal analysis was used to explain the bases upon which supply and demand are founded, marginal utility underlying demand, and the concepts of marginal revenue and marginal cost being employed to determine supply. These same tools of economic analysis can be applied also to the pricing of the factors of production. The entrepreneur's costs consist of payments made for the services of various factors, the quantity of each factor he employs depending largely on its price. Instead of the term, price, for the payments made to factors of production, the terms rent, wages, interest and profit, are used. Demand in the market for consumers' goods is the demand of consumers; demand in the factor market is the demand of entrepreneurs for the services of factors of production. The basis of demand in the market for consumers' goods is the marginal utility of the commodity to consumers in the market; the basis of demand in the factor market is the marginal productivity of the various factors to the entrepreneurs. The demand for factors, however, is a derived demand, being derived from the demand for the commodities in the production of which they are employed.

(2) THE MARGINAL PRODUCTIVITY OF A FACTOR

Marginal productivity is similar to the other marginal concepts previously considered. The marginal product of any factor is the addition to output and income[1] of the entrepreneur arising from the employment of an additional unit of that factor. If perfect competition is assumed a large output can be sold at the same price as a small output, and so if the employment of one more man in an enterprise results in the production in a week of (say) fifteen units of a commodity that can

---

[1] The increase in income is sometimes called marginal *revenue* productivity to distinguish it from an increase in output (marginal *physical* productivity).

be sold for £1 each, then the marginal productivity of the factor, labour, in this enterprise is £15 per week. The employment of more men will reduce the marginal productivity of labour in exactly the same way that an increase in a consumer's supply of a commodity reduces its marginal utility to him. The more labour (or any other factor) the entrepreneur employs, the lower will be the marginal productivity of that factor. The following table shows the marginal productivity of labour when different numbers of men are employed:

Table XXXVIII

The Marginal Productivity of Labour

Price = £1 per unit

Number of men	Units of output	Total revenue	Marginal productivity (output)	Marginal productivity (income to firm)
40	589	£589	—	—
41	604	£604	15	£15
42	617	£617	13	£13
43	629	£629	12	£12
44	640	£640	11	£11
45	649	£649	9	£9

When forty-one men are employed, the marginal physical productivity of labour is fifteen units of the commodity and the marginal revenue productivity is £15. If forty-two men are employed, marginal productivity falls to thirteen units, or £13. How much a consumer will buy of a commodity depends on its price, more being bought the lower the price, so that the demand curve for the commodity slopes downwards. Similarly, how much labour the entrepreneur in the above example will employ will depend on the price—that is, wages—of labour. If he has to pay labour a wage of £11 per week he will employ forty-four men, but if the wage is £15 per week he will employ only forty-one men, since he will never pay more for a factor—whether it be land, labour or capital—than the value of its marginal product. It is obvious that this must be so. If he paid more than this his net revenue would be less. For example, if he already employs forty-four men, and is considering the employment of an additional man, he will not pay him more than £9, that being the value of the marginal product. If he were to pay more his total profit would be less than before.

Under perfect competition then, according to this theory, no factor will receive more than the value of its marginal product, and in fact the price paid by the entrepreneur will be equal to its marginal productivity. A similar demonstration to the above can be made to show that the price paid for land or capital will be equal to the value of its marginal product. A fall in the price of any factor will increase entrepreneurs' demand for it, just as a rise in the price of a factor will decrease entrepreneurs' demand for it. This line of reasoning formerly led economists to believe that employment varied inversely with wages, unemployment being the result of wages being too high, but Lord Keynes disagreed with this view. In any case, the theory applies only to perfect competition, and at most marginal productivity influences only the demand for a factor; the influence of supply must also be taken into account when the determination of a factor's price is being considered.

The marginal productivity theory has been subjected to much criticism. The concept is highly theoretical, since the employment of one more unit of a factor may be impossible, so that in practice the value of its marginal unit cannot be calculated.

II. THE SUPPLY OF AND THE DEMAND FOR FACTORS OF PRODUCTION

(3) THE DEMAND FOR FACTORS

The demand for factors is a derived demand. The demand for the services of factors of production is not due to the factors being desired for their own sake. Factors of production are required only for the production of other goods and services, and it is the demand for these other goods which determines the strength of the demand for the factors used to produce them. Land is not wanted for itself, but merely as a site where some form of production can be carried on—for a factory, shop or house, road or railway, or on which to grow crops or rear animals. The demand for labour is derived from the demand for things made in factories or grown on the land and from the demand for commercial and direct services, such as those provided by the medical and legal professions. The various forms that capital takes—factory buildings, machinery, raw materials, etc.—are obviously not wanted for their own sake, but only because of the demand for things they help to produce. Since production takes place in anticipation of demand, the demand for factors of production in the present will depend on the anticipated future demand for the commodities in the production of which they are to be employed.

(4) INFLUENCES ON THE ELASTICITY OF DEMAND FOR FACTORS

Three important influences on the elasticity of demand for factors of production can be distinguished:

(i) *The elasticity of demand for the final product.* By elasticity of demand for factors is meant the response of demand for their services to changes in their prices. The demand for a factor will be elastic if a slight fall in its price results in a large increase in its employment. Since the demand for factors is a derived demand, the elasticity of demand for the commodity, for the production of which the factors are required, will determine the elasticity of demand for the factors. If the demand for the commodity is elastic, then the demand for the factors required in its manufacture will be elastic; if the demand for the commodity is inelastic the demand for the factors also will be inelastic. For example, fluctuations in employment will be greatest in those occupations where the labour is engaged in the production of commodities for which there is an elastic demand.

(ii) *The amount of the factor required.* A second influence on the elasticity of demand for factors is the extent to which a factor is required in a particular form of production. If a factor plays only a small part—that is, if its payment forms only a small percentage of the total cost of producing a commodity—the demand for that factor will be fairly inelastic. For example, the cost of building an ocean liner will not be appreciably affected by the price of chronometers, and so the demand for chronometers and the factors required to make them is likely to be fairly inelastic.

(iii) *Substitutability between factors.* The greater the ease with which factors can be substituted for another, the more elastic is likely to be the demand for them, for a slight rise in the price of one factor will result in more of the alternative factor being employed. High wages may result in less labour and more machinery being employed if the work is of a kind that can be done by machinery. Or if machinery becomes relatively dear more labour may be employed. The more specific the factor, however, the more inelastic will be the demand for it.

(5) THE SUPPLY OF FACTORS

Consider now some of the influences on the supply of factors of production:

(i) *Land.* The supply of commodities depends on their cost of production, and so the higher the price, the larger the quantity that will be put on to the market. On the supply side it is more difficult to carry the analogy of the commodities market into the factor market. Land, for instance, has been described as a "gift of Nature," and as such it has no cost of production. Though the total supply of land is more or less fixed, the supply for a particular purpose is rarely fixed. The total available supply of land in England amounts to 50,874 square miles, and this is distributed among a variety of uses (Table XXXIX). Although the total area has varied little over the past 150 years, that given up to permanent pasture has greatly increased during the period, at the expense of land devoted to arable farming. The expansion of large cities, their suburbs encroaching more and more upon the countryside, the building of new towns, the construction of motorways with their huge intersections and junctions, other wide main roads with dual carriageways, and the building of large airports have all taken

TABLE XXXIX

Land Utilisation in England

Use	Per cent of total
Woods and plantations	5
Rough grazing	11
Permanent pasture	43
Arable land	26
Other (including urban) land . . .	15

land from other uses, a not inconsiderable amount having previously been good farm-land. In the past much woodland has been cleared, and more recently the Forestry Commission has undertaken the planting of trees. Variations in the distribution of crops on the arable land are also possible, less grain being grown and more root crops produced, or vice versa. Thus there are often many competing uses for land, and though a high price cannot call more land into existence, the offer of a high price for land for a particular use will increase the supply coming into the market for that purpose. Nevertheless, it has to be recognised that the supply of some kinds of land is strictly limited, as for example the number of sites facing on to the main street in a city centre; in this case a high price cannot call forth an increased supply.

(ii) *Labour.* With regard to the supply of labour, it is doubtful whether high wages will increase the total supply, though the early economists thought that any rise in wages above subsistence level would inevitably lead to an increase in population by reducing deaths from malnutrition. High wages may, however, lead to earlier marriages, and even if the average size of family remains unchanged, the shortening of the period between generations will increase total supply.

As with land, there are many competing demands for labour, and high wages in one occupation will cause more labour to seek employment there. It requires no real extension of the meaning of words to apply the term *cost of production* to labour. Even if no special training is required, children have to be kept at school at least until the statutory leaving age, and though family allowances, cheap or free milk and school meals, free education and maintenance grants have reduced the cost somewhat, the bringing up of a family still involves considerable expense. Where special training is required, especially if this entails a university education, membership of an Inn of Court or a long period as an articled clerk, with little or no remuneration, the cost of production of such labour may be very heavy. The supply of a particular type of labour can be increased in either of two ways: more workers may be drawn away from other occupations, or people not previously working —for example, married women and men who had retired—drawn into employment; or the number of hours worked by each person may be increased.

(iii) *Capital.* The supply of capital presents little difficulty because, like consumer goods, capital goods have to be made by the ordinary processes of production, and so generally the higher the price, the greater the supply that will be forthcoming. A change in costs of production will affect the quantity supplied at each price. The basis of supply in this case is saving, for without saving in some form there can be no production of capital goods at all.

(6) ELASTICITY OF SUPPLY OF FACTORS

The elasticity of supply of a factor of production means the responsiveness of its supply to changes in price. The more specific the factor, the more inelastic will be its supply, for in the short period the supply of most specific factors cannot be increased, though the supply of some factors may be fixed in both short and long periods. Let us consider each factor of production in turn:

(i) *Land.* An increase in the demand for milk will raise the price of milk, and the higher price will call forth a bigger supply. To increase the supply of milk more dairy cattle and grazing land will be required, and to bring this about will take time. The supply of grazing land may be fairly elastic in the long period, for other farm-land can be turned over to grass. It would not be so easy, however, to increase the supply of some kinds of fruit or rubber, for several years must elapse (five in the case of rubber) before new trees begin to yield any return. No price, however high, can increase the total frontage for shop sites in London's Bond Street or Regent Street.

(ii) *Labour.* Two things influence the elasticity of labour: its occupational specificity and its geographical mobility. The longer the period of training, the more specific the labour becomes, and this not only causes a period to elapse before supply can adjust itself to a higher price, but the possibility that price may fall again during the period of training will tend to check the number of new entrants. It may be, too, that the number of new entrants is limited. In some professions this occurs when members are restricted in the number of articled clerks they may employ. Or numbers may be limited by the accommodation available in the training establishments. Only very slowly has the supply of university graduates been increased in spite of a great increase in the demand for them, since to do so required the establishment of many new universities. Where special aptitude is required, an increase in supply is even more difficult to bring about. Similarly, where labour is specific, a fall in wages does not quickly lead to a reduction of supply.

Even if the work is not highly specific, men become less mobile between occupations as they become older. This is a serious problem in the case of declining industries; men who have spent their lives in one occupation are too old, or may be too obstinate, to train for another. The older coachmen clung to the roads in the early nineteenth century, though it was plain to everyone else that the railways had sounded the death-knell of the coach. A hundred years later, when motor buses replaced trams, some of the older tram-drivers were too old to learn to drive motor omnibuses, and were often reluctantly compelled to accept other jobs.

Though wages may be higher in one area than another, labour is often unwilling to move. Further, it is not always true that the higher the wage, the more hours the worker is prepared to work. The marginal utility of leisure increases steeply as the working day lengthens, and if the work is unpleasant, the higher the wage per hour, the fewer the number of hours the worker may be willing to work. Absenteeism increases in many occupations as the wage rate increases. This provides an example of what is sometimes called "the regressive supply curve." It shows that after a certain point the higher wage calls forth a smaller supply in terms of the number of hours worked (Fig. 67).

The vertical scale represents the wage rate per hour, increasing from O towards Y; the horizontal scale represents the number of hours the worker is willing to work, increasing from O to X. At a wage OP he is willing to work OH hours; at any lower wage he is willing to work only for a shorter period; if, however, his wages rise above OP his willingness to work again declines, and at the wage OP^1 he would work only OH^1 hours.

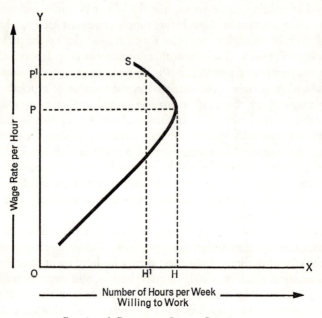

FIG. 67.—A REGRESSIVE SUPPLY CURVE.

(iii) *Capital.* With capital, too, its elasticity of supply depends to a certain extent on its specificity, though in most cases a rise in the price of capital will increase the amount produced. In the case of a simple machine, an increase in supply may be brought about very quickly— that is, its supply will be elastic. For a raw material such as flax a longer period will be required to increase supply; for a raw material such as wool it may take even longer. In the case of a very large and costly unit of capital, such as a blast-furnace or an ocean liner, a rise in price will not immediately result in an increase in supply. Indeed, it may require a very steep rise in price, maintained over a considerable period, to bring about an increase in supply in such cases.

(7) SUPPLY AND DEMAND CURVES FOR FACTORS

It thus becomes possible to construct supply and demand curves for factors of production. The intersection of the supply and demand curves for any factor, as in the case of a commodity, gives the equilibrium position at which supply equals demand, and shows the amount of the factor supplied at the equilibrium price. For example, if the

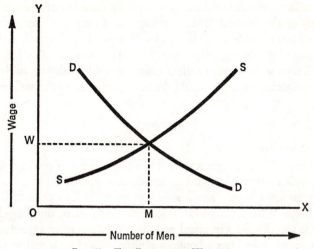

FIG. 68.—THE EQUILIBRIUM WAGE.

supply and demand curves for a particular type of labour are as shown in Fig. 68 it means at the wage *OW* the number of men willing to undertake this kind of work will be *OM*. The steeper the supply curve—that is, the more inelastic the supply—the smaller the difference in the number of men employed at different levels of wages.

The effect of changes in supply or demand can be shown by inserting a second supply or demand curve. An increase in the demand for this kind of labour would therefore result in more men being employed, and at a higher wage than before.

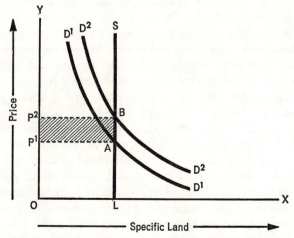

FIG. 69.—CHANGE IN DEMAND FOR A FACTOR IN FIXED SUPPLY.

Similar diagrams could be drawn to show the effect of changes in the supply or the demand for land or capital. If supply is fixed, as in the case of some urban sites, the price will depend on demand, a change in demand producing a very considerable rise in price (Fig. 69).

OL represents supply of sites. Under the old conditions of demand the equilibrium price was OP^1; the new equilibrium price will be OP^2.

III. RENT

(8) ECONOMIC RENT

Since rent is no longer restricted to a single factor of production, it is appropriate to consider it in a general chapter on distribution. In everyday speech the word "rent" is used to mean the hire price of land or buildings. When a person hires a car or a television, or anything else, he has the use of it for a specified period on payment of an agreed sum of money; when he hires a house or a piece of land he is said to rent it, and the periodic payment is termed rent. In the ordinary sense, then, rent is merely a price for the use of the services of a factor of production, land, or land together with capital (buildings), paid by the tenant to the owner. Rent, as the hire price of land, however also includes interest on capital.

The early economists restricted the term rent to land, but it is now used in relation to any factor. It has, too, been given a more precise connotation. Rent can be defined in slightly different ways, but its main characteristic is that it is a surplus, that is, additional income, accruing to a factor which was not foreseen when the factor entered that line of production. One form of the definition of economic rent comes from the economist Pareto, who considered rent to be the surplus received by any factor of production above its opportunity cost—that is, any surplus over and above what was necessary to keep that factor in its present employment. Rents can therefore be received by labour, capital or the entrepreneur, as well as by land.

Consider the demand schedule for a certain type of labour given in Table XL. The higher the wage, the more labour will offer itself for employment. If the wage offered is 3s. per hour only fifty men offer themselves for employment; at 3s. 6d. seventy men offer themselves; at 4s. a hundred men are willing to do this kind of work, and so on. Suppose now that the actual wage agreed upon is 5s. 6d. per hour. At this wage three hundred and eighty men are available for employment, and although two hundred and fifty men would have accepted a lower wage, 5s. 6d. per hour must be paid to all. Some men, therefore, will receive more than is necessary to keep them in that particular kind of employment, and so part of the wages can be considered to be economic rent. Fifty of these men will be paid at the rate of 5s. 6d. although willing to work for 3s., and so their remuneration really consists of 3s. wage, plus 2s. 6d. rent. In this sense most labour receives

TABLE XL

A Demand Schedule for Labour

Wage offered per hour	Number of men offering their services
3s.	50
3s. 6d.	70
4s.	100
4s. 6d.	160
5s.	250
5s. 6d.	380
6s.	540

wages and rent as payment for its services. The payment of this labour force will be made up as follows:

TABLE XLI

Rent in Wages

Number of men	Per hour		Payment received
	Wages	Rent	
50	3s.	2s. 6d.	5s. 6d.
20	3s. 6d.	2s.	5s. 6d.
30	4s.	1s. 6d.	5s. 6d.
60	4s. 6d.	1s.	5s. 6d.
90	5s.	6d.	5s. 6d.
130	5s. 6d.	—	5s. 6d.
380			

Transfer earnings. The more difficult it is for a factor to secure alternative employment—that is, the more specific it is—the less it will be necessary to pay it in order to retain its services, once it has been put to a particular use. For example, a blast-furnace cannot be used for any other purpose other than that for which it was originally intended, and so in one sense its entire earnings can be considered to be rent. The amount that a factor could earn in its best-paid alternative employment is sometimes known as its *transfer earnings.* Any payment in excess of this amount is a surplus above what is necessary to retain the factor in its best-paid employment, and so is a rent. In the above example, to obtain the services of three hundred and eighty men it was necessary to offer 5s. 6d. per hour. If this type of employment were not available some of them might be able to obtain alternative employment at 5s. 4d. per hour, others at 4s. 8d. per hour, etc., and so another table might be constructed to show how much of their remuneration is rent, as shown by their transfer earnings:

TABLE XLII

Transfer Earnings and Rent

Number of men	Transfer earnings	Rent	Payment received
80	5s. 4d.	2d.	5s. 6d.
180	4s. 8d.	10d.	5s. 6d.
90	4s.	1s. 6d.	5s. 6d.
30	3s. 4d.	2s. 2d.	5s. 6d.
380			

The more specific the factor, the greater the proportion of its earnings that consist of rent.

(9) RENT, PRICE AND COST OF PRODUCTION

A test to discover whether the earnings of a factor contain rent or not is to answer the question: does this extra payment arise *because* higher prices are being offered, or does it *cause* prices to be higher? Rent-income *results from* the high price of the product or service, and does not *cause* the high price. The rent of a piece of land depends on the price of the product of the land; if the rent of agricultural land is high it is because the price of the crop grown on the land is high, and the price of the crop will be high if the demand for it is strong. If the price of the product is high, then the price of the land will be high. Similarly, the rent of city sites is high because the demand for them is high. If there was a vacant site near the centre of a large city there might be competition to acquire it for a department store, a cinema, an hotel or an office block. If each firm made a bid for it the size of the bid would depend on each firm's estimate of what its customers and clients would be willing to pay. If eventually the site were to be used for an hotel the charges for hotel accommodation will be high, not because of the high rent, but the other way round, because of the high demand for hotel accommodation in that locality. Therefore it is the fact that people are prepared to pay high charges for hotel accommodation on that site that makes the rent of that site high.

An entrepreneur who requires the services of a specific factor of production, the supply of which cannot easily be increased, will have to pay a scarcity price or rent if he wishes to employ it. To the entrepreneur, of course, such rent payments form part of his costs of production. But if he were relieved of the payment of rent the price of the product would not fall because, owing to the scarcity of the factor, supply could not easily be increased, and price in the short period is determined principally by demand.

(10) HOW RENTS ARISE

It may perhaps be thought that rent as considered above is not a very useful concept. Rent can, however, be defined in terms of its origin. Rent can be said to be the surplus accruing to any factor of production, the supply of which cannot easily be increased, and arises from an increase in the demand for the services of that factor. Rent is, then, the result of dynamic or changing conditions; and under perfect competition it would not persist for long. It can be seen, therefore, why rent was formerly restricted to land, for land is a factor some kinds of which are permanently fixed in supply. The number of corner sites at the intersection of the two principal shopping streets in a town is definitely limited to four. With the development of the town the demand for these sites will increase and the price to be paid for their use will rise. Any increase in the earnings of such land is due to its scarcity and the impossibility of increasing its supply in response to an increase in demand.

Consider the diagram (Fig. 69) on page 289. This shows the effect of a change in demand on the price of a factor, the supply of which is fixed. Before the increase in demand took place the factor's income was represented by the rectangle OP^1AL; as a result of the increased demand for it the factor's income became OP^2BL, the shaded portion P^1P^2BA representing the rent now accruing to this factor.

(11) QUASI-RENT

This term is really no longer required. Following Marshall, it was used to describe all rents received by factors other than land, but it is unusual now to differentiate between land and other factors in this way. If the factor is highly specific it will receive rent so long as its supply falls short of the demand for its services. Since in the long period the supply of most specific factors can be increased, rent is often of temporary duration. The higher incomes of such factors will attract factors from other employments wherever possible, and so with the increase in the supply of the factor the rent will eventually disappear.

L

If the supply of a factor is perfectly elastic supply will immediately adjust itself to changes in demand, and so no rent will arise; if the supply of a factor is less than perfectly elastic an increase in demand will enable it to earn a rent, at least for a time. Thus, a second feature of quasi-rents is that they tend to be temporary, received by the factors concerned in the short period only until supply catches up with demand.

Rent in wages. Many kinds of labour are highly specific because of the long period of training or the special ability required. As with land, the supply of some kinds of labour may be almost perfectly in-elastic. Just as perfect substitutes cannot be found for particular sites in a city centre, so there may be no perfect substitutes for a prima donna, a great violinist, a film star, some comedian or heavy-weight boxer. The incomes of such people consist mostly of rents, which will persist so long as the demand for their services remains, for supply cannot be increased. The supplies of most kinds of specific labour are not generally so inelastic as this, for usually in the long period the supply can be increased, though the period of training may be of many years' duration. An increased demand for the services of barristers would enable them to raise their fees (and so receive rent), but the possibility of high earnings would eventually attract more people into the profession, so that perhaps in four or five years' time the supply would again equal demand, with the result that rent would disappear and the level of barristers' fees would fall. The special ability required of a successful barrister may be rare and not capable of being deliberately trained, and such a person would then be in a similar position to the prima donna or a famous violinist who, because close substitutes could not be found, would continue to command high remuneration—that is, would still receive rent. This is sometimes known as a "rent of ability."

Rent in interests and profits. The supply of some forms of capital is in-elastic in the short period, and so an increase in demand will give rise to additional income or rent. The supply of large, expensive plant will not immediately respond to an increase in the demand for the com-modities in the production of which it is required. The initial cost of erecting additional plant will tend to restrain the entry of new firms into the industry until there is some indication that the increased demand for the commodity is likely to be maintained. If high profits persist, new firms will eventually enter the industry, but meanwhile such capital will receive rent payments. High profits earned by a railway serving two cities will not immediately lead to the construction of a second railway to connect them, but if the expansion of traffic is more than the first railway can cope with, and if the increase seems likely to be per-manent, sooner or later a second railway will be built. An increase in the demand for houses—due perhaps to people getting married earlier—cannot easily be met, for the building of a large number of new houses takes time, and so houses will become scarce and the high prices paid for them may include a substantial amount of economic rent.

(12) MONOPOLY PROFIT AND RENT

Rent arises as a result of an increase in demand, where the supply of a factor cannot readily be increased. The monopolist makes a profit above normal (that is, a surplus profit) because he deliberately restricts output in order to keep up price. In the one case scarcity is due to an increase in demand; in the other scarcity is artificially created. The monopolist's profit is a surplus; so is rent. Neither monopoly profit nor rent is necessary in order to retain factors of production in their present employment. There is, then, a strong similarity between rent and monopoly profit. There is, however, an important difference: rent is the *result* and not the cause of high prices, whereas the monopolist's restrictionist policy is the *cause* of the high price of his product. Many professional bodies and some trade unions (particularly unions of skilled workers) deliberately restrict entry to their professions or trades by examinations, definite restriction of numbers or insistence on a lengthy period of apprenticeship, so that their additional incomes resulting from these practices are more akin to monopoly profit than to rent.

(13) THE RICARDIAN THEORY OF RENT

The English economist best known for his theory of rent is Ricardo, whose book *The Principles of Political Economy and Taxation* was published in 1817. Like the other classical economists, he thought that the value of a commodity depended on the amount of labour put into its production. The cost of production of farming products, however, presented difficulties, for it appeared to vary according to the fertility of the soil—wheat, for example, being grown at much lower cost on fertile land than on land of inferior quality. It was this problem that led him to formulate his theory of rent—that part of his work for which he came to be best known. Ricardo defined rent in what he called the strict sense (to distinguish it from the popular or ordinary sense in which Adam Smith and others used the term) as "that portion of the produce of the earth which is paid to the landlord for the use of the original and indestructible powers of the soil."

Rent, according to Ricardo, then arises in the following way. If a country has an "abundance of rich and fertile land," there will be no rent, for no one will be willing to pay for the use of land if there is a greater supply of it than is required for all purposes. There would thus be no rent if all land was of best quality and unlimited in quantity. Rich and fertile land, however, is not unlimited in quantity in any country, nor is land uniform in quality. It is because of this that rent arises, for says Ricardo, "when land of the second degree is taken into cultivation, rent immediately commences on that of the first quality, and the amount of that rent will depend on the difference in the quality of these two portions of land." Land at the margin of cultivation—that is, land that it is only just worth while to cultivate—Ricardo considered yielded no rent. More fertile land will yield a greater return, and the value of this excess yield over that of land at the margin of cultivation ("no-rent" land) is its rent. The greater the difference between a country's poorest and the best-cultivated land the higher then the rent of the best land.

Suppose the value of the crops from four pieces of land of equal area, and equal distance from the market but of different fertilities, to be £60, £48, £40 and £35. Assuming that the £35 yield comes from the land that is only just worth cultivating, that is "no-rent" land, and the rent on the other three pieces of land will be the excess yield over £35, that is, £25, £13 and £5 respectively:

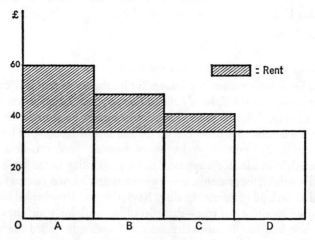

FIG. 70.—THE RICARDIAN THEORY OF RENT. (A, B, C, D represent equal areas of land.)

As population increases, ever less fertile land will be drawn into cultivation, and the rent of previously cultivated land will rise, and with the operation of the law of diminishing returns, profit from the cultivation of land will tend to fall.

Rent, Ricardo thought, could also arise if land is cultivated more intensively. Two pieces of land may be of equal quality, but if more capital and labour are applied to one, this will earn rent equal to its excess return. As land is cultivated more intensively, each additional amount of labour and capital applied to it will yield a less return—and therefore less rent—than the previous application, again giving diminishing returns.

(14) SOME CRITICISMS OF THE RICARDIAN THEORY

The following are some of the criticisms levelled against Ricardo's theory:

(i) His theory is based simply on the natural variation in the productivity of different pieces of land as a result of differences in their fertility.

(ii) He ignored the fact that there might be competing uses for a particular piece of land—that a piece of land might be farmed or built upon—though he did admit the possibility of advantageous situation with regard to the market.

(iii) Marginal land is not necessarily land at the margin of cultivation, since it is not always the least fertile land that is the first to go out of cultivation if the supply of a commodity is to be reduced. Whether a certain piece of land ceases to grow wheat depends not only on its fertility but also on the alternative uses to which it can be put. An airport, for example, might be built on the most fertile land of all just because that particular site is the most suitable for this purpose. Ricardo ignored the important fact that land can be put to uses other than farming. Nor, in a developing country—like the United States in Ricardo's time—is land necessarily brought under cultivation in order of its quality. The first land to be cultivated was more likely to be the most accessible rather than the most fertile.

(iv) According to Ricardo, there would be no rent at all if all land were of equal fertility, equally well situated with regard to markets, and farmed with the same degree of intensity.

(v) Not unnaturally, perhaps, in view of his definition, he restricted rent to land. As it is defined by modern economists, rent becomes a much more useful concept, since it can apply to any of the factors of production.

(vi) Ricardo asserted that rent was not a cost of production, since the cost of producing a commodity on the poorest land determined its cost of production.

(15) RENTS AS AN OBJECT OF TAXATION

Since rent is a payment over and above what is necessary to keep a factor in its present employment, it has been argued that economic rent is an unearned increment, and therefore a suitable object of taxation, for, provided that the tax does not exceed the rent, it will have no adverse effect on production. Henry George and others have, for example, advocated the taxation of any increased value in land sites, on the ground that such increased value owes nothing to effort on the part of the owner. This is quite true, but in equity, if rent accruing to land is taxed, rents accruing to other factors should also be taxed. The main difficulty, however, is to distinguish between that part of a factor's income that is unearned economic rent and that part of its income that is earned. It would be difficult, if not impossible, to devise a satisfactory scheme for the taxation of all forms of economic rent. However, an attempt was made by the British Government in 1948 to acquire increases in the site value of land resulting from its re-development. This scheme failed, but another attempt was made in 1966 by the setting up of a Land Commission under the newly established Ministry of Land and Natural Resources.

RECOMMENDATIONS FOR FURTHER READING

K. Boulding: *Economic Analysis*, Chapters 9–12.
P. Wicksteed: *Common-sense of Political Economy*, Vol. I, Chapters 8 and 9.
A. Marshall: *Principles of Economics*, Book VI, Chapters 1–2, 9, 11.

QUESTIONS

Theory of Distribution.

1. Examine the causes of inequalities in the real income of individuals. What are the present-day tendencies? (R.S.A. Adv.)

2. (*a*) How were the factors of production allocated among industries in the days of *laissez-faire*?

(*b*) On what principle are they allocated when the central authority has the determining voice? (A.C.C.A. Inter.)

3. "It has now become certain that the problem of distribution is much more difficult than it was thought to be by earlier economists, and that no solution of it which claims to be simple can be true." (Marshall.) Discuss. (A.C.C.A. Final.)

Rent

4. Explain the statement "Rent is a surplus." Why are rents in the city higher than in the country? (R.S.A. Inter.)

5. Is rent a cost of production? (C.I.S. Inter.)

6. "The prices at which I sell are high because my rent is high," says a shop-keeper. Is this correctly stated? (I.H.A.)

7. Distinguish between agricultural rent, site rent and house rent. How do developments in transport affect site values? (I.T.)

8. Discuss the theory of rent with special reference to (a) a tobacconist shop, (b) a ladies' dress shop, both in a fashionable centre of a large city. (I.B.)

9. What warrant is there for extending the concept of rent to the factors of production other than land? (I.H.A.)

10. State (a) the similarities, (b) the differences between the rent of land and the rent of houses. (C.C.S. Inter.)

11. "The profits of monopoly are most properly regarded as rents." Discuss this statement. (C.I.S. Final.)

12. What economic forces help to determine the annual rent of a plot of land in the centre of a city? (G.C.E. Adv.)

CHAPTER XVIII

WAGES

I. THEORIES OF WAGES

(1) REAL AND NOMINAL WAGES

Wages and salaries. In ordinary speech a distinction is frequently made between wages and salaries, though there is no clear line of demarcation between them. Some people would say that wages are payments for manual work, salaries for non-manual work; others that wages are paid weekly, salaries at longer intervals; others, again, that wages are paid for a definite amount of work, as measured by time or piece, so that if less than a full week is worked a proportionate deduction from the weekly wage will be made, whereas those "on the staff" receive salaries and suffer no such deductions. Only the last distinction is of any economic importance; wages are a variable cost, varying with output, whereas salaries are in the short period a fixed cost, and so do not vary with output. This distinction is made in book-keeping, wages being included in the Trading Account, drawn up to enable gross profit to be calculated, and salaries being included in the Profit and Loss Account, as one of the expenses to be deducted from gross profit in order to arrive at net profit. Except in discussions of variable and fixed costs, the economist does not distinguish between wages and salaries, the two terms being taken as alternative terms for the share of labour in the national income—that is, income received from work.

It is important, however, to distinguish between real and nominal wages. Nominal wages are wages in terms of money, and the term *money wages*, which is sometimes used, is perhaps to be preferred. In comparing wages at different periods of time it is not sufficient to know that in 1913 few men received more than £1 per week; that their average earnings were £3 9s. per week in 1938, £12 in 1955 and £19 10s. in 1965. Such statements are frequently made, the inference being that the economic position of these men had improved by nineteen times between 1913 and 1965. Wages are wanted only for what they will buy. Real wages are wages in terms of the goods and services that can be bought with them. "The labourer," says Adam Smith, "is rich or poor, is well or ill rewarded, in proportion to the real, not to the nominal price of his labour."

In comparing the nominal wages of people in different occupations account must be taken of payments in kind, such as free uniform for policemen, railway workers and many others, free travel to and from work for those engaged in passenger transport undertakings, the use of a car by some business executives, free board and lodging for some hotel workers.

It is further necessary to distinguish between wage rates and earnings. During the period 1956–65 wage rates in Great Britain rose by 48% but earnings rose by nearly 60%, for in most industrial occupations overtime was being worked. The introduction of the five-day week in many industries has often merely meant that work on Saturday mornings has ranked for overtime.

(2) THE MARGINAL PRODUCTIVITY THEORY OF WAGES

In the previous chapter the marginal productivity theory of distribution was considered. According to this theory, it will be remembered, the entrepreneur will pay no more for any factor of production that he employs than the value of its marginal product, since to do so will increase his costs of production by more than the increase in his revenue (pp. 281–3).

The following are some of the principal criticisms levelled against the marginal productivity theory of wages:

(i) It is too theoretical a concept, since it does not appear to agree with what actually takes place.

(ii) In practice, too, it is generally impossible to calculate either the amount or the value of the marginal product of labour or of any other factors of production.

(iii) The employment of one more or one fewer man may completely upset the method of production in use at the time. To employ an extra man may simply mean that there will be more labour than is necessary; to take away a man may remove a vital link in the chain of production. For this reason a small rise or fall in wages is not likely to bring about an immediate change in the amount of labour employed.

(iv) The productivity of labour does not depend entirely on its own effort and efficiency, but very largely on the quality of the other factors of production employed, especially capital and the entrepreneur.

(v) According to this theory, the higher the wage, the smaller the amount of labour the entrepreneur will employ. Surveys that have been taken appear to indicate that few employers take account of the wage rate when considering how many men to employ, being influenced more by business prospects.

(vi) Lord Keynes said the theory was valid only in static conditions, and therefore, to lower the wage rate in a trade depression would not necessarily increase the demand for labour.

(vii) In any case the marginal productivity theory is applicable only in conditions of perfect competition.

(3) THE MARKET THEORY OF WAGES

Another approach to the problem of wage determination is to regard wages as a price—the price of labour—and, therefore, like all other prices determined by the interaction of the market forces of supply and demand. In Chapter XVII it was seen that it is possible to conceive of factor markets as well as commodity markets, the price of a factor of production then depending on the demand for it in relation to its supply. Therefore, in the case of wages, it is necessary to consider the labour market.

(i) *The supply of labour.* It has already been pointed out that there is some ambiguity in the concept of a supply of labour, since supply can be taken to mean either the total number of people available for employment or the total number of hours worked. In the case of a commodity its supply depends on its cost of production. Though it is more difficult to apply cost of production to labour in general, it can more easily be applied to the various forms of specific labour which require a sacrifice of earnings during a long period of training.

(ii) *The demand for labour.* In the factor markets demand is a derived demand. It is, too, an anticipated demand, since commodities must be produced in anticipation of a future demand for them. Thus the demand for labour is derived from the anticipated demand for the goods and services in the production of which it assists. Expectations of favourable conditions of business activity, therefore, will stimulate a demand for labour. Another influence on the demand for labour is the possibility of substitution. For example, the entrepreneur may be able at any time to substitute capital for labour, and whether he does so depends on the relative prices of these two factors of production. Conditions for substitution, however, may change—a new machine or a new development, such as automation, may reduce the demand for labour. An increase in real capital investment, public or private, will therefore increase the demand for labour.

(iii) *The price mechanism and the labour market.* Through the price mechanism supply is brought into equality with demand. An increase in demand in relation to supply, therefore, should raise the price of labour and so push up wages; on the other hand, a fall in demand in relation to supply should cause wages to fall. A rise in price can be expected to increase the supply of a factor coming on to the market.

Though this may be generally true, it is not certain, however, that the supply of labour can always be increased by an offer of higher wages, since after wages have reached a certain level leisure may come to be preferred to further income, thus providing an example of a regressive supply curve (see p. 288).

The Market Theory of Wages does not run counter to the Marginal Productivity Theory. In the same way that marginal utility forms the basis of individual demand, so marginal productivity forms the basis of demand for labour and other factors of production. It has been said that marginal productivity acts as "a regulator of wages, but it does not determine their precise magnitude."[1]

(4) THE BARGAINING THEORY OF WAGES

Earlier theories of wages, some writers believe, have been rendered invalid, or at least inadequate, as a result of collective bargaining by trade unions. The Marginal Productivity Theory rests on the assumption of perfect competition, whereas collective bargaining makes competition imperfect, so that it becomes necessary to study the determination of wages in both conditions in the same way that one has to study production in terms of both perfect and imperfect competition. The forces that determine wages under perfect competition continue to influence wages even though competition is imperfect. Collective bargaining provides an example of what is sometimes called bi-lateral monopoly, the trade union being the monopolist supplier and the employers' association the monopolist (or more correctly, monopsonist) buyer of a particular kind of labour.

Those who support the Bargaining Theory of Wages assert that the level of wages in an industry depends on the bargaining strength of the trade union concerned, so that, they say, differences in wages in different occupations are the result of differences in the strength of the respective trade unions. Salaried workers have called in this theory to support their view that salaries have lagged behind wages during the past twenty-five years. The power of a trade union depends on a number of thing—the size of its membership, the size of its "fighting" fund and the extent of the dislocation it can cause to the national economy by a strike. Clearly, a strike of milliners is going to inconvenience the community less than a strike of transport workers at a popular holiday period. Nevertheless, however great may appear to be the bargaining skill of some trade-union leaders, this is of less importance than the prevailing economic conditions. In times of full

[1] J. R. Hicks: *The Theory of Wages*, p. 86.

employment the trade unions will be in a strong position; in a depression they will be weaker. The apparent success, however, of the more powerful industrial unions has led to a demand for stronger action from employees in less-well-organised occupations.

To what extent, then, can a trade union raise the wages of its members? In this connection it is necessary to distinguish between real and nominal (money) wages. Adherents of the Marginal Productivity Theory of Wages argue that real wages can be increased only if they are below the value of the marginal product of labour, since real wages can never for long exceed this. They also point out that real wages can be increased only by employing less labour in relation to other factors of production or by increasing the efficiency of labour. In inflationary conditions it is easy to increase nominal wages but not so easy to raise real wages. Thus, if a trade union obtains an increase in wages the benefit to its members tends to be short-lived, since other wage increases follow and prices rise. A permanent increase in real wages can be achieved only by an increase in the volume of production, that is, as a result of economic growth, and recently Great Britain has found it difficult to maintain the average annual rate of growth of 3–4% achieved over the past fifty years.

Since 1945 efforts have been made on several occasions to increase real wages and not merely nominal (money) wages. During 1948–50 the Government tried to persuade the trade unions for a time to accept a "wage freeze"; in 1961–62 an attempt was made to effect a "pay pause"; and during 1964–66 the Government struggled to persuade the unions to agree to an "incomes policy" with increases in wages dependent on increases in productivity.

(5) WAGES IN SERVICE OCCUPATIONS

Associations representing workers providing services—clerical, postal, teaching, etc.—have generally been less successful in securing increases in wages for their members than the large, powerful trade unions. This fact seemed to add point to the Bargaining Theory of Wages. These associations have generally attempted to apply the "principle of comparability" with wages of those in similar occupations, though it is often very difficult to compare work in different occupations, since no two jobs are alike. The laws of the market, however, have an important influence. When labour is plentiful in relation to the demand for it their wages tend to be low. Only when there is a strong demand for labour are people in service occupations able to secure increases in wages. At such times alternative openings for employment are often available to them.

The Priestley Commission which inquired into pay in the Civil Service was in favour of "a fair comparison with comparable work"; the Guillebaud Committee accepted the same principle for railway workers; the Pilkington Committee, which undertook a similar task for doctors and dentists, stressed that earnings in these professions should be compared with the incomes of people in other professions with equivalent qualifications, and the Willinck Committee, which considered the pay of the police, emphasised the necessity for higher wages than in similar occupations in order to attract more recruits to the police service. To offer more than is paid in other occupations in inflationary conditions can only lead to demands from others for parity of treatment.

In the case of the self-employed, it should be remembered that their earnings generally include some interest on the capital employed to enable them to set up on their own account.

Bargaining strength is clearly an important influence on wage determination, but, though the market has been rendered imperfect, the influence of the market forces of supply and demand continue to be of great importance.

(6) THE EFFECTS OF INVENTIONS

Ever since the Luddites took to smashing machinery during 1811–16, workers have generally been suspicious of the introduction of new machines, which it was thought inevitably reduced the demand for labour, and so caused unemployment. Sometimes it has been impossible to introduce new inventions until the trade union concerned has been satisfied that the interests of its members would not be adversely affected. Instances could be quoted of new machines that would have increased production not being used for several years, for fear of the workers going on strike. On another occasion the use of new machinery for loading and unloading ships was permitted only on condition that as many men as previously were employed on this work!

There is no doubt that in the long run new inventions are to the advantage of labour, though it has to be admitted that the immediate effect of the installation of a new machine often causes some frictional unemployment. In the end, however, additional employment will be created, for the machines themselves have to be made, while the effect of using them has generally been to increase output and to lower prices, with the result that the real wages of other workers has risen and in consequence their demand for all kinds of goods. As a result, employment in other industries, and perhaps also in the industry in which the new machinery has been introduced, is thereby stimulated. During the Great Depression of 1929–35 this view was challenged, and it was seriously suggested that a halt should be called to scientific progress. The ultimate benefit of new techniques was admitted, but it was feared that if technical progress was too rapid further unemployment would be created before those previously thrown out of work had found other jobs. This fear has been revived with the development of automation, which makes it possible to employ even less labour.

The effect of a new invention or innovation on employment and wages depends on whether it is a *labour-saving* or a *capital-saving* invention. Possibly there may be a third group where the effect is neutral. An invention may be labour-saving if it reduces the demand for labour, whereas a capital-saving invention will reduce the demand for capital. If the wages of labour are high, as in times when the demand for labour tends to exceed the supply, this will act as a stimulus to the invention of labour-saving machinery. Only by the adoption of the most up-to-date techniques, however, can productivity be increased; this is a prerequisite of higher real wages. The ultimate effect of most inventions has therefore been a rise in real wages and in the standard of living.

II. DIFFERENCES IN WAGES

(7) NO SINGLE LABOUR MARKET

It was seen in Chapter XII that an equilibrium distribution of expenditure in the market was achieved by a housewife when the marginal utilities of all the commodities she had purchased were equal, for only then would she have no incentive to dispose of a little of one commodity in order to obtain a little more of another. An equilibrium distribution of labour among different occupations might then be expected to occur when the wages of labour in all occupations are equal.

Why, then, do wages vary between one occupation and another? The reason is that there is no such thing as a single labour market, for there are as many markets for labour as there are types of labour, for labour is not a homogeneous commodity. If there is a shortage of doctors the services of plumbers cannot be enlisted, nor can butchers be employed to make good a deficiency of accountants. One kind of labour may differ from another because of its ability to undertake certain work, or because of the special training required for certain occupations. Where a special aptitude is needed, little can be done to meet any shortage of supply, though sometimes, even in such a case, training may improve the aptitude of a lower-grade worker. The special training required for some occupations makes it difficult to increase the supply of labour in the short period. The better-paid occupations might be expected, however, to attract more new entrants than those that are poorly paid. This would increase the supply of labour and reduce wages in these better-paid occupations, and at the same time, because of the reduced supply of labour in the poorer-paid occupations, wages there would rise. Equilibrium would eventually be achieved only when wages in all occupations were equal.

There are several reasons why this does not happen. The period of special training may be long and expensive. Attendance at a university for three, four or five years may be required, and the necessity to pass an examination at the end of the course adds a measure of uncertainty. Though the salaries paid to those who successfully complete such periods of training generally amply compensate for the expense incurred, many parents, even when they can afford it, are unwilling to allow their children the opportunity of qualifying for these better-paid occupations because they may feel that at (say) sixteen years of age, when a decision has to be made, it is time for their children to begin to earn their own living. Many blind-alley jobs are well paid for beginners, just as most well-paid posts can be obtained only by those who have been willing to accept low wages in the early years of their careers. Some differential payment for skilled work is necessary in order to encourage people to undertake the period of training required. Many people too would be unwilling to accept posts carrying responsibility if such posts did not carry higher pay.

The main influence on the separation of labour markets, therefore, is lack of occupational mobility. The fact too that labour is not completely mobile in a geographical sense helps still further to keep labour markets separate. The question of mobility of labour was considered in Chapter III. However, in times when the demand for labour greatly exceeds the supply, as in inflationary conditions, many people change their jobs frequently.

(8) NON-MONETARY CONSIDERATIONS

Another influence on wages is that some occupations possess advantages of a non-monetary kind. Consider first non-monetary (or net) advantages. Some kinds of work are more congenial than others and are carried on under pleasanter conditions; in some employments the worker has a greater degree of independence than in others; in some occupations there is a high degree of security from dismissal except for serious misconduct—for example the Civil Service and Local Government. Other occupations are subject to non-monetary advantages: in some cases an occupation may carry a degree of prestige that gives satisfaction to the worker—or, at any rate, to his wife—as in most professions, and to some extent even in the more lowly white-collar occupations. Some work is dangerous—for example, that of steeplejacks—some occupations are more subject to unemployment than others, especially seasonal unemployment—for example, bricklayers; sometimes the hours of work are inconvenient, requiring very early or very late attendance, or shifts may have to be split, as with those employed in public transport; in some occupations it may be necessary to work on Saturdays or public holidays—as for example in a public utility service; for some kinds of work it may be necessary to spend long periods away from home—for example, fishermen and commercial travellers.

Wage differences can arise from all these causes. Generally, the greater the non-monetary advantages of the occupation, the lower the wages, and the greater the non-monetary disadvantages of the occupation, the higher the wages. The reason for this is that non-monetary considerations affect the supply, which tends to be greater when there are non-monetary advantages and less when there are non-monetary disadvantages. However, it is not always necessary to offer higher wages in order to persuade people to do disagreeable work. If the work requires some measure of skill, then it will probably be better paid than the more congenial work requiring an equivalent amount of skill, but disagreeable work often requires little skill, and generally the supply of labour available for this kind of work is greater than the demand for it, and so it is often poorly paid. Nevertheless, in times when the general demand for labour is tending to outrun the supply many of the more disagreeable jobs become difficult to fill unless higher wages are offered.

(9) WOMEN'S WAGES

Women on the average earn less than men. The fact that many women, especially married women, are not entirely dependent on their own earnings has often in the past made them willing to work for much lower wages than they otherwise would. In the textile industries, in the earliest days of the factory system, it was customary for all adult members of the family to go out to work, and the family income was often of greater importance than the incomes of the individual members. The effect of this was to depress men's wages in these industries. Apart from the textile industries and domestic work, there were formerly few openings for women, and so the supply of this type of labour tended to exceed demand, with the result that payment was low. The demand for women in many industries was low because their productivity was thought to be low. Many kinds of work, done by the men of the same class, were considered to be unsuitable for women, and in occupations requiring considerable physical strength this was largely true, but the experience of two World Wars has shown that women are capable of many kinds of work formerly considered to be suitable only for men, such as transport and engineering, to quote only two examples.

In most of the professions, especially those that until fairly recently were closed to women, there is no differentiation between men and women with regard to payment, but in these occupations there may often be a wide difference in the earnings even of different men. Women barristers can earn as much as the male members of the profession if they can obtain a sufficient number of briefs. Similarly, women doctors' incomes can equal those of their male colleagues if patients come in sufficient numbers to seek their advice. In the Civil Service, Local Government and the teaching profession (except at university level) there used to be lower scales of salary for women, but equal pay now prevails in these occupations. In some kinds of factory work, however, there are still two rates of pay. If men and women are doing equal work with equal efficiency there seems to be no economic reason why they should not receive equal pay. An increasing number of women now take up clerical posts in commerce, which were once looked upon as men's occupations, the main reason for the change being that employers formerly found it cheaper to employ young women.

Most girls still look upon the period of employment after leaving school as a temporary interval until they marry, and so do not remain long enough at work to consider making it their career. The average age of girl clerks is thus low, as also are their average wages. For this reason most employers do not consider it to be worth while to train women for the more responsible positions, as so frequently this training would be wasted. Most men—and some women, too—dislike working under a woman. Some employers think that men are more reliable than women, and if men and women receive the same pay, prefer to appoint men. It frequently appears that many highly efficient women are less tolerant of human short-comings in others than equally efficient men, and so make less-capable managers.

It is particularly difficult, however, to decide what is equal work. Superficially two posts may seem to be alike, and equally well filled in the one case by a man and in the other by a woman, and yet one of them may be far more efficient in that particular type of work than the other. For example, a woman may be able to perform her duties as a bus conductor for most of the time as efficiently as a man, but if she has trouble with an obstreperous passenger the driver may have to come to her assistance. One reason why women are generally paid less than men is that trade-union organisation is still weaker among women, and so less effort is made to improve their conditions of work. It has long been customary for women to be paid less than men, and old customs are sometimes difficult to change.

Some men's organisations oppose equal payment for men and women, even if it is clear that they are doing equal work, on the ground that most men have family responsibilities, and equal pay would result in many women being able to enjoy a higher standard of living than was possible to married men. It was pointed out that the Armed Forces recognise the married man's position by granting him a marriage allowance. This, however, is a social rather than an economic question, and not unrelated to the population problem. The payment of different rates to the married and the unmarried employee would be impracticable in industry, for if this were so, in a trade depression married men would be the first to lose their jobs. The payment of a marriage allowance under the National Insurance scheme would, too, require a huge increase in the weekly contribution. An extension of the present system of Income Tax allowances might be more feasible. The difference in the standard of living between married couples and single women has been lessened as a result of an increasing number of women continuing to go out to work after marriage.

The Royal Commission on Equal Pay (1946) published Majority and Minority Reports. The Majority Report favoured differentiation between the earnings of men and women on the ground that men possess greater physical strength and are generally more efficient than women, that the sickness rate was higher among women, that they were more likely than men to absent themselves from work for trivial reasons, and were generally less ambitious than men and in crises showed less initiative. The Minority Report admitted that where physical strength was concerned, men were more capable than women, but it was claimed that with this exception women were equally efficient as men, the fact that in the past women had been promoted to few posts of responsibility being ascribed to the prejudice of employers and the jealousy of male employees.

The increasing acceptance of the principle of equal pay in many

occupations has been less a triumph of principle than of expediency—
shortage of labour.

III. EARLY THEORIES OF WAGES

(10) THE SUBSISTENCE THEORY OF WAGES

According to this theory, wages tend to keep to a level that will
provide the workers only with a bare subsistence. If wages for a time
rise above this level it inevitably leads, it is said, to an increase in the
population, and increased competition among workers for employment causes wages to fall again. If wages fall below subsistence level
fewer children are born and malnutrition raises the death rate, so that
competition for employment is reduced and wages tend to rise. This
"iron law" of wages was looked upon as a natural law by the French
School of economists, known as the Physiocrats, who based it upon
their observations of conditions of life among the French peasants of the
eighteenth century. "Wages are fixed and reduced to the lowest level
by the extreme competition of the workers," said Quesnay (1694–
1774), who first put forward this theory. The theory of population,
expounded by Malthus nearly half a century later, was based on this
"iron law."

A number of objections to this theory of wages can be brought
forward:

(i) Is it based on correct facts? Even if it were generally true in
eighteenth-century France, and though it may still be true of some
densely populated countries with a low standard of living, it was
certainly not true of England in the nineteenth century. During that
century real wages almost doubled, while the population increased
over two and a half times. Nor did rising real wages after 1850 lead to
a rise in the birth rate, for the exact opposite occurred, the birth rate
falling from 35 per thousand in 1850 to 28·7 per thousand in 1900.

(ii) Like the Labour Theory of Value, the Subsistence Theory of
Wages approaches the problem entirely from the side of supply, the
demand for labour being completely ignored. If a rise in wages led to
an increase in population the larger supply of labour might be more
than balanced by an increase in the demand for labour.

(iii) The most serious objection to this theory, however, lies in the
ambiguity of the term "subsistence level." What is considered to be
the bare minimum for human existence varies between one period and
another, and things at one time looked upon as luxuries of the rich
often eventually became necessaries even for the poor. Tea and coal-
fires are two examples. At the present day most households take at

least one daily newspaper, and very few are without radio and television sets. What is considered to be bare subsistence in the 1960s would have been thought a very substantial standard of comfort in the 1840s.

(11) THE WAGES-FUND THEORY OF WAGES

If the Subsistence Theory were valid all efforts to raise wages would be doomed to failure, since according to that theory wages were bound to remain at subsistence level. The Wages-fund Theory was an attempt to show, without discarding the Malthusian theory of population, that in certain circumstances wages could rise. This theory, which is generally somewhat unjustly associated with the name of J. S. Mill, approached the question more from the side of demand, the demand for labour depending on the amount of capital available for the payment of wages. Since production takes time, entrepreneurs have to pay wages in advance of the marketing of their products. At the time when the Wages-fund Theory was developed it was thought that a fund of capital had to be accumulated in advance before wages could be paid. Thus the size of the fund at any given moment limited the total amount of wages that could be paid. The size of this fund was determined by past accumulations of capital, and so the level of wages could be calculated by dividing the wages fund by the number of people seeking employment.

Wages then were not fixed, as the earlier theory seemed to show, but depended on the relation between the wages fund and the size of the population. An increase in population would lower wages unless this was accompanied by a corresponding increase in capital accumulation. Wages could be improved (i) by restricting the growth of population, (ii) by an expansion of the wages fund. Taxation of employers, by reducing their ability to accumulate capital, would thus result in lower wages. Though the wages fund was capable of expansion or contraction over a period, yet at any given time its size was fixed, and so, therefore, was the total sum available for the payment of wages. Though the theory did not specifically say so, it appeared to imply that if one group of workers obtained a rise in wages it could be only at the expense of other workers, whose share of the fund was thereby reduced. Wages therefore could rise in one industry only at the expense of another, since it was impossible for the general level of wages to rise unless capital increased more rapidly than the population.

Though somewhat crudely expressed, there are elements of truth in this theory. The proportion between the factors of production is an important influence on production, and by increasing the productivity of labour the accumulation of capital tends to raise wages. There is, however, no such thing as a fixed fund set apart for the payment of wages that has to be accumulated in advance, for modern credit facilities enable production to be financed in advance. In conditions of full employment, however, with production at a maximum, one aspect of the theory appears to come into its own, since in these conditions (assuming no increase in productivity takes place) one group of workers can obtain a rise in their *real* wages only at the expense of all other workers, since if a rise in prices results, then the *real* wages of all other workers will fall.

IV. SYSTEMS OF WAGE PAYMENT

(12) WAGES RATE

Standard rates. The payment of a standard rate to all workers engaged on similar work is an advantage to both employer and employee. Without standard rates an employer would have to make an individual wage bargain with each employee before engaging him, and this would take up too much of his time. The calculation of the cost of employing labour becomes easier to the employer when he knows exactly how much each additional hour of labour will cost. Standard rates, whether per hour or per piece, are essential to collective bargaining, for otherwise it would be impossible for a trade union to make an agreement with the employers regarding wage rates.

Time-rates and standard rates. Various methods of calculating wages are in operation, but of these the best known are the time-rate and the piece-rate systems of payment. Where time-rates are in operation all employees engaged on similar work are paid an agreed sum per hour. Good, bad and indifferent workers receive equal payment if they work the same number of hours. Under this system it becomes necessary to keep records of the number of hours worked by each employee, and in most factories and workshops a time-clock is installed, workers having to "clock in" and "clock out," their times of arrival and departure being recorded on cards. It is a further necessity of this system that workers have to be kept under constant supervision in order to prevent slacking. The quicker and more efficient workers may receive the same pay as those who are slower and less efficient, but the better workers may have greater security of employment, for if it becomes necessary to curtail production the first to be dismissed will be the less-efficient workers—those who, because of their poor physique, carelessness, unreliability, or temperament (the bad-tempered and the man with a grievance), have a low net productivity.

Piece-rates. In order to give the workers an incentive to work harder, a number of different systems have been tried, all of which aim at making the wages received by the worker dependent on the amount of work done. Of these, the simplest, and therefore the most favoured system, is the straight-forward piece-rate method, where the employee receives a fixed payment for a definite, measurable amount of work. If he receives 6s. for each unit of work and in a week completes fifty units his wages for that week will be £15; if the following week he accomplishes fifty-two units of work his pay will be £15 12s. Such a system is easy for the workers to understand, since he himself can easily check his earnings. Piece-rates can, however, be operated only where each individual's work can easily be measured, though where groups of employees work together the principle can be extended to the group. If the work is of a continuous nature, and cannot easily be standardised and measured, such as the work of shopkeepers, teachers and bus drivers, payment by piece-rates is not possible, though attempts have sometimes been made to pay shop assistants a bonus based on the value of their sales, and in the nineteenth century teachers in inspected schools were paid according to the number of "passes" in examinations conducted annually in the schools by H.M. Inspectors. But chaos would result if bus drivers were paid according to the number of journeys they were able to accomplish per hour between two points! If the quality of the work is more important than the quantity piece-rates are an unsuitable method of payment.

Advantages of piece-rates.

(i) The quicker workers can earn more than those who are slow or inclined to waste time.

(ii) Output will probably be increased and the cost per unit reduced. The employer's variable costs (including expenditure on wages) will increase as output increases, but his fixed costs (rent, rates, etc.) will remain as before. His total costs, therefore, will not increase proportionately with output. Wherever the type of work makes their introduction possible, employers prefer to pay piece-rates.

(iii) The cost of supervising employees while they are working will be reduced, because any slacking will affect the employees themselves by reducing their earnings.

(iv) The work of costing becomes easier, for the employer knows the exact cost of the labour required for a given unit of output.

Disadvantages of piece-rates.

(i) The attempt to increase earnings may result in work being rushed. Thus it will be necessary to employ "passers" or inspectors to check the quality of the work done and to reject unsatisfactory work.

(ii) The more careful and conscientious workers, who take a longer time over their work, will earn less than those whose work is just satisfactory. The highest earnings will generally go to those whose work is just good enough to be accepted.

(iii) Workers may be induced by the possibility of higher earnings to speed up their work to such an extent that overstrain may injure their health. Employees new to the system often tend to overwork in the early part of the day or week, and then fatigue may slow down their output so much that their eventual earnings are lower than those of a steady worker. Though most employees might be expected to find out from experience the most remunerative speed at which to work, some advice to the beginner from the supervisor is required. Working at excessive speed also increases the liability to accident, and in their own interest men may have to be warned to work more slowly and more carefully.

(iv) A complaint made by workers in the past against the piece-rate system was that the wage rate per piece was reduced when it was found that workers were earning considerably more than they previously earned on time-rates. Piece-rates, however, are difficult to fix, and a "fair" rate can be determined only by experiment. A change too in the market conditions for a commodity may necessitate some adjustment of the rate. Considerable attention has been given in recent years to the question of fixing the rates of pay for particular work, especially where the work varies greatly in difficulty. The time taken by workers has been scientifically evaluated by time-and-motion studies.

(v) In the past, piece-rates often led to dissatisfaction on the part of the employees because they had no proof that they were being paid for all the work they had done. This led in 1872 to the coal-miners obtaining the right to appoint a check-weighman at each colliery to see that each miner was credited with his correct output. In 1891 the textile trades adopted the "ticket" system, which entitled each worker to a "ticket" showing the work to be done and the payment for it.

(13) BONUS SYSTEMS

From time to time various modifications of the simple piece-rate system have been adopted, all of them aiming at reducing the additional amount to be paid in wages for increased output on the part of the worker. A serious drawback to many of the bonus systems that have been tried is that they are more complicated than the straightforward piece-rate system, and more difficult for the employee to understand.

There are three main types of bonus systems: the premium-bonus, the task-bonus systems, and the Bedaux system:

(i) *Premium-bonus systems.* In the *Rowan* system (so called because David Rowan of Glasgow first introduced it) each unit of work has a standard time assigned to it. Time-rate wages, say, 8s. per hour, are in operation, and if the worker completes the work in the "standard" time (say, eight hours) he will be paid 8 × 8s., that is, 64s. On a straight piece-rate system this would be the payment received whether the time taken was less or greater than eight hours. If, however, he works very hard and finishes this particular job in six hours, he will be paid at 8s. per hour for six hours (48s.), with in addition a bonus equal to the percentage of time saved. In this case the time saved is two hours out of eight hours, and so the bonus will be 25 per cent., that is 12s. He will thus receive 60s. for six hours' work.

Under the *Weir* or *Halsey* system the bonus is half the hourly rate for the time saved. In the above example if the bonus is calculated on the Weir system payment would be for six hours at 8s. per hour—that is, 48s. + two hours at 4s. per hour = 56s. The following table compares earnings under these two systems, where the standard time is eight hours and the rate 8s. per hour.

TABLE XLIII

Rowan and Weir Bonus Systems

Time taken (hours)	Rowan System			Weir System			Ordinary piece-rate
	Time payment	Bonus	Full payment	Time payment	Bonus	Full payment	
7	56s. +	7s.	= 63s.	56s. +	4s.	= 60s.	64s.
6	48s. +	12s.	= 60s.	48s. +	8s.	= 56s.	64s.
5	40s. +	15s.	= 55s.	40s. +	12s.	= 52s.	64s.
4	32s. +	16s.	= 48s.	32s. +	16s.	= 48s.	64s.
3	24s. +	15s.	= 39s.	24s. +	20s.	= 44s.	64s.

(ii) *Task-bonus systems.* In these systems piece-rates are paid, but in addition a bonus is payable only if the task is completed within a certain standard time. The severity of the task varies, sometimes, as in the *Gantt* system, being double that of the average worker, and no bonus is paid if the worker just fails in his task. In other systems such as the *Emerson*, a more reasonable task is set, and the bonus payments vary according to how near the worker approaches it.

(iii) *The Bedaux system.* Invented in New York in 1911 by Charles Bedaux, and introduced into England in 1926, this system attempts to apply a uniform system of bonus payment to work of varying degrees of difficulty and strain in the same factory. Each type of work is analysed, and according to the strain involved a proportion of time is allowed as "rest." For all kinds of work there is a standard unit of time, known as a B-unit (B for Bedaux), but in an easy job this may consist of fifty-five seconds of work and five seconds of rest, whereas in a more difficult job it may comprise forty-five seconds of work and fifteen seconds of rest. These standard times are calculated by experts supplied by the Bedaux Company. In this way standard times are worked out for all types of work carried on in the factory. The bonus is calculated as in the Weir system, as a percentage (usually 75) of the hourly rate for the time saved.

(14) PROFIT-SHARING

Profit-sharing is another method by which some firms have tried to give their employees a more direct interest in the prosperity of the firm. Workers are permitted to hold a certain number of shares, so long as they remain in the employment of the firm, and so they receive a share in the profits. Profit-sharing schemes have been inspired by two motives: (i) an incentive to increase output, and (ii) in order to stimulate good relations between management and employees. Though some 400 profit-sharing schemes are still in existence, the number of such schemes has steadily declined during the past thirty years or so. Trade unions have always been suspicious of them, since in the early schemes it was often made a condition that the employees should not be members of trade unions. The addition to wages is really a collective bonus depending on the profits earned by the firm. Some of these schemes have been carried on successfully for long periods, and many of the firms operating them proudly boast that they have never been concerned in either a strike or a lock-out. It is claimed, too, that where profit-sharing is in operation less supervision is necessary, and that workers are more careful in their handling of the firm's equipment. A serious objection to profit-sharing is that the bonus is paid only at long intervals: there is too long a time lag between putting forward an extra effort and being paid for it.

(15) WAGES AND THE COST OF LIVING

Some trade unions have secured agreements whereby the wages of their members are on a sliding scale varying with the cost of living, and a number of such agreements are in existence. The Index of Retail Prices will be considered later. Its main feature, however, is that a certain date is selected as a base year and given an Index Number of

100, a rise in the cost of living of 5% over the base year giving a new Index Number of 105. When wages are linked to the Index of Retail Prices it is agreed that if the index rises a certain number of points wages are to be increased by a certain amount, and similarly if the index falls, wages are to be reduced. This gives wage rates a certain degree of flexibility, but there are two main objections to linking wages to the Index of Retail Prices:

(i) The original Index (known then as the Cost-of-living Index Number) was based on the expenditure of a working-class family, and had July 1914 as its base. Since 1956, however, the index has included people with incomes of up to £1,000 a year. People in different income-groups distribute their expenditure differently, and changes in the Index Number may affect one income group only to a slight extent, whereas other terms of expenditure, not allowed for in the Index, may affect them to a much great extent.

(ii) If wages rise or fall proportionately to the rise or fall in the cost of living, and assuming the Index Number to be representative of the standard of living of the workers concerned, real wages become stabilised. For this reason many trade unions are opposed to having wages linked to an index, as their aim is to raise the standard of living of their members.

VI. INDUSTRIAL RELATIONS

(16) THE DEVELOPMENT OF TRADE UNIONS

The Industrial Revolution made possible the development of organisations of employers and of employees, whose interests seemed to diverge the larger industry grew. In the Middle Ages the gilds included within their membership not only masters but also journeymen and apprentices both of whom had good hopes of themselves eventually becoming masters, so that there was no real difference in outlook or cause of antagonism between masters and men. The decline of the gilds left both employers and employees unorganised, but the State intervened to regulate wages and working conditions, the Justices of the Peace being empowered to fix wages in their own localities. By the time of the Industrial Revolution this system had lapsed, and each employer decided for himself what wages he would pay. Not unnaturally, employees began to combine together in order to try to improve the conditions under which they worked. The *Combination Acts* of 1799 and 1801, however, prohibited combinations formed for the purpose of raising wages, on the grounds that such associations were in restraint of trade. These Acts remained in force until 1824, when, largely as a result of the efforts of Francis Place, they were repealed, only to be restored in a modified form the following year. Employees, however, obtained the right to hold meetings and to strike.

A great increase in the number and membership of trade unions followed upon the Acts of 1824 and 1825 and many strikes occurred, but after 1845 disturbances became less frequent, though a recurrence of violence on the part of the trade unions in 1867 led to the setting up of a Royal Commission to inquire into their organisation. The immediate result was the passing of the *Trade Union Act* of 1871, which, with the Acts of 1875 and 1876, clarified the position of trade unions and defined their legal position more precisely, giving them protection for their property, and the right to "peaceful picketing" and freeing of their members from possible charges of conspiracy. The last decade of the nineteenth century saw the development of what was called the New Unionism, which widened the trade-union movement to include the unskilled. As a result of the admission of unskilled workers the membership of the unions greatly increased.

In 1900, however, the position of trade unions was again challenged when the Taff Vale Railway successfully sued a trade union because some of its members had induced other employees to break their contracts, but the *Trade Disputes Act* of 1906 freed the unions from a repetition of such charges. If proper notice is given a strike is not a breach of contract, but in the case of *Rookes v. Barnard*, the House of Lords in 1965 found that in certain circumstances a threat to strike was unlawful.

Then in 1909 the right of a trade union to use its funds for political purposes was put to the test in the Osborne case, when a member objected to part of his subscription being applied to that purpose. The decision of the courts was that it was illegal for trade unions to engage in political activity. The *Trade Union Act* of 1913 permitted unions to contribute to the support of a political party, but members who wished were allowed "to contract out."

The Trades Union Congress in 1926 called a general strike of all the unions in support of the coal-miners, who had been on strike for some time. The general strike failed, and this type of strike was made illegal by the *Trades Disputes and Trade Unions Act* of 1927. This Act was, however, repealed in 1947.

(17) ORGANISATION OF TRADE UNIONS

Trade unions are combinations of employees formed for the purpose of collectively bargaining with employers. The oldest trade unions were the craft unions, which restricted their membership to skilled workers engaged in a particular craft. These tend to be the smaller unions. They are especially concerned about the enforcement of apprenticeship regulations in order to restrict entry. The large unions are generally industrial unions, which admit both skilled and unskilled workers, and include all types of workers in the various branches of a particular industry. For example, in the wool textile industry there are small craft unions of warp dressers, twisters, loom tuners, etc., but nearly three-quarters of the employees in the industry are members of the National Union of Dyers, Bleachers and Textile Workers, an industrial union. Many unions are grouped together in federations (for example, the National Association of Unions in the Textile Trades), and most unions (369 in 1960) are affiliated to the Trades Union Congress. There are some unions with barely a hundred members, others with over a million.

Each union has local branches which send representatives to district and national committees. Before the development of national insurance many unions offered their members sickness benefit, and some of them (generally the craft unions) also provided unemployment benefit. Total membership of the trade unions in Great Britain increased from one and a half million in 1900 to over ten million in 1966, though as a result of amalgamations the number of unions has declined by about one-third.

(18) EMPLOYERS' ASSOCIATIONS

The break-up of the medieval craft gilds came about when separate masters' and journeymen's associations were formed. The development and expansion of trade unions in the nineteenth and twentieth centuries have been paralleled by a similar development and expansion of employers' associations. Some exist primarily for the purpose of enabling employers to negotiate collectively with trade unions; others exist principally for the discussion of questions relating to particular trades. As with trade unions, there are often small associations, grouped into federations and affiliated to a national body—in this case the Confederation of British Industry. Thus in the wool textile industry there are four large federations covering the main branches of the industry—the British Wool Federation, the Wool Combing Employers' Federation, the Worsted Spinners' Federation and the Woollen and Worsted Trade Federation. These are linked together in the Wool (and Allied) Textile Employers' Council.

The International Labour Organisation, set up in 1919 under the Treaty of Versailles, carries the discussion of labour questions to the international level, each member country being represented by four delegates—two appointed by the Government and one each by employers' and employees' organisations. The diagram on page 322 shows the general structure of the trade unions and the employers' associations in the wool textile industry, and their relationship to national organisations.

(19) COLLECTIVE BARGAINING AND INDUSTRIAL DISPUTES

The existence in an industry of bodies representative of employers and of employees makes possible collective bargaining. The individual employee is by himself in a weak position for bargaining with his employer, but when he combines with his fellows in a trade union his interests can be watched more effectively. Employers, too, nowadays prefer that there should be some organisation representing their employees with which they can negotiate, for individual bargaining would waste too much time. The existence of trade unions and employers' associations is useful to the State if discussions with representatives of an industry are necessary. Though many other matters are often the subject of discussion between trade unions and employers' associations, the most frequent cause of dispute between these two bodies is, of course, wages. The early trade unions were often over-anxious to support their claims for increased wages by taking collective action against the employers by calling strikes. The unions, however, found the strike to be a double-edged weapon, for the employers were able to retaliate by a lock-out if the union refused to accept a reduction in wages. The strike, however, came to be recognised mainly as a weapon of last resort, to be used only when negotiations have failed and deadlock has been reached.

Collective bargaining depends, however, for its success on the willingness of each side to accept whatever agreement may be made on their behalf by their representatives. In recent years, however, there have been many "unofficial" strikes called by discontented groups of members with their own particular local grievances, and frowned upon by the officials of the union concerned. Some of these unofficial strikes have occurred when the local branch of a union has insisted on a "closed-shop" policy—that is, that all employees should be members of a union, or when some of the members have been unwilling to accept an agreement negotiated by the unions.

Conciliation and arbitration. The State for over half a century has shown itself anxious to provide machinery for settling industrial disputes to avoid a recourse being made to the strike. In 1896 a *Conciliation Act* gave powers to the Labour Department of the Board of Trade

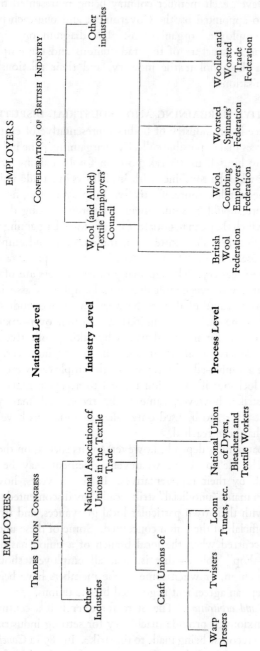

Fig. 71.—Associations of Employers and Employees in the Wool Textile Industry

(later the Ministry of Labour) to inquire into causes of disputes, to bring the two sides together, and upon the application of one of them to appoint a conciliator, or, if both sides were agreeable, an arbitrator. In industries where no machinery previously existed for negotiation between employers and employees Joint Industrial Councils have been set up. They are generally known as Whitley Councils, because the Rt. Hon. J. H. Whitley was chairman of the committee which in 1916 recommended their establishment. Both trade unions and employers' associations are represented on these committees, which meet at regular intervals. There are also Whitley Councils for those in the Civil Service, and in the employment of Local Authorities. Since 1919 there has been in existence a permanent Industrial Court with independent members, as well as representatives of employers and employees, to which reference can be made in the case of specific problems, but its decisions are not enforceable.

RECOMMENDATIONS FOR FURTHER READING

M. Dobb: *Wages.*
J. R. Hicks: *Theories of Wages.*
Report of the Royal Commission on Equal Pay. (1946.) (H.M.S.O.)
Ministry of Labour: *Industrial Relations Handbook.* (H.M.S.O.)
E. H. Phelps Brown: *A Course in Applied Economics,* Chapter VIII.

QUESTIONS

1. "The labourer is rich or poor, is well or ill rewarded in proportion to the real, not to the nominal, price of his labour." (Adam Smith.) Elucidate this statement in the light of conditions at the present time. (R.S.A. Inter.)

2. Why do wages vary between different occupations? (C.I.S. Inter.)

3. What do you understand by the "net advantages of an occupation"? To what extent is there a tendency for all occupations to offer equal net advantages? (I.B.)

4. Why are some dirty and disagreeable jobs paid less than many pleasant jobs? (G.C.E. Adv.)

5. What are the main causes of the inequality of personal incomes in a country? (G.C.E. Adv.)

6. Why do solicitors earn more than their clerks? (G.C.E. Adv.)

7. Does the fixing of wages by collective bargaining, as is common in Great Britain, supersede the market mechanism? (C.I.S. Final.)

8. What are the economic consequences of automation? Would you advocate that automation should be accelerated in this country? (C.I.S. Final.)

9. By what means, if any, can a government effectively influence the rate of change of money wages? (C.C.S. Final.)

10. "The main case for an incomes policy rests on post-war experience suggesting that full employment, price stability and free collective bargaining are inconsistent policies." Discuss. (I.B.)

11. What is meant by "incomes policy"? Describe its objectives and the difficulties that are likely to emerge in its use. (G.C.E. Adv.)

12. Salary claims by trade unions are often made on the grounds of higher salaries in "comparable occupations." What analytical arguments might be used in support of such a case? (G.C.E. Adv.)

13. "Marginal productivity theory cannot explain the salaries of civil servants." Explain. (Final Degree.)

14. Discuss the contention that rates of wages should be adjusted to take account of alterations in the cost of living. (Final Degree.)

Trade Unions.

15. What is a trade union? In what manner and to what extent does it differ from other types of economic associations? (I.B.)

16. In what circumstances might a trade union bring about a permanent increase in the wage rate of the workers in a particular occupation? (G.C.E. Adv.)

17. Explain what you understand by collective bargaining. How does it affect the wage structure in the United Kingdom? (G.C.E. Adv.)

18. Discuss the relative merits of trade union organisation based on (*a*) the craft, or (*b*) the industry, from the point of view of the efficiency of a country's economic life. (C.I.S. Final.)

CHAPTER XIX

INTEREST AND PROFIT

I. THE NATURE OF INTEREST

(1) THE PAYMENT OF INTEREST

Income, it has been seen,[1] is payment for services rendered to production, and is derived from either direct personal service or the ownership of property providing impersonal services. Wages are the payment for labour, and are generally easily distinguished. Rent, interest and profits are not so easily assigned to particular factors of production. This difficulty has already been considered in the case of rent, elements of rent being found in each of the other forms of income. Interest and profit are often difficult to distinguish from one another in practice. Interest may be looked upon as a payment for the use of capital, and profit as the reward of the entrepreneur for his services; or interest may be regarded as income from *money* capital, and profit as income from *real* capital, but interest and profit are often inextricably mixed. Interest is a payment for the use of a certain sum of money for an agreed period of time. If a person borrows £100 at a rate of interest of 5% per annum he will in one year's time have to repay £105—that is, the £100 that he borrowed together with £5 interest.

The medieval Church, following the Mosaic Law[2] and the Greek philosophers, condemned usury. For the lender to receive back from the borrower more money than he had lent was considered unjust, and yet no objection was raised in the later Middle Ages to the payment of rent for land, although money may have been borrowed for the purpose of buying the land. This attitude to the payment of interest is, however, more readily appreciated if the difference between borrowers today and borrowers in ancient or medieval times is taken into consideration. At the present time the most important lenders are the commercial banks. The people who find it easiest to borrow are those whose financial position is basically sound. The business man borrows only because he thinks he can use the money in a way that will yield him more in profit than he has to pay in interest. In less industrialised societies those who sought loans were usually poor people who found themselves in difficulties as a result of some misfortune—perhaps

---

[1] Chapter XVI, p. 268. [2] Exodus xxii. 25.

a fire or a bad harvest—so that by accepting interest the lender appeared to be taking advantage of another man's misfortune. The money-lender of today who does business with the poor is no more respected a member of society than was Shylock, but even so he provides a service for clients who would be unable to borrow elsewhere. From the time of Henry VIII onwards many statutes were passed regulating the rate of interest. The Usury Laws, however, were not repealed until 1854, though they had not been enforced for some time. The rates charged by pawnbrokers continue to be regulated, and moneylenders' charges are subject to review by the courts.

Some opposition to the payment of interest was based on the view that it cost the lender nothing to make a loan, and Karl Marx and his followers maintained this opinion. Since, however, the purchaser of a motor car expects to pay for it, and since too a person who hires a motor car also expects to pay for the use of it for an agreed period of time, it appears to be reasonable to pay for the use of a sum of money for a period, since both the owner of the car and the owner of the sum of money are providing a service and forgo something when the two things are temporarily lent out. Interest is paid because a loan provides a service, and because loanable funds are scarce relative to the demand for them.

(2) PRESENT-DAY BORROWERS AND LENDERS

Borrowing and lending are indispensable adjuncts to an advanced economic system. At the present day the chief lenders are:

(i) Commercial banks, which lend to business men and private individuals (on loan account or overdraft) and to the Government (by the purchase of Government securities).

(ii) Building societies, which assist private individuals and business to purchase house or business property.

(iii) Finance companies, whose main business is to finance hire-purchase transactions.

(iv) Moneylenders, who lend to private individuals.

All the above make lending their main function.

(v) Insurance companies, which lend to the Government (by the purchase of Government securities) and to business (by the purchase of debentures and shares).

(vi) Individuals, who lend to the Government and to business (in a similar manner as do insurance companies) and to banks, building societies and finance companies (by making deposits).

(vii) Business men, who may lend part of their reserves to the Government (by the purchase of Government securities) or to banks (on deposit account).

All these lenders, except individuals, obtain funds for lending by borrowing in their turn, so that the extent of their borrowing determines the amount they are able to lend.

The chief borrowers, therefore, are the Government, business men and private persons; banks and building societies borrow by accepting deposits. The following diagram shows the intricate pattern of present-day borrowing and lending:

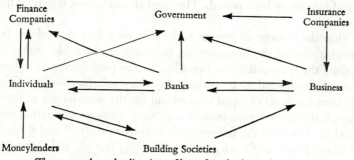

(The arrows show the directions of loans from lenders to borrowers.)

(3) ELEMENTS OF INTEREST

There are three elements in gross interest:

(i) *Payment for risk.* In one case £5 may have to be paid for the use of £100 for a year; in another case £7 may have to be paid for a similar loan. Why should there be any difference in the "hire price" of two equal sums of money for the same period of time? Why do insurance companies charge higher premiums for insuring motor cars to some people than to others. The reason is exactly the same in both instances: more risk is involved in one case than in the other. Part of the interest charged on a loan is therefore a payment for risk—the risk that the loan may not be repaid. Generally, some sort of security has to be given for a loan—something that the lender can turn into cash if the loan is not repaid. In such cases the risk to the lender is reduced, and so the risk payment will be smaller. The person who offers to lend without security will charge a higher rate of interest because his risk of loss is greater.

(ii) *Payment for the trouble involved.* When goods are sold on the hire-purchase system the price to be paid will be higher than that charged to a person who pays cash. Again part of the higher price is a risk payment, but a charge is also made for the inconvenience which this type of sale causes the retailer. The reason why a pawnbroker charges a high rate of interest on loans is partly because there is a great risk that the loan will not be repaid, and partly because of the work the granting of such loans entails. Lending money, then, causes the lender a certain amount of work; he has to keep a record of the transaction and he may have to collect the interest. Thus part of the interest payment is a charge for the lender's trouble.

(iii) *Pure interest.* Any charge additional to payment for risk and for the trouble involved in making the loan must therefore be for the use of the money, to compensate the lender for allowing the borrower the use of his money for a period. This third element, then, is pure or net interest.

Thus the amount of interest to be paid on a loan depends on (*a*) the character of the borrower, (*b*) the expenses the lender incurs in making the loan, and (*c*) the prevailing rate of pure interest. Of these three factors (*a*) and (*b*) are variable, but at a particular time (*c*) will be the same for loans of equal amount and for the same length of time, though the rate of pure interest may vary between one period and another. Consider the following three borrowers, A, B and C, each of whom borrows £100 for a year, A at $4\frac{1}{2}\%$, B at 5% and C at 10%.

	Amount of loan	Rate of Interest	Elements of Interest			
			Payment for use of money (Pure Interest)	Expenses of lender	Payment for risk	Total payment
	£	%	£	£ s.	£ s.	£ s.
A	100	$4\frac{1}{2}$	4	5	5	4 10
B	100	5	4	5	15	5 0
C	100	10	4	1 0	5 0	10 0

Although different rates of interest are paid by the three borrowers, the pure interest is the same in all three cases. If the rate of pure interest rises it will increase the cost to all borrowers.

(4) THE RATE OF INTEREST AND THE RATE OF YIELD

In order to raise a new loan, the Government may have to offer 5% interest to persuade a sufficient number of people to subscribe to it. New stock or bonds to the required amount will be issued, and these may bear some such name as Five per cent. National Bonds 1980–84. The name is required to distinguish the bonds from other issues, and the dates signify that the bonds are not redeemable—that is, repayable —before 1980 or later than 1984, the Government having the option of repaying at any time convenient to itself between these two dates. If the bonds are issued at par this means that £100 of bonds can be bought for that amount, and 5% is the rate of interest to be paid on them. A person purchasing £100 of bonds will therefore acquire an income of £5 per annum. Some time later the Government, again wishing to borrow, may find that now it can obtain the sum required by paying only 4%, and a new issue of (say) Four per cent. State Bonds 1992-98 may be offered to the public. The Stock Exchange— the market for securities—will then experience an increased demand for Five per cent. National Bonds because they carry a higher rate of interest. This increased demand will push up the price, so that more than £100 will have to be paid for £100 of these bonds. In this case the price will probably rise to about £125, for at that price the rate of yield (£5 on £125) will be 4%, the same rate of interest as on the new issue. On the Stock Exchange the prices of bonds and other securities fluctuate daily, and the rate of yield varies with each change of price. If the price of £100 of National Bonds fell to £90 the rate of yield would rise to just over $5\frac{1}{2}$% (£5 on £90). The important feature of all such securities is not the fixed rate of interest they bear, but the rate of yield at any given time, for it is this that reflects the prevailing rate of interest.

II. SAVING

(5) BORROWING AND SAVING

People borrow money not because they want it for its own sake but only because it gives them command over goods and services. Nobody will seek a loan unless he considers that the value of the satisfaction to be derived from the goods or services on which the money is to be spent is at least equal to the interest that he has to pay. Most loans are wanted by business men to finance production. The essential feature of a loan, therefore, is that the lender for an agreed period forgoes in favour of the borrower his claim to a quantity of goods and services. The supply of loanable funds depends on the amount of saving that has previously taken place,[1] the saver forgoing the consumption of a certain quantity of goods and services, which then become available to the borrowers. It is important, therefore, to consider

---

[1] Bank credit complicates this question, but its consideration must be reserved until later. See Chapter XXII.

the different types of saving and the reasons for saving before considering the factors that determine the rate of interest.

Types of saving. The importance of saving lies in the fact that it makes possible real investment—that is, the accumulation of capital goods. Saving reduces the demand for consumers' goods, and so enables more of a country's resources to be devoted to the production of producers' goods or capital goods. Any course of action, therefore, that makes possible capital formation can be considered to be saving. Thus there are a number of types of saving:

(i) *Individual saving.* This is the type of saving ordinarily associated with the word. For a variety of reasons, some of the more important of which are considered in the next paragraph, people are prepared to abstain from current consumption in order to build up a fund of purchasing power for use at a later date, or in order to provide themselves with a future source of income.

(ii) *Corporate saving.* Only about half the total amount of saving comes from private individuals, most of the remainder being provided by the undistributed profits of joint-stock companies. By the decision of the directors, the shareholders have to forgo this amount of profit, which otherwise might have been distributed among them.

These two types of saving are both voluntary.

(iii) *Compulsory saving.* In ordinary speech, saving and taxation are regarded as two quite separate and distinct things, but the economic effect of each can be similar, since each results in a curtailment of consumption, and so makes possible capital investment. If individuals are unwilling to save it may be necessary for the State to compel them to curtail their consumption, and to do this it would impose additional taxation to bring in the amount to be "saved."

(iv) *Forced saving.* The demand for consumers' goods may be checked by a moderate inflation if this results in a rise in prices without a corresponding rise in incomes. By curtailing consumption, resources are released for the production of capital goods, and this has the same economic effect as other kinds of saving. It is sometimes called "forced saving."

(6) REASONS FOR SAVING

It is probably true on the whole that the higher the rate of interest, the greater the amount that will be saved, for it is generally agreed that a low rate of interest discourages saving and encourages spending. Though, by and large, this may be true, there are many exceptions, for in some cases the rate of interest has little effect on saving, and sometimes a lowering of the rate may actually result in more being saved.

It is necessary, therefore, to consider why people save, for the extent to which the rate of interest affects saving will depend on their motives for saving. The following, then, are some of the reasons for saving:

(i) *For unforeseen contingencies.* Most people prefer to have some reserve of cash which they can fall back upon in time of need. In the past the most likely occasions when such a reserve would be useful have been periods of ill-health. The extension of National Insurance to all classes in 1948 has reduced the necessity for this type of saving. It is extremely unlikely that saving of this kind will be affected by the rate of interest.

(ii) *For some future purpose.* In the past one of the most urgent reasons for saving was the desire to put something by for old age. In Great Britain Old Age Pensions were first paid in 1908, and though they were increased after each of the two World Wars, they provide little more than a safeguard against destitution. More generous retirement pensions were provided under the National Insurance scheme for everyone, and these also have been periodically increased. Even when these pensions are supplemented by other contributory schemes, as in the Civil Service, Local Government and many large firms, saving for old age does not appear to have declined. People save in the hope on retirement of being able to continue to enjoy the standard of living to which they have been accustomed. Many people, too, desire for their children a form of education different from that provided by the State, and often begin saving for this purpose from the time of their birth. If a definite sum is required by a certain date more will have to be saved if the rate of interest is low, so that a fall in the rate may actually increase saving for this purpose.

(iii) *For the purchase of expensive goods.* In some ways this purpose is similar to the previous type, as it is merely deferred spending. Things such as motor cars, houses (even if building societies lend a high percentage of the purchase price) and furniture are expensive, and so to a lesser extent are holidays and many durable household goods. For those who find it difficult to save, because to them present satisfaction far outweighs future satisfaction, there are the clothing club, the Christmas club and the holiday club. The effect of hire-purchase is to discourage saving (apart from the initial deposit) and to encourage spending. Some people, however, still prefer to save up in advance for things they wish to buy. The rate of interest has no direct bearing on such saving, which often merely brings forward or puts back a little the date when the particular satisfaction can be enjoyed.

(iv) *To raise social status.* Power, influence and social prestige depend to some extent on personal wealth and income. By saving, it is possible for a man to build up a source of future income either for himself or his descendants. It is doubtful how far the rate of interest will affect this kind of saving. A low rate may discourage some, but for others it may merely lead to a redoubling of effort.

(v) *As a matter of principle.* Some people may look upon thrift as a virtue, and so consider self-denial a desirable thing in itself. In such cases saving is obviously independent of the rate of interest, but there is less of this kind of saving than formerly.

(vi) *For speculative purposes.* Saving for this purpose is directly related to the rate of interest. If the rate is high there is a strong inducement to save, whereas if the rate is low saving ceases to be worth while.

(vii) *Some saving is not planned.* The very rich may save the surplus that remains from their incomes after they have spent all they wish, though heavy taxation of high incomes has reduced the amount saved in this way. The rate of interest clearly has not much effect on this saving. All saving is, however, to a greater or less extent dependent on the saver's wealth and income, for the rate at which wealth increases is cumulative. The more that is saved, the larger the income, and so the easier it is to save still more.

III. THE DETERMINATION OF THE RATE OF INTEREST

(7) THE SUPPLY AND DEMAND ANALYSIS

The subject of interest is one of the most controversial in the whole of economics. According to one school of thought, the rate of interest, being the price of loans, is determined by the demand for loans, on the one hand, and the supply of loanable funds, on the other, so that the equilibrium rate (or natural rate, as Wicksell called it) is the rate that equates demand with supply.

Time-preference. The supply of loanable funds comes from saving. As with other things, more will generally be supplied the higher the price, so that a high rate of interest will increase the supply of loanable funds. This is probably largely true, though it has been seen above that much saving is independent of the rate of interest. Time preference theories, including that of Böhm-Bawerk, stress the idea that the supply of loans depends on the fact that most people prefer to have a certain sum of money now than at some future time. Interest, therefore, arises because one person prefers £100 now, to (say) £104 a year hence, while another prefers £104 a year hence to £100 now, lending and borrowing being possible only because the satisfaction of immediate wants occupies a higher place on the borrower's than on the lender's scale of preferences.

Capital is productive. There is a demand for loans because capital is productive. A greater output is achieved if a more capitalistic method of production is adopted, but this increases the time interval between the taking of the decision to produce and the beginning of the outflow of goods. The more capitalistic the method of production, the longer this time interval will be. In order, then, to be able to undertake a more capitalistic method of production the entrepreneur has to sacrifice a smaller immediate gain for a future greater gain. He is willing to pay interest because he hopes that his gain from *waiting*, that is, extending the time interval of production, will more than compensate him for what he has paid. Interest can therefore be regarded either as the reward of waiting or as a payment for not waiting.

The holding of stocks—generally financed by borrowing—makes possible a more even flow of goods to the market, particularly in the case of agricultural products, merchants buying large stocks of wheat, for example, when supplies are plentiful, storing the commodity and releasing it gradually. In a somewhat similar way the wholesaler eases the distributive process by holding stocks of goods turned out in large quantities by manufacturers and wanted by retailers in smaller quantities only when their stocks are in need of replenishment.

Marginal productivity of capital.[1] Capital can never receive more than the value of its marginal product, because the entrepreneur will employ a little more capital only if the additional income arising from its employment exceeds what he has to pay for it. If the entrepreneur can borrow £100 at 4% and use it productively so as to yield him a return of £10 he will gain £6 by borrowing. The incidence of the Law of Diminishing Returns may mean that a further £100 (assuming that he can continue to borrow at the same rate) yields a return of £8, a third £100 a return of £6, a fourth £100 a return of £4, and a fifth only £3. He can increase his profit by borrowing up to £400, because at that point the interest he has to pay is equal to the value of the marginal product of the capital. The demand for business loans depends therefore on the marginal productivity of capital in relation to the rate of interest, and the greater the amount of capital employed, the lower generally will be its marginal productivity. In the same way there is a tendency towards equality of wages in all occupations, so there is, similarly, a tendency for the marginal productivity of capital to be the same in all forms of production. This being so, capital will be attracted into those kinds of production where it would yield a higher

[1] Lord Keynes used the term "marginal efficiency of capital," which he defined as "the relation between the prospective yield of one more unit of that type of capital and the cost of producing that unit." (*General Theory of Employment, Interest and Money*, p. 135.)

return, being drawn away from those employments where the return is lower, so that equilibrium will be achieved only when marginal productivity is in all cases equal. Some capital, of course, cannot easily be transferred to alternative use, but it need not be replaced when it becomes worn out.

The importance of interest to production. The rate of interest is important because it influences capital accumulation. If a new machine costing £500 will add £30 a year to the income of the firm installing it it will be to the advantage of the entrepreneur to borrow the necessary £500, provided that the rate of interest is less than 6%. As the rate of interest falls, some forms of production previously unprofitable can be undertaken. Since production is undertaken in anticipation of demand, it is the prospective yield of capital, and not its current yield, that influences entrepreneurs. Capital is scarce relative to the demand for it, and so it is the purpose of interest (as with other prices) to distribute it among all the various uses competing for it; and such a rationing of capital by means of the rate of interest is necessary even under a communist régime.

(8) THE MONETARY THEORY OF INTEREST

Liquidity-preference. The view that the rate of interest equates the demand for loans with the supply of savings is too simple, for the question is complicated by the fact that banks can create credit and by the public's demand for holding money balances. People require to hold money for everyday purposes—bus fares, for example—with a little in reserve to meet any unforeseen calls upon them. If more is held than is necessary for these purposes it must be because they prefer to keep their resources "liquid"—that is, in the form of money rather than in the form of some other assets, such as stocks and shares. To keep liquid, however, involves a loss of interest. But if the prices of securities are expected to fall in the future it will be advantageous to postpone purchasing them, since a fall in their prices will increase their yield. In such circumstances, then, more money will be held—that is, liquidity-preference will be strong. If the prices of securities are expected to rise, it will be advantageous to purchase them without delay, and so less money will be held—that is liquidity-preference will be weak. Liquidity-preference and the rate of interest affect one another. The banks, by their credit policy, decide what the total quantity of money shall be, but the general public's liquidity-preference determines how much money will be held—that is, the demand for money. According to this theory, the rate of interest is not determined by people's willingness to save, but by their attitude towards liquidity. The rate of interest can therefore be considered as the reward for parting with liquidity. This question will be discussed further in Chapter XXI in connection with the demand to hold money.

It is likely that each one of these explanations of the determination of the rate of interest contains some truth, for it may be partly determined by real forces such as the productivity of capital, and partly by monetary forces such as liquid-preference. Controversy is largely the result of difference of emphasis.

(9) LONG- AND SHORT-TERM RATES OF INTEREST

Differences in the liquidity of securities affect their rates of yield. $2\frac{1}{2}$ per cent. Consols are an example of a non-liquid security, for there is no date when they are due to be redeemed. Many Government Stocks are dated, two dates usually being given, the Government having the option to redeem them at any time between these two dates. Generally the longer the period to the date of redemption, the higher is the rate of yield, though there have been exceptions to this when the short-term rate of interest has been very high, as, for example, on the occasions when Bank rate has been 7%. The following were the Stock Exchange quotations for some Government Stocks on 23rd March 1966:

3% British Electricity Stock, 1968–73	$78\frac{3}{4}$
3% Savings Bonds, 1965–75	$73\frac{7}{8}$
3% British Transport Stock, 1978–88	$58\frac{1}{4}$
3% British Gas Stock, 1990–95	$54\frac{3}{4}$
$2\frac{1}{2}$% Consols	$37\frac{1}{4}$

The quotations in all cases refer to stock of £100 nominal value. The yields on these stocks vary inversely with their prices. On the 3% British Gas Stock 1990–95 the yield is over 6·8%, whereas on the 3% British Electricity Stock, 1968–73 the yield is 6·6%, calculated to the latest date.

There are, however, securities that fall due within a very short period of time, such as bills of exchange (trade bills and Treasury bills), which generally mature in three months. Since these bills are fairly liquid, they generally bear only a low rate of interest. This is the short-term rate of interest. The two rates—long-term and short-term—generally follow one another up and down, though the short-term is more liable to fluctuations. On account of the greater risk of a change of yield over a long period of time, the long-term rate is usually higher than the short-term, except when the short-term rate is very high. That the two rates tend to rise or fall together is largely the result of the action of speculators, who sell their long-term securities if their price is high and buy short-term securities with the proceeds, reversing this process later if the prices of short-term securities rise. The yield on bills is generally likely to be small (except when bank rate is high) because they are a fairly liquid form of asset. The cost of keeping one's assets liquid, therefore, is the short-term rate of interest, and so this, depending largely on liquidity-preference, is generally regarded as the fundamental rate, the long-term being determined by it.

IV. PROFIT

(10) GROSS PROFIT AND NET PROFIT

Suppose that Pecksniff is the sole proprietor of a small retail drapery business. In order to show his gross profit he periodically draws up a trading account:

TABLE XLIV

Trading Account

For the period 1st January to 30th June

			£			£
Jan. 1.	To opening stock	.	1,030	June 30. By sales . .	.	3,020
June 30.	„ purchases	.	1,340	„ 30. „ closing stock	.	1,050
„ 30.	„ gross profit	.	1,700			
			£4,070			£4,070

This shows that his gross profit for this period of six months is £1,700. Pecksniff will then proceed to draw up a Profit and Loss Account in order to find his net profit:

TABLE XLV

Profit and Loss Account

			£			£
June 30.	To wages	. .	300	June 30. By gross profit	.	1,700
„ 30.	„ rent	. .	180			
„ 30.	„ rates	. .	140			
„ 30.	„ lighting	. .	40			
„ 30.	„ heating	.	50			
„ 30.	„ depreciation	.	50			
„ 30.	„ net profit	.	940			
			£1,700			£1,700

Pecksniff's net profit for this period of six months is therefore £940, and this has been calculated by deducting his expenses from his gross profit. Even this simple illustration shows one important characteristic of profit, namely that, unlike wages, it is not a fixed sum, but a residual amount received after all payments have been made. A sole trader he will probably regard as profit the whole of the amount that the business yields him—£940 in the above example.

(ii) ELEMENTS OF PROFIT

Before setting up in business on his own account, Pecksniff may have been employed as branch manager of a multiple-shop, saving a portion of his income each year for the purpose of accumulating the capital necessary for a business of his own at some future date. Suppose that as manager of the Northampton branch of Multiple Drapers Ltd. his salary was £1,200 per annum, and that his savings finally amounted to £6,000 which he had invested in Government Stock at 5%. At that time his income for six months would be:

	£
Salary as manager of the shop	600
Interest on his savings	150
Total income for six months . . .	£750

In business on his own account his income for six months is his net profit of £940. As a sole trader he has been acting as manager of his own shop, and also using his own capital, which otherwise would have yielded him interest. His net profit can therefore be split up as follows:

Salary as manager of his own shop (assuming his services to himself to be worth as much as Multiple Drapers Ltd. paid him)	600
Interest on his capital	150
Pure profit	190
	£940

Thus three elements in profit can be distinguished: wages of management, interest on capital and pure profit.

If Pecksniff's business had been a limited company his salary would have been reckoned as part of working expenses, and the company's profit would have been shown as £340. Assuming the profit for the next six months to be the same, and that the whole amount was distributed among the shareholders (a most unlikely event), the company would have been able to declare a dividend of 11% for the year. The distributed profit of a company, therefore, contains two elements: interest on capital and pure profit.

Pure profit. This is a payment for taking risk. People would be unwilling to provide capital for business enterprises if there was no possibility of a greater return than could be obtained from "safe" investments such as Government Stock. At the beginning of this chapter it was said that interest can be considered as income from money capital, and profit as income from real capital, but it is clear now that income from real capital also includes an element of interest.

Some writers look upon pure profit as the peculiar reward of the entrepreneur for his share in the work of production; others, who refuse to recognise the entrepreneur as a factor of production, stress the concept of profit as the surplus remaining after all the expenses of production, including wages of management, have been met. These two concepts are, however, not nearly so divergent as might at first appear. Profit goes to the owners of the business, who risk holding assets in that form. In both cases profit appears as a payment for bearing risk. In Chapter III it was seen that uncertainty-bearing was the principal function of the entrepreneur, uncertainty covering all risks that could not be insured against, whereas contractual payments are made for the services of labour. The income of the entrepreneur is residual and also, unlike wages, it can be negative—that is, a firm may make either a profit or a loss.

Under perfect competition a certain level of profit is necessary if capital is to be retained in a particular line of production, and this has been called *normal profit*. Apart from this, pure profit would tend to disappear under static conditions. Profit arises, then, under dynamic conditions. In the more extreme forms of imperfect competition— those forms that approach most nearly to monopoly—profit above normal arises as a result of restriction of output, so that monopoly profit is more in the nature of a rent than a true profit, since it has its origin in the scarcity of the product, even though in this case scarcity is created by the monopolist himself.

(12) CAUSES OF UNCERTAINTY

Pure profit, then, occurs in dynamic conditions, since there will always be uncertainty when conditions are liable to change. The entrepreneur may be fully conversant with the state of the markets for his factors, and for his final product, at the time when he embarks upon production, but since production takes place in anticipation of demand, and a time interval must elapse between the taking of his decision to produce and the beginning of the outflow of his goods to the market, no entrepreneur can be sure what will be the eventual demand for his product. In other words, uncertainty is present. In static conditions there would be no pure profit, for uncertainty is the result of dynamic change.

Some of the influences liable to produce uncertainty are as follows:

    (i) changes in population, either in numbers or in its distribution among different age-groups, with consequent changes in demand;

    (ii) changes of fashion which can cause sudden changes of demand;

(iii) a rise or fall in total money income or a change in the distribution of income among consumers;

(iv) the introduction of new forms of capital, with consequent changes in the technique of production;

(v) ignorance of the price and output policy of rival firms.

If any of these changes takes place uncertainty will arise, and entrepreneurs may earn pure profit. If for any reason uncertainty declines, then pure profit will also decline.

(13) DIFFERENCES IN PROFIT

While uncertainty exists there can be no general rate of profit, for profit will vary between different industries according to the extent of uncertainty in each line of production. Therefore, in well-established industries, where conditions are less subject to change, uncertainty is at a minimum, and so pure profit tends to be low. In such industries there will also be only slight differences in the amount of pure profit earned by different entrepreneurs. Wherever differences in pure profit earned by entrepreneurs occur in the same industry these differences can be explained only by variations in entrepreneurial skill. The greater the uncertainty, the greater will be the possibility of profit, but also the greater the risk of loss. People are willing to put their capital into risky undertakings only because of the possibility of high profit. Uncertainty is always high in the case of new products, and so the expectation of high profit is the inducement to capital to enter new fields of activity. If an industry yields high profit this will encourage new firms to enter, and so tend to lower profit in that industry. The entrepreneur aims at maximising his profit, and this induces him to adopt new techniques. Profit, therefore, encourages enterprise.

Differences in profit in different industries are therefore the result of differences in uncertainty; differences in profit between firms in the same industry are due to differences in the skill of entrepreneurs in bearing uncertainty.

(14) PROFIT AND COST OF PRODUCTION

The residual character of profit has already been stressed. This being so, two questions may be asked. Is profit a cost of production? Does profit enter into price? Wages of management are clearly a cost of production, as was shown in the case of a joint-stock company. If capital is provided in the form of debentures these are a charge on the firm, and so interest on this capital becomes a cost of production. In the case of the dividend on ordinary shares it is difficult to distinguish between interest and pure profit, but the interest element is clearly a cost. Unless entrepreneurs receive what is regarded as the "normal profit" for an industry, capital will move elsewhere, and so normal profit, the minimum reward the entrepreneur is prepared to accept, too, must also be regarded as a cost of production. Any further profit, however, is due to the entrepreneur's own skill and judgment in overcoming uncertainty, and is a surplus earned only by the more successful entrepreneurs. This element of profit is not a cost, and therefore it does not influence the price of the commodity. High profits, therefore, are not the cause, but the result of high prices, which in turn are the result of a high level of demand.

Both profit and rent, then, are surpluses, but rent is a surplus accruing to any factor of production as a result of a condition generally outside the factor's control—the difficulty in the short period of increasing the supply of a specific factor to meet an increase in the demand for its services. Rent is therefore unearned, for no factor can as a result of its own exertions obtain rent. Profit, however, is the reward for the successful bearing of uncertainty.

RECOMMENDATIONS FOR FURTHER READING

F. H. Knight: *Risk, Uncertainty and Profit*, Chapters 1, 2, 7–10.
A. Marshall: *Principles of Economics*, Bk. VI, Chapters 6–8.
P. Wicksteed: *Common-sense of Political Economy*, Vol. I, Chapter 7.

QUESTIONS

Interest

1. What reasons may be advanced for and against the payment of interest? (R.S.A. Inter.)

2. "The rate of interest is the reward for parting with liquidity for a specified period." Assess the adequacy of this definition of the rate of interest. (C.I.S. Inter.)

3. What are the factors that tend to link together the movements in long-term and short-term rates of interest? How far are these factors operative in present conditions? (I.B.)

4. "The rate of interest is not the 'price' which brings into equilibrium the demand for resources to invest with the readiness to abstain from present consumption." (Keynes.) What do *you* think determines the rate of interest? (A.C.C.A. Final.)

5. What factors influence the level of savings in an economy? (G.C.E. Adv.)

6. Illustrate the interaction of Demand and Supply in determining the rate of interest. (C.C.S. Final.)

7. What place does the Keynesian theory of interest leave for thrift and the productivity of capital? (Final Degree.)

Profit

8. Distinguish between profits, rent and interest. (I.M.T.A.)

9. How would you distinguish between interest and profits? (C.I.S. Inter.)

10. What is meant by the "profit-motive"? In your answer bring out carefully the nature and genesis of profits. (I.H.A.)

11. Examine the contention that if profits were reduced wages could be increased in any given industry. (I.T.)

12. "Profits are the reward for risk-taking." Discuss this statement with reference to the present-day financial structure of industry. (Exp.)

13. "Profits tend to equality." Point out the ambiguities in this statement and submit a clear statement about the relations between profits in different industries. (I.B.)

14. On what factors does the profitability of an enterprise depend? (Final Degree.)

15. "Super-normal profits are a rent and may be taxed away without affecting business enterprise." Discuss. (Final Degree.)

PART SIX

BANKING AND FINANCE

CHAPTER XX

THE ORIGIN AND FUNCTIONS OF MONEY

I. THE ORIGIN OF MONEY

(1) DISADVANTAGES OF BARTER

The use of money facilitates exchange. Under the most primitive conditions of human existence each family provided for its entire needs, though even then there would probably be some division of labour among the members. In so small a group, held together by family ties, each member might make a contribution to the common tasks and be content to receive a share from the common pool according to his needs. As soon as peaceful intercourse took place between different groups of people the possibility of exchange would arise if one group were able, by reason of differences of climate or geology, to produce something another group lacked. Division of labour, by making it possible for people to specialise in those occupations for which they are best fitted, raises the standard of life, but makes exchange necessary. The man who devotes his whole time to working in iron is compelled to exchange some of the things that he has made for food and clothing. Before money came to be used goods had to be exchanged for goods; the smith, for example, might exchange a spade perhaps for a quantity of meat or wheat, just as a modern schoolboy might exchange a penknife for a handful of marbles.

The exchanging of goods for goods is known as *barter*. It has three serious drawbacks. In the first place, it makes exchange dependent on what is called a "double coincidence of wants." Thus it is not sufficient for the smith to find someone requiring a spade; if he wants wheat in exchange for the spade he must find a farmer who not only wishes to dispose of wheat but who at the same time requires a spade. Since farmers are likely to want spades, this might be less difficult than the task of a goldsmith in search of a butcher who is in want of a gold trinket of some kind. Even after two men who are able to satisfy each other's wants have been brought together, there is the further difficulty of deciding how much wheat has to be given for a spade or how much meat for a gold ornament. Different rates of exchange have to be determined to cover every transaction before it can take place. A third problem arises if one party to a transaction has only a large commodity,

345

such as a table, to offer, but requires only a small quantity of something
—perhaps a stone of potatoes in exchange. Barter, therefore, involves
a waste of human effort and is a clumsy method of exchange, but even
under a system of barter there is need of some unit of account in which
to assess the values of different commodities, even though no medium
of exchange has been agreed upon.

(2) EARLY FORMS OF MONEY

The difficulty of bringing two people together, each of whom was
able to supply something the other desired in exchange for what the
other could offer him, led to the development of an intermediate stage.
There would be some things that were in general demand, and so
instead of seeking out a farmer in need of a spade, the smith might, for
example, exchange his spade for a quantity of salt, and then exchange
the salt for wheat. Anything in common use and generally acceptable
could serve as a medium of exchange. Thus goods which first served
as money were those that were most marketable—that is, those
considered to be valuable for their own sake.

To be generally acceptable, goods have to be either useful or orna-
mental, and so cattle, hides and leather, furs, tea, salt, cowrie shell
and many other things have at different times and in different places
served as money. Adam Smith declared that in his own day salt was
still being used as money in Abyssinia, shells in some parts of India,
dried cod in Newfoundland, tobacco in Virginia and sugar in the
West Indies. Immediately after the Second World War cigarettes
for a time served as a medium of exchange in Western Germany. All
these things, however, have serious drawbacks. Cattle are not all of
equal quality; they are bulky and not easily taken around by a shopper;
the units are too large, and so can be used only for large purchases; and
their owners would suffer loss if the cattle were to die. Tea and salt are
more easily divisible, but both are liable to deterioration when stored.
Cowrie shells, though used as money in China, are fairly abundant in
the Indian Ocean, and there are places where one's stock could easily be
replenished.

Qualities of good monetary media. A good medium of exchange must
not only be (i) generally acceptable, but must also be (ii) fairly durable,
(iii) capable of being divided into reasonably small units, and (iv) easy
to carry about. A fifth necessary quality is that it should be relatively
scarce, though not too scarce. The precious metals, at first silver and
later gold, fulfilled all these conditions, and they quickly superseded
other things as money, silver being in use for this purpose in the earliest
days of recorded history. Though there has been considerable varia-

tion at different times in the output of gold and silver from the mines, the amount mined in any one year has never formed more than a small percentage of the total amount in existence. Commodities more valuable than gold, such as diamonds and platinum, have never been used as money because the amounts required for the purchase of cheap things would be too small to handle. In early times a sixth quality was required before a commodity could be used as money—namely, that it should be valuable for its own sake. Once a commodity had been selected for use as money its value tended to increase. When, during the nineteenth century, many countries replaced silver by gold as their monetary standard the value of silver fell considerably, while the value of gold rose.

II. TYPES OF MONEY

(3) COINS

One of the main advantages of using the precious metals as money was their divisibility, and at first merchants paid for what they purchased by weighing out an agreed amount of the metal. Though the use of the precious metals in this way was a great improvement on previous media of exchange, the disadvantages of this method of making payments must soon have become apparent. In time coins came into use. A coin is nothing more than a definite amount of metal, its weight and fineness being guaranteed by the official stamp of the issuing authority. At first, for example, the Jewish shekel was a certain weight of metal, but later it came to mean a coin, and similarly, the pound sterling was originally a pound by weight of silver. Coins were the most convenient form of money yet used, but there was always the danger that the issuing authority might make them of less weight than they were reputed to be. The responsibility for the issue of coins soon came to be regarded as the prerogative of the State, and monarchs in financial straits were often tempted to debase the coinage by reducing the amount of precious metals in them. Henry VIII had recourse to debasement of the coinage on an extensive scale, the coins issued between 1543 and 1551 containing each year less silver than the year before, until eventually the amount of silver in the coins was only one-seventh of the amount they had originally contained.

Merchants in those days looked upon coins simply as a convenient means of handling quantities of the precious metals, and they were not to be deceived by such unscrupulous behaviour, for whenever the issuing authority resorted to debasement the value of the coins fell. In such cases the merchants would have recourse to weighing the coins themselves. Thus an article priced at 3s. would require 4s. in payment if the silver content of the coins had been reduced by 25%. If the debasement was the result of mixing base metal with the silver the value of the coins would be proportionately reduced, and this again would result in a rise in prices. During the reign of Henry VIII prices, therefore, for this—and other[1]—reasons rose steeply, but since the debased coins were still legal tender, the king and other debtors were able to pay their debts more easily—so long as creditors would accept them.

Gresham's Law. With each debasement of the coinage by Henry VIII the better coins passed out of circulation, thus providing an example of Gresham's Law, which states that "bad money drives out good." This so-called law takes its name from Sir Thomas Gresham, Elizabeth I's finance minister, to whom fell the task of putting the currency on a sound basis again. It is not, however, universally true that bad money drives out good. The base coins may not circulate at all if people refuse to accept them, for the fact that coins have been declared to be legal tender will not make them serve as money unless they are generally acceptable. If there are insufficient of the inferior coins in circulation to meet the needs of trade some of the good coins will circulate along with the bad. As people come to regard money merely as a medium of exchange, and not as something desirable in itself, they may continue to accept a form of money of less value than it purports to be, either from habit or a realisation that any commodity can serve as money if it is generally acceptable and relatively scarce.

(4) LEGAL TENDER

Any means of payment that a debtor can legally compel his creditor to accept is legal tender. In Great Britain at the present time Bank of England notes—£10, £5, £1 and 10s.—are full legal tender up to any amount, but £10 and £5 notes are legal tender only in England and Wales. Coins, however, are only limited legal tender—copper to a maximum of 1s. silver up to 40s. and the twelve-sided three-penny pieces up to 2s. The reason for this limitation is now largely historical. Before 1914 the gold sovereign and half sovereign were worth their full face value, and so were full legal tender. The silver and copper coins were even then worth less than their face value—that is, they were merely token coins. Since 1946 cupro-nickel coins have replaced silver coins in Great Britain, and as metal these are worth little more than one-sixth of their face value. Inconvertible paper money, in circulation in

---

[1] The discovery of silver in Central and South America resulted in a further rise in prices.

this country since 1931, has little value apart from its use as money, so that all money now in use in Great Britain is token money, and it has been said that our coins are really "bank-notes printed on metal."[1] The most commonly used means of payment—the cheque—is not legal tender, nor are bills of exchange, postal orders or money orders. For a short time in 1914 and 1939, in each case during the early months of war, postal orders became legal tender.

Bi-metallism. If both gold and silver coins of full face value were minted supporters of bi-metallism believed money would be more stable in value, though difficulties would arise if a change took place in the relative values of the two metals. For example, if the price of silver rose, while that of gold remained unchanged, the silver coins would become worth more than their face value, and would tend to be driven out of circulation in accordance with Gresham's Law. Fluctuation in market prices occur daily, and so it is impracticable to have both gold and silver coins of their full face value in circulation at the same time.

(5) PAPER MONEY

Paper money had its origin in the receipts given by goldsmiths to clients who deposited money and other valuables with them for safe custody. The nature of the goldsmith's business made it necessary for him to have a strong room in which to store his valuable stock, and in times when acts of violence were of common occurrence it was natural for people to make use of the goldsmiths' facilities for storing things of great value. For this service a charge was made. If a client, Tigg, deposited £50 in silver coins he would receive from Tapley, a goldsmith, a receipt for that amount. When some time later Tigg, in the course of business, made a purchase from Pinch for £50 he could either take his receipt to Tapley, obtain his £50 in cash and then hand it over to Pinch, or instead he might endorse the receipt with instructions to Tapley to pay the £50 to Pinch, who in turn might pass on his claim to yet another merchant. It would be unusual at first for receipts to cover such convenient amounts as the £50 of this example. More often they might be awkward amounts, such as £98 10s. or £43 16s. 5d.

When the usefulness of these goldsmiths' receipts for making payments was realised it became the practice to issue receipts in smaller denominations. Instead of a receipt for £50, Tigg, perhaps, might accept ten separate receipts each for £5. In this way the bank-note came into existence. In London the goldsmiths became the first bankers, and they soon found the issue of bank-notes to be a profitable

[1] G. Crowther: *An Outline of Money*, p. 16 n.

business. Thus the bank-note was a receipt for a debt, an IOU, show-ing that the banker owed the bearer of the note a stated sum of money, the banker being expected to redeem the promise printed on his note and exchange it on demand for actual cash. Confidence in the early bankers grew only slowly, but as people became more accustomed to bank-notes the banker eventually found it unnecessary to keep a stock of cash equal to the total value of all the bank-notes that he had issued, and so he could employ some of his cash profitably. At the present time the only bank in England that possesses the power to issue bank-notes is the Bank of England, though several banks in Scotland, Northern Ireland and the Isle of Man are permitted to issue a limited amount in notes.

(6) CONVERTIBLE AND INCONVERTIBLE MONEY

If a bank-note can be exchanged on demand for gold or silver coins it is said to be convertible. The earliest bank-notes had to be con-vertible, because people were willing to use only a medium of exchange which was of value for its own sake, and it was a long time before people were willing to accept as money something of no value in itself. The convertible bank-note was not, in the strictest sense, itself money, but merely a substitute for money, or a claim to the sum of money named upon it. On the other hand, there is no compulsion on the issuing authority to exchange inconvertible paper money for gold or any other form of money of full face value.

Inconvertible paper is the final stage in the development of the bank-note. So long as it can be used to purchase what people want to buy, it is not necessary for the medium of exchange to be valuable in itself. So long as people have confidence in the medium, so long will it be generally acceptable, but once this confidence is lost it can no longer serve as money—a fact of which people living in a country that has suffered a major inflation are only too painfully aware. Confidence in a currency will be lost if an excessive amount of it is put into circulation. If paper money has to be convertible on demand this limits the amount that can be issued; but if notes are inconvertible States may be tempted to choose the easy way of covering expenditure by merely printing more notes. That is the great danger associated with the use of incon-vertible paper money.

The issue by private institutions of paper money—whether conver-tible or not—has always been regulated in some way by the State. Regulation may take the form of limiting the issue to a definite fraction of one or more of the issuing authority's assets. For example, in the United States of America the Federal Reserve Banks were at one time legally compelled to hold gold certificates up to a minimum of 40% of their note issue.

In England the *Bank Charter Act* of 1844 limited the power of the Bank of England to issue notes. Except for £14 million, the Bank's notes were to be backed in full by gold, additional notes being issued only if the bank acquired an equivalent additional amount of gold. That part of the note issue not backed by gold is known as the *fiduciary issue*. Before 1914 Bank of England notes in denominations of £5 and multiples of £5 were convertible and circulated along with gold sovereigns and half-sovereigns. During 1914–25 Bank of England notes ceased to be convertible, but in 1925 they, as well as the £1 and 10s. Treasury Notes issued by the Government during 1914–28, again became convertible, but only in large amounts—in exchange for gold bars each weighing 400 oz. and worth approximately £1,560 each. Since 1931 bank-notes in England have been inconvertible, and the promise of the Bank of England printed on them now has little meaning.

(7) BANK DEPOSITS SUBJECT TO WITHDRAWAL BY CHEQUE

The final stage in the development of money is the use of bank deposits as money. The cheque as a means of payment is most widely used in Great Britain and the United States. The greater political stability of these two countries and the greater confidence of business men in banks—in spite of some banking crises—have been responsible for this development. The use of cheques is, however, rapidly expanding now in most countries.

In Great Britain the Act of 1844 restricted the note issue to an amount insufficient for the needs of a rapidly expanding economy, and so bank deposits were used to make good this deficiency. In order to obtain the right to draw a cheque it is necessary to open a current account at a bank. A cheque-book is then obtained, and if a payment has to be made a cheque can be drawn for the required amount. The person receiving the cheque deposits it with his own banker, who collects the amount for him from the bank on which the cheque has been drawn.

It is to be noted that it is the bank deposit that is considered to be money, and not the cheque, for the cheque itself is merely an order from the owner of a bank deposit to his banker to transfer a certain sum to the payee named on the cheque. The validity of a cheque therefore depends on whether the drawer of the cheque has a sufficient amount in his current account to meet the cheque. If he draws a cheque for £80 when his bank account shows that he has only £5 to his credit the bank will dishonour the cheque and the payee will find that he has been given a worthless piece of paper. Cheques therefore are not legal tender and so a creditor has the right to refuse to accept this method of payment. Cheques, however, are often acceptable, and by permitting bank deposits to be transferred from one person to another, enable bank deposits to serve as money.

In one way cheques resemble bank-notes: they both have to do with bank debts. The bank-note is an acknowledgment by a bank that it owes the bearer a certain sum, and as the bank-note passes from hand to hand, the bank's debt is transferred from one person to another; similarly, a bank deposit is an acknowledgment of the bank's debt to a particular depositor, who by means of the cheque can transfer the bank's debt to some other person. The bank-note may be more generally acceptable because the bank is more widely known and enjoys the public's confidence to a greater degree than do many drawers of cheques. At the present time it is estimated that approximately 90% of all business payments made in Great Britain are made by cheque. When calculating the total of bank balances that can be drawn upon by cheque, and so used as money, it is usual to include sums on deposit account as well as sums on current account, the assumption being that transfers can easily be made from one account to the other. The total of bank deposits in Great Britain at the present time is more than five times as great as the total cash in the country. It is clear, therefore, that bank deposits now form the chief type of money in this country.

The principal stages in the development of money have therefore been the use of:

(i) commodities in general demand, such as cattle;
(ii) precious metals by weight;
(iii) definite weights of metal in the form of coins;
(iv) goldsmiths' receipts for deposits of cash;
(v) bank-notes convertible into cash on demand;
(vi) inconvertible paper money; and lastly
(vii) bank deposits, transferable from one person to another by cheque.

III. FUNCTIONS OF MONEY

(8) ADVANTAGES OF USING MONEY

The following advantages can be claimed on behalf of money:

(i) It enables a person who receives payment for his services in money to obtain in exchange for it the assortment of goods from that particular amount of expenditure *which will give him maximum satisfaction*. No two persons have exactly the same wants, and so any other system of distribution would yield less satisfaction to most people. For example, a system of rationing will give some people more and others less than they want of some commodities. Rationing does not enable a person to forgo one thing in order to enjoy more of another. Without money, wages would have to be paid in kind, and for most people this would be even worse than rationing.

(ii) Without the use of money, *division of labour* would be difficult, if not impossible, to sustain. Exchange is the essential corollary of division of labour, and exchange is simplified if money is employed rather than a system of barter. It is only when money is used that it becomes possible for people to specialise.

(iii) When money is employed it becomes *easier to make loans*. A borrower never wants money for its own sake, but only to give him command over real resources. Lending can, of course, take place without the intervention of money, as when a person borrows his neighbour's lawn-mower, but in business it is not often possible to borrow a machine from the makers. One firm specialises in making machinery, another in making loans. The use of money makes this possible.

(iv) Deferred spending, too, would be impossible without money. By refraining from spending some of one's current income for a period it becomes possible to save up a sum of money to spend later.

(9) FUNCTIONS OF MONEY

Money performs four main functions:

(i) *A medium of exchange.* Money comes into use because of the inconvenience of barter. A system of exchange which requires the bringing together of two people who have "a double coincidence of wants" will reduce the exchange of goods to a minimum. It has been seen that the use of a medium of exchange occurred at quite an early stage in the development of trade. By acting as a medium of exchange, money facilitates the exchange of goods, and historically, this was probably the earliest function of money.

(ii) *A measure of value and a unit of account.* A second drawback to barter is the difficulty of determining a rate of exchange between goods of different types, especially in the case of large, indivisible articles. It is possible, therefore, that even while a barter system was still in operation this difficulty may have led to the use of some commodity as a means of assessing the relative values of a heterogeneous group of things. It is probable that some commodity was serving as a unit of account even before a medium of exchange was in use, and so in point of time money may have fulfilled this function even before it became a medium of exchange, for it is not necessary for a commodity to be generally acceptable—the first characteristic of money—in order for it to be used for making calculations. The unit of account, however, could have been used merely to assign prices to commodities, and not as a means of payment.[1] Almost anything, therefore, can serve as a unit of account, since goods will still be exchanged for goods, and it will not be necessary to handle the unit of account.

Commodities that would be inconvenient as money because they lack divisibility or portability can quite well serve as units of account. For purposes of calculation it is possible, for instance, to speak of hundredths of a cow or fractions of a sea-shell; or even such intangible things as hours of labour could be used. Some unit of account would be required even if the State, on the grounds that "money is the root of all evil," determined to do without money. It would still be necessary to find some means of deciding which of two methods of producing a commodity was the more economical; it would be necessary to decide between the production of a little more of one commodity and a little more of another. For such purposes of calculation a unit of account would be needed. Where a medium of exchange is in use, this is obviously the most convenient unit of account, and so money generally fulfils this second function. If, however, people for any reason lose confidence in their money, as in Germany in 1923 or Hungary or China in 1946, the national currency may cease to serve as the unit of account and be replaced perhaps by a foreign currency or some acceptable commodity.

Some writers point out that the value of a good cannot be measured, since it is subjective and determined by each person for himself. Commodities therefore can be arranged only in order of preference. Therefore, they say, money cannot be regarded as a measure of value. They have to admit, however, that it is a great convenience to be able to assign money-prices to goods, and money-prices are partly determined by market demand, which is made up of a large number of individual subjective demands.

(iii) *A store of value.* Without the use of money it would be impossible to build up for the future stores of many things. Money, therefore, makes it possible for a person to provide for old age. By forgoing current consumption he can accumulate a reserve of purchasing power for use in the future, though it provides no certainty that the things he wants will be available when he wants them. While a person keeps his assets in the form of money—a liquid asset—he is free to turn them

---

[1] The Anglo-Saxon shilling was merely a unit of account, since no such coin was minted at that time.

into whatever fixed assets he pleases. In a period of falling prices, however, the money-value of real assets falls; at such times money gains in value. But if prices are rising, the value of money will fall. In a period of inflation money therefore becomes a very poor store of value, as many people in Europe found in the years following each of the World Wars. In Great Britain £1 would buy five times as much in 1913 as in 1966.

(iv) *A standard for deferred payments.* The use of money makes it possible for payments to be deferred from the present to some future date; it also enables contracts to be made in the present for the future delivery of goods. Credit transactions cannot easily be carried out unless money is used. The vast credit structure of the modern world is based on the use of money, and much of production today depends on credit facilities being available. Just as money, however, ceases to be a store of value in times of severe inflation, so it will cease to be a standard for deferred payments once people's confidence in it has been lost, and future contracts will cease, or will be made in some other currency or commodity.

RECOMMENDATIONS FOR FURTHER READING

G. Crowther: *An Outline of Money,* Chapter 1.
D. H. Robertson: *Money,* Chapter 1.

QUESTIONS

1. Why has the use of money and credit become necessary in modern economic life? (R.S.A. Inter.)

2. Explain the terms (*a*) legal tender, (*b*) token money, (*c*) the gold standard. (C.C.S. Inter.)

3. What do you understand by the quantity of money? How does the quantity of money influence prices? (C.I.S. Inter.)

4. Describe the functions of money, and examine critically the extent to which the various forms of money in use today fulfil these functions. (Exp.)

5. It has been stated that anything generally acceptable will serve as money. Examine this statement. (I.M.T.A.)

6. What is money? (A.C.C.A. Final.)

7. Indicate the main functions of money, and state the extent to which, in your view, it is satisfactory in fulfilling these functions at the present time. (C.I.S. Final.)

8. Describe Gresham's Law and indicate the restrictions to which it is subject. I.B.)

9. In what ways does money differ from all other economic goods? (D.P.A.)

10. What are the functions of money? Show that they can be efficiently discharged only when its general purchasing power is secured against violent changes. (L.G.B.)

11. What functions are performed by money? What things perform these functions in the United Kingdom? (G.C.E. Adv.)

12. "The most important invention ever made for the development of civilisation was that of money." Discuss this dictum. (Final Degree.)

CHAPTER XXI

THE VALUE OF MONEY

I. THE PRICE LEVEL

(1) THE VALUE OF MONEY AND THE PRICE LEVEL

Price is the relation between a quantity of money and a quantity of goods. Even if it is agreed that value is subjective and therefore cannot be measured, so that price and value are not the same thing, it is convenient to regard market prices as indicators of the relative value of commodities in terms of money at a particular time. Since money itself is used as the measure of value, its own value can be seen only indirectly through the prices of other things. If the prices of goods rise, this is equivalent to saying that the value of money has fallen, for fewer goods than before can then be obtained in exchange for a given sum of money. If a basketful of commodities costs £3 in 1939, whereas a similar assortment of goods in 1945 cost £6, this shows that between 1939 and 1945 the value of money fell by a half.

Between 1939 and 1969 the value of money in Great Britain fell to a third of its former value—that is, prices on average increased by three times during these thirty years. On the other hand, between 1925 and 1931 prices in Great Britain were falling, and so during that period the value of money therefore was rising. By 1966 the value of money in France had fallen to $\frac{1}{240}$ of its value in 1914, prices in France having risen by 240 times during that period. The value of money is thus shown by the level of prices, a general rise in prices indicating a fall, and a general fall in prices indicating a rise, in the value of money. The price of a commodity is the amount of money that has to be given for it; the value of money is the quantity of goods it will buy.

(2) CHANGES IN THE VALUE OF MONEY

The study of changes in the value of money is thus a study of prices. Indeed, it is easier to understand this problem from the angle of price rather than from that of the value of money. It must, however, be constantly kept in mind that prices vary inversely with the value of money.

Three distinct trends in price movements can be noticed: a long-period, a medium-period, and a short-period movement:

(i) *A long-period movement of prices.* Over the centuries there has been a general tendency for prices to rise, that is, for the value of money to fall. In the eleventh to fourteenth centuries money was scarce and most people handled very little of it, most payments being in kind or by so many days' labour per week on the lord's demesne. In the fourteenth century a few pence would buy a sheep or a cow. The level of prices, however, was higher at the end than at the beginning of almost every century from 1100 to 1900, and there is little doubt that the twentieth century will see the largest increase in prices of any century. The exceptions to this were 1400–1500, when prices were fairly steady, and 1600–1700 when slight falls in prices occurred.

The following diagram illustrates the general long-term trend of prices in Great Britain to rise:

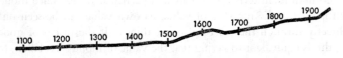

FIG. 72.—THE LONG-PERIOD RISE IN PRICES.

(ii) *A medium-period movement of prices.* A second feature of price fluctuation was noticeable during the nineteenth century. Periods of from twenty-two to twenty-nine years succeeded each other during which there was first a general tendency for prices to fall, followed by a period of approximately similar length during which there was a general tendency for prices to rise. The relation between the rate of increase in the quantity of money and the rate of increase in the production of goods available for the money to buy seems to have been the basis of these price movements. During the nineteenth century the monetary importance of gold increased, and the quantity of money was therefore closely related to the amount of gold available. Generally the amount of gold mined each year forms only a small percentage of the total supply, and so is not likely seriously to affect prices, but on occasions when new gold-mining areas are being developed the influence of the new supplies on prices is much greater. A large increase in the supply of the monetary metal may be expected, other things being equal, to cause a rise in prices. As more countries substituted gold for silver as their monetary standard, there was relatively less gold available for each, and so there was a tendency for prices to fall. The nineteenth century, too, saw a vast expansion of production, but, like the output of gold, the rate of expansion was more rapid at some periods than at others. If the supply of gold was increasing more rapidly than the supply of other goods prices tended to rise; if the output of other goods increased more rapidly than gold prices tended to fall.

Four periods of medium-term fluctuation of prices can be distinguished:

(a) *1820–49.* This was a period during which prices were generally falling, the output of goods increasing more rapidly than the output of gold.

(b) *1849–74.* This was a period of generally rising prices. In 1847 gold was discovered in California and in 1849–51 in Australia. After 1844 there was also a gradual extension of the use of cheques, the Bank Charter Act of that year restricting the issue of bank-notes. The output of goods failed to keep pace with the increase in the quantity of money.

(c) *1874–96.* This was a period of falling prices. Germany adopted a gold coinage in 1873, and France in 1878. Production of commodities had again been speeded up relatively to the output of gold.

(d) *1896–1914.* This was another period of rising prices. Gold was discovered in South Africa in 1884–85, and in time this area produced half the world's annual output.

The following diagram illustrates the medium-term movement of prices:

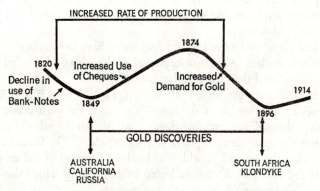

FIG. 73.—THE MEDIUM-TERM MOVEMENT OF PRICES.

(iii) *A short-period movement of prices.* The short-period variation in prices is associated with the trade cycle, but discussion of this phenomenon must be reserved for a later chapter.[1] At the moment it is sufficient to note that during the nineteenth and early twentieth centuries the ups and downs of business activity showed certain regular

[1] See Chapter XXIX.

recurring features. Booms and depressions succeeded one another at regular intervals; on average a period of eight years separated one depression from the next, the interval never being less than five years and never greater than eleven. Once a depression had set in, recovery at first was slow, but after a few years boom conditions would develop. During this upswing of the cycle prices at first would remain steady, but at the height of the boom they would rise more rapidly. The down-swing of the cycle was characterised by a fall in prices and trade activity, often after an economic crisis of some kind. The value of money, therefore, increases in a depression and falls in a boom, although graphs of fluctuations in production and prices do not entirely coincide. The following is a graph of a portion of the trade cycle in the latter part of the nineteenth century:

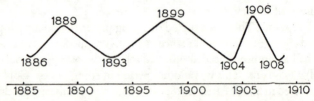

FIG. 74.—THE SHORT-PERIOD MOVEMENT OF PRICES.

Booms occurred in 1889, 1899 and 1906, depressions in 1886, 1893, 1904 and 1908. Between the booms of 1889 and 1899 there was an interval of ten years, but the boom of 1906 occurred only seven years after its predecessor.

These three tendencies to price fluctuation have to be superimposed upon one another. As a result, each peak of the trade cycle tended to be at a higher level than the one that preceded it.

The rhythm of the trade cycle was upset by the two World Wars. The Great Depression of the inter-War years was both deeper and more prolonged than previous depressions, though the value of money did not rise as much as might have been expected. The feature of the years after the Second World War has been a period of full employment and inflation of unprecedented length, during which there has been a continuous fall in the value of money.

II. THE DETERMINATION OF THE VALUE OF MONEY

(3) THE QUANTITY THEORY OF MONEY

In the seventeenth century it was noticed that there was a connection between the quantity of money and the general level of prices, and this led to the formulation of the Quantity Theory of money. In its

THE VALUE OF MONEY

crudest form it stated that an increase in the quantity of money would bring about a proportionate rise in prices. After being long discarded, the theory was revived in the 1920s by Prof. Irving Fisher, who introduced into it the concept of the velocity of circulation. Money circulates from hand to hand. Micawber, the greengrocer, spends 5s. at Bumble's, the tobacconist; Bumble uses the 5s. to make a purchase from Swiveller, the grocer, who in his turn spends it at Cuttle's, the confectioners; Cuttle then buys 5s. worth of greengrocery from Micawber. The 5s. has returned to where it was before the first transaction took place. In this case the same coins were used for four separate transactions; five shillings did the work of twenty shillings. In the course of a year each unit of money is used many times. If one unit of money is made to serve four transactions this is equivalent to four units of money each being used in only one transaction.

As modified by Irving Fisher, the Quantity Theory came to be expressed by the equation of exchange:

$$MV = PT$$

The symbol M represents the total amount of money in existence—bank-notes, etc., and bank deposits.

The symbol V represents the velocity of circulation. This is difficult to calculate, though the combined totals of the bankers' clearing houses in relation to the quantity of money at the time gives some indication of it.

MV therefore represents the amount of money used in a period.

On the other side of the equation, P stands for the general price level, a sort of average of the prices of all kinds of commodities—producers' goods as well as consumers' goods—and services.

The symbol T is the total of all the transactions that have taken place for money during the period.

The equation of exchange shows us that the price level, and therefore the value of money, can be influenced not only by the quantity of money but also by (i) the rate at which money circulates, and (ii) the output of goods and services. Thus prices might rise without any change taking place in the quantity of money if a rise occurred in the velocity of circulation. On the other hand, prices might remain stable in spite of an increase in the quantity of money if there was a corresponding increase in the output of goods and services.

(4) SOME CRITICISMS OF THE QUANTITY THEORY

The Quantity Theory, however, has been subjected to severe criticism ever since it was revived by Fisher:

(i) In the first place, it is said, it is not a theory at all, but merely a convenient method of showing that there is a certain relation between four variable quantities—M, V, P and T. It merely shows that the total quantity of money, as determined by the actual amount of money in existence and the velocity of circulation, is equal to the total volume of trade transactions multiplied by their average price. As such it is obviously a truism, since the amount of money spent must be equal to the amount received from sales. In other words, not only must MV be equal to PT, but MV is PT, since they are only two different ways of looking at the same thing.

Even if it is agreed that the equation of exchange is nothing more than a truism, it would not be quite correct to say that it demonstrates nothing. For example, it shows that it is possible for there to be an increase in the quantity of money without a general rise in prices. It informs us too that if there is a change in one of the variables of the equation, there must also be a change in one or more of the other variables. It would, however, probably be wrong to read into it much more than this.

(ii) The four variables, M, V, P and T, are not independent of one another as the equation of exchanges implies. For example, a change in M is likely of itself to bring about a change of V or of T or both. It is probable that a rise in prices will follow an increase in the quantity of money, but this will most likely be brought about because the increase in the quantity of money stimulates demand and production.

(iii) There is a serious defect in the representation by the symbol P of the *general* price level. Price changes do not all keep in step with one another. The equation in its original form has been criticised as implying that an increase in the quantity of money will bring about a proportionate increase in all prices. A study of price changes between 1939 and 1966 shows that though some prices increased during these years by as much as three times, others rose by only 50%. Clearly, then, there is no such thing as a *general* price level, but instead, as the Index of Retail Prices now shows, there is a number of sectional price levels, one for food, another for clothing, another for fuel and light, and so on.

(iv) The Quantity Theory only attempts to explain *changes* in the value of money, and does not show how the value of money is in the first place determined, that is, it takes a certain value of money as given.

(v) It is said, too, that the Quantity Theory approaches the question of the value of money entirely from the side of supply, completely ignoring the influence of demand. Though this was true of the original theory, it was not true of Irving Fisher's modification of it. Since the demand for money is the demand to hold money, the greater the strength of the demand to hold money, the lower will be the velocity of circulation. Thus, the desire to hold money varies inversely with the velocity of circulation, and so the introduction into the equation of V to some extent disposes of this criticism.

(vi) Finally, the most serious criticism levelled against the Quantity Theory is that it is quite inadequate as a theory of money, since it takes no account of the influence of the rate of interest.

Large falls in the value of money during periods of severe inflation, however, can probably be explained by the quantity equation, since it does contain at least one fundamental truth—namely, that there is a connection between the quantity of money and its value. Though few modern writers would go further than grudgingly admit this, Prof. K. Boulding, however, thinks the quantity equation is more useful than most present-day writers are prepared to recognise.[1]

(5) THE SUPPLY OF MONEY AND THE DEMAND FOR MONEY

It has been shown earlier in this book that the value of a commodity depends on the relative strength of the forces of supply and demand. Since this provides a satisfactory theory of value, it has been suggested that it should be employed also to explain the value of money.

Caution, however, is required in applying this technique to the determination of the value of money, since unlike commodities, money is not wanted for its own sake, and the term, *demand for money*, therefore, is not used to mean demand in quite the same sense as (say) the demand for a commodity such as butter. By demand for money is meant the demand to *hold* money as distinct from investing it. The concept of the supply of money presents less difficulty, though again, unlike other commodities, its supply is not related to its cost of production.

(i) *The supply of money.* In this country at the present day there are two main kinds of money: (*a*) cash in the form of inconvertible Bank of England notes and coins; and (*b*) bank deposits transferable by cheque. Today bank deposits form about four-fifths of the total supply of money in Great Britain, and how much money there is of this kind is dependent on the credit policy of the commercial banks, the Bank of England and the monetary authorities, as we shall see in the next chapter. The size of the Bank of England's note issue nowadays depends primarily on the volume of bank deposits.

(ii) *The demand for money.* The demand for money is a more difficult concept than the demand for goods and services. As stated above,

[1] K. E. Boulding: *Economic Analysis*, Chapter 15.

the demand for money means the demand to hold money, that is, to keep one's resources in liquid form instead of in some less liquid form of investment. First of all, therefore, it is necessary to inquire why people hold money, since, clearly, this involves a loss of the interest it might otherwise have earned. According to the late Lord Keynes, there are three motives for holding money, which he distinguished respectively as the "transactions motive," the "precautionary motive" and the "speculative motive."

(a) *The transactions motive.* A certain amount of money is needed for everyday requirements, the purchase of food and clothing and other ordinary expenses. How much is it necessary to hold for these purposes will depend on two factors: a person's income and the interval between one pay-day and the next. Generally, the higher the income, the more money will be held, though millionaires are notorious for declaring that they are short of cash. The weekly wage-earner will need to hold less than a person who receives his salary monthly, for in the one case sufficient has to be held to cover expenses for only one week, whereas the other man has to make provision for four weeks. Similarly, in business, cash has to be held to cover expenses, such as wages, during the period of production.

(b) *The precautionary motive.* Most people like to keep something in reserve, in case an unexpected payment has to be made. One of the commonest of unforeseen contingencies is sickness, and formerly this was probably the main reason for people keeping a little money in reserve. The introduction of the National Insurance scheme, however, made it less necessary to hold money for this purpose. Certain household expenses—for example, those due to breakages—are also of this nature, though again, so far as these contingencies can be covered by insurance, there will be less need to hold money for renewals.

(c) *The speculative motive.* Holding money involves the sacrifice of the interest it would have yielded if it had been invested. In considering the functions of money, however, it was noticed that it can serve as a liquid asset. To have an asset in the form of money means that whenever one so wishes, it can be exchanged for some other asset. Because there are advantages in keeping one's assets liquid, some inducement in the form of interest is necessary to make people forgo liquidity. As we have already seen in our consideration of the monetary theory of interest,[1] the strength of the desire for liquidity is called *liquidity-preference*, and it is this that decides what proportion of their assets people will hold in the form of money.

How much is held for the transactions motive and the precautionary

---

[1] pp. 334-35.

motive depends on daily needs and habit, and, in the short period, the amount is unlikely to vary very much. The demand for money for the first motive is fairly inelastic, somewhat less inelastic for the second, and most elastic for the third. If more is held than is required for the first two purposes it must be held for speculative reasons—that is, it will depend on expectations regarding the future trend of the rate of interest. If people think the rate is likely to rise—that is, if they think the price of stocks will fall in the future—they will hold money, since any loss of interest which this involves will be counter-balanced by the lower prices to be paid later. On the other hand, if they think the rate of interest is likely to fall they will invest their money at once, while the prices of stocks are low. Expected future prices of other assets will determine how much money is held. Many consumers will postpone some of their purchases—particularly of durable consumers' goods—if they think there is a possibility of a fall in prices in the near future. In a boom, then, when prices are rising, less money will be held; in a depression, when prices are falling, more money will be held.

The advantage of this theory of the value of money is that it employs the general theory of value. Secondly, unlike the Quantity Theory, it gives a prominent place to the influence of the rate of interest.

A second equation of exchange. It is possible to construct a second equation of exchange which makes allowance for the demand to hold money.

$$p = \frac{M}{kR}$$

The symbol k is used to represent the proportion of a community's total income held in money; R stands for the country's output of goods and services—that is, *real* income; M, as in the previous equation, represents the country's stock of money (cash and bank deposits) at a given time; p is the general price level of consumers' goods. (P in the former equation, it will be remembered, represented the general price level of all kinds of goods, including producers' as well as consumers' goods.) This equation takes account of the total volume of production (R) and the demand to hold money (k). An increase in either of these will reduce the general price level of consumers' goods. If other things remain the same an increase in the demand for money will bring about a fall in prices. The greater the proportion of money that is held, the lower will be the velocity of circulation; the less money that is held, the greater will be the velocity of circulation. The symbol V of the first equation thus varies inversely with k of the second equation.

III. INDEX NUMBERS

(6) MEASUREMENT OF CHANGES IN THE VALUE OF MONEY

The usual method adopted to measure changes in the value of money is by means of index numbers of prices. A number of these indices have been compiled, but the main principle in all cases is the same: a group of commodities is selected, their prices noted in some particular year which becomes the base year for the index number and to which the number 100 is given. If the prices of these commodities rise by 1% during the ensuing twelve months the index number next year will be 101. A fall in price of 1% would be shown by an index number of 99. Indices of wholesale prices have been compiled by the Board of Trade, *The Economist* and the *Statist*. The index number of *The Economist*, with 1929 as base year, shows a fall to 80 in 1939, followed by a rise to 172 in 1945. The Monthly Digest of Statistics, compiled by the Central Statistical Office, now takes 1954 as its base year for wholesale prices, the index number for manufactured goods being 113 in 1960 and 128 in 1965.

The best-known index number is the former Cost-of-living Index Number, compiled by the Ministry of Labour. This took July 1914 as its base. In 1921 it stood at 240, falling to 100 in 1929 and to 85 in 1933, after which date it began to rise again, reading 96 in 1939 and 132 in 1945. It was superseded by a new Interim Index of Retail Prices, for which 1947 was selected as base year. It was revised again in 1952 and 1956 and, following a new survey, the index was completely revised with January 1962 as the base.

(7) THE PROBLEM OF WEIGHTING

The greatest difficulty facing the compiler of an index number is to decide how much of each commodity to select. This is the problem of weighting. Different "weights" will yield different results, as the following example illustrates. Assume that there are only three commodities, A, B, C, the prices of which are 5s., 2s. and 4d., respectively. By taking one unit of each—that is, without any weighting—the index number for the base year is constructed as follows:

Base Year

Commodity	Price	Weight	Index
A	5s. 0d.	1	100
B	2s. 0d.	1	100
C	4d.	1	100
		3	300

Index for all items = 100

Assume that one year later the price of *A* is 4*s*. 6*d*., *B* 2*s*. 6*d*. and *C* 6*d*.:

Commodity	Price	Weight	Index
A	4*s*. 6*d*.	1	90
B	2*s*. 6*d*.	1	125
C	6*d*.	1	150
		—	—
		3	365

Index for all items = 121·6

The index-number in the second year is 121·6, showing an increase in price of 21·6% over the base year.

If the commodities *A*, *B*, *C* are differently weighted a different result will be obtained. For example, suppose that one unit of *A*, four of *B* and twenty of *C* are taken. The index number will then be compiled as follows:

	Base Year				Second Year		
Commodity	Price	Weight	Index	Commodity	Price	Weight	Index
A	5*s*. 0*d*.	1	100	A	4*s*. 6*d*.	1	90
B	2*s*. 0*d*.	4	400	B	2*s*. 6*d*.	4	500
C	4*d*.	20	2,000	C	6*d*.	20	3,000
		—	—			—	—
		25	2,500			25	3,590

Index for all items = 100   Index for all items = 143·6

By weighting *C* heavily this index shows a rise in prices of 43·6%, *although individual prices show only the same change as before.* By weighting commodity *A* heavily an index number can actually be compiled from the same data to show a *fall* in prices!

	Base Year				Second Year		
Commodity	Price	Weight	Index	Commodity	Price	Weight	Index
A	5*s*. 0*d*.	10	1,000	A	4*s*. 6*d*.	10	900
B	2*s*. 0*d*.	1	100	B	2*s*. 6*d*.	1	125
C	4*d*.	1	100	C	6*d*.	1	150
		—	—			—	—
		12	1,200			12	1,175

Index for all items = 100   Index for all items = 97·9

The importance of correct weighting will now be clear. The choice of weights is, however, no easy matter. The method employed in the case of the old Cost-of-living Index Number was to make a survey of the distribution of expenditure of working-class families, the 1914 index being based on a survey taken in 1904. For the 1947 index number the survey took place in 1937–38, and the weighting was based upon the assortment of goods purchased by families with annual incomes of less than £250. In 1952 the weighting of the index was again revised.

A new inquiry was undertaken, and following this the weighting, introduced in 1956, was based on the expenditure of people with incomes up to £1,000 a year. A revised index was introduced in January 1963 with January 1962 as 100. Since 1962 the weighting has been modified each year.

The collection of data presents difficulties, for many people resent inquiries into the ways in which they spend their money, and even when people are prepared to give this information they are often unwilling to admit the full amount they spend on things such as drink, tobacco and entertainments.

It is instructive to compare the weights used in the 1914, 1947, 1952, 1956 and 1962 indices:

Commodity groups	1914 index	1947 index	1952 index	1956 index	1962 index
	%	%	%	%	%
I. Food	60	34·8	39·9	35·0	31·9
II. Alcoholic drink . .	—	} 21·7	} 16·8 {	7·1	6·4
III. Tobacco . . .	—			8·0	7·9
IV. Housing	16	8·8	7·2	8·7	10·2
V. Fuel and light . .	8	6·5	6·6	5·5	6·2
VI. Durable household goods .	—	7·1	6·2	6·6	6·4
VII. Clothing and footwear .	12	9·7	9·8	10·6	9·8
VIII. Transport and vehicles .	—	—	—	6·8	9·2
IX. Miscellaneous . . .	4	3·5	4·4	5·9	6·4
X. Services	—	7·9	9·1	5·8	5·6
	100	100	100	100	100

The changes in the weights of the various groups of goods and services is of particular interest in showing how people's distribution of expenditure changes as their standard of living rises. For example, Groups I, IV, V and VII, covering the basic wants of food, clothing and shelter, formed 96% of the total expenditure of a family in 1914, but less than 60% in 1947 and 1962. The most striking change is the fall in the proportion of expenditure on food and housing—from 60% and 16% in 1914 to 35% and 8·7% respectively in 1962. The changes in weighting show clearly how as the standard of living rises, expenditure on things other than basic necessaries increases. The heavy allowance for Groups II and III in the 1947 index is of interest in showing how people in the lower-income groups actually spend their incomes, but if it is used as a basis for claims for higher wages increases in the prices of semi-luxuries and less necessary things have an undue influence on the index. Similarly, a fall in the prices of less-necessary things will bring about a fall in the index number, perhaps to the disadvantage of people in the lowest income groups.

(8) OTHER PROBLEMS OF INDEX NUMBERS

The weights to be given to different commodities and services having been determined, the next problem is to decide what grades and quantities to take into account. Again an attempt is made, by including more than one grade, to make a representative selection. An even greater difficulty occurs when the price of a commodity remains unchanged, although the quality has declined. In recent revisions of the index, however, adjustments have been made for changes in quality, account being taken, for example, of changes in the strength of beer! On account of seasonal variation in their prices, green vegetables and fresh fruit were excluded from the 1914 Index, but since 1947 they have been included during the months when they are in season.

Other difficulties associated with the construction of index numbers are:

(i) The choice of a base year. This should preferably be a year when prices are reasonably steady, and so years during periods either of severe inflation or deflation are to be avoided. The first half of 1914 was quite a good date to select, as would have been 1938 or the early part of 1939. The outbreak of war in 1939 caused the postponement of a new index number, at first because of the abnormal conditions of the war period and later because of the difficulties of the immediate post-war years.

(ii) Index numbers are of little value for comparisons over long periods of time because (a) new commodities come on to the market; (b) changes in taste or fashion reduce the demand for some commodities and increase the demand for others; (c) the composition of the community is liable to change; (d) changes may occur in the distribution of the population among the various age-groups; and (e) the rise in the standard of living. The 1914 price index was probably representative of upwards of 60% of the population, but by 1938 it was applicable to less than 30%. It is for this reason that periodic revision of the Index of Retail Prices is essential if it is to retain any degree of accuracy.

(iii) Even people in the same income groups do not distribute their expenditure over the same range of commodities or buy similar proportions of them. The higher the general standard of living, the greater these differences are likely to be. Thus an Index of Retail Prices can be used to show variations in the cost of living only for the particular income groups on whose expenditure it is based. For example, the higher the income, the smaller the proportion of it that will be spent on food. The 1914 index was appropriate to a more homogeneous group than the 1962 index with its relatively high upper-income limit.

Though index numbers are the best means at our disposal, they do not provide a very satisfactory method of measuring the value of money. They are mainly of interest in showing how much people within a specified income range distribute their expenditure.

On account of the many difficulties associated with their compilation, and their many drawbacks, and in spite of the great care now taken in compiling the index, economists attach little importance to index numbers for comparing changes in the value of money over long periods of time. They do, however, give an approximate indication of changes over short periods—month-to-month fluctuations, for example—or for comparing one year with the preceding year.

(9) THE INDEX OF RETAIL PRICES[1]

TABLE XLVIA

Index of Retail Prices

	Group and Sub-group weights (1965)	Base: Jan. 1962	Jan. 1964	Aug. 1965	Jan. 196–
ALL ITEMS	1,000	100	104·7	112·9	
I. Food	311	100	105·4	110·3	
Bread, etc.	47	100	—	112	
Meat and bacon	82	100	—	113	
Fish	10	100	—	118	
Tea, coffee, cocoa	18	100	—	105	
II. Alcoholic drink	65	100	103·2	109·0	
III. Tobacco	76	100	100·0	112·4	
IV. Housing	109	100	110·9	121·7	
V. Fuel and light	65	100	110·1	112·7	
Coal and coke	27	100	—	104	
VI. Durable household goods	59	100	101·2	112·1	
Furniture	27	100	—	111	
VII. Clothing and footwear	92	100	104·0	107·2	
Men's outer clothing	15	100	—	110	
Women's outer clothing	20	100	—	107	
VIII. Transport and vehicles	105	100	100·6	107·6	
IX. Miscellaneous goods	63	100	102·9	109·3	
Books, newspapers, etc.	17	100	—	126	
X. Services	55	100	105·0	107·6	
Postage and telephones	6	100	—	114	
Entertainment	22	100	—	112	

Source: Monthly Digest of Statistics (H.M.S.O.)

The data for this index is collected in three ways:

(i) The prices of some foodstuffs, clothing and household goods are

[1] See 'Interim Index of Retail Prices: Method of Construction and Calculation,' published by Her Majesty's Stationery Office, for an excellent account of the method of compiling the 1947 index-number.

ascertained by inquiry of shops in each of 200 places, selected as representative of different population groups—for example, twenty-five are in Greater London, twenty-five are towns with populations over 200,000, fifty are towns with populations between 50,000 and 200,000 and so on.

(ii) The prices of branded goods, tobacco and beer are obtained by inquiry of the manufacturers of these commodities.

(iii) Information regarding rent and rates is obtained from Local Authorities and Property-owners' Associations.

Commodities and services are divided into ten groups, each of which is further subdivided into a number of sections. Group I (food), for example, includes nineteen sections covering such items as bread, beef, fish, etc. Separate indices are calculated for each group and even for individual items within each group, as well as an overall index for all items. Table XLVIA shows the Index of Retail Prices for All Items, the ten main Groups and also for a few typical items within some of the groups. This table shows how necessary it is to think in terms of sectional price levels.

The following table shows the rise in the index number of retail prices since 1956 and inversely, therefore, the fall in value of money:

TABLE XLVIb
Index of Retail Prices
(1956–65)

1956	100·0
1957	105·8
1958	109·0
1959	109·6
1960	110·7
1961	114·5
1962	117·5
1962	100·0
1963	103·6
1964	107·0
1965	112·9

IV. INFLATION

(10) EFFECTS OF CHANGES IN THE VALUE OF MONEY

(i) *On the level of production.* If prices are rising, business activity will be stimulated. Since production is carried on in anticipation of demand and as all costs do not increase immediately as prices begin to rise, profit margins will be greater than anticipated. There is therefore less risk to the entrepreneur. In order to take advantage of rising prices it is to his interest to increase his output to its maximum, for so long as rising costs lag behind rising commodity prices the entrepreneurs' profits will be greater than before.

If, however, prices are falling, profit margins will be smaller than was anticipated when production was undertaken. A severe fall in prices may result in a loss for the entrepreneur, for costs of production will not fall proportionately with commodity prices, wages being particularly difficult to adjust. To the entrepreneur the outlook will appear black, and therefore he will tend to become more cautious and restrict his output.

If it is desired to maintain a high level of production gently rising prices are then to be preferred to falling prices.

(ii) *On the distribution of incomes.* The incomes of different groups of people are not equally affected by price changes. As Mises points out, any advantage accruing to one group of people as a result of a change in the value of money must be at the expense of other groups. Those who suffer from rising prices are people with fixed money incomes and to a lesser extent wage-earners. Those who suffer when prices are falling are the profit-receivers.

Consider first those people whose incomes are derived from profits. It has been noticed above that when prices are rising profits are generally higher than was anticipated. A rise in prices, therefore, immediately results in higher profits, and so profit-receivers tend to be better off than before—that is, their *real* incomes rise. A fall in prices also immediately affects their incomes, which fall as profits fall, and if the fall in wages is severe losses may be incurred.

Wages generally do not rise immediately, but prices continue to rise, production is stimulated and entrepreneurs become willing to pay higher wages in order to maintain production. Thus though wages eventually rise, wage increases tend to lag behind prices. In times of rising prices wage-earners may find their real wages are lower than before, but since demand for labour will be high, there will be less unemployment, and so the total amount of real income distributed among them will probably be greater than before. When prices are falling there is a similar time lag with wage decreases, and so those who succeed in keeping their jobs may gain in real income, but unemployment will be greater, and so the total distributed in wages will be less. In a prolonged period of rising prices such as the one that has occurred since 1945 wages may eventually increase more rapidly than prices.

The third section of the community comprises those who receive fixed incomes. Among these will be retired people. If they are living on annuities bought with past savings their money incomes will remain unchanged. If they have invested their savings in gilt-edged securities their position will be similar; but if their savings are in shares in companies or in unit trusts they will have joined the profit-receivers. People in receipt of pensions also have the same money income whether prices are rising or falling. Again, however, in a prolonged period of rising prices some pensions may be slightly increased. National Insurance pensions have been increased on several occasions during recent years. In a period of rising prices all people on fixed incomes find that their real incomes decline, but when prices are falling, as during 1925-31, their real incomes increase.

In many occupations incomes are fixed for long periods, adjustments being made only after great changes have occurred in the value of money. During the short periods of rising and falling prices in the past salaried workers could be regarded as fixed-income receivers, but since 1950 most salaries have almost kept pace with the rise in prices. In Great Britain the salaries of judges varied little during the 100 years before 1953; the highest grades in the Civil Service obtained their first adjustments of salary in 1950, after eleven years of rising prices. In most of these cases salary increases generally fail to keep pace with the fall in the value of money, although, like all those with fixed incomes, they benefit from falling prices. Those who gain when prices are rising are the ones who lose when prices are falling, and vice versa. It has been seen, however, that there is a long-period tendency of prices to rise, and present-day economic policy is likely to encourage this. On balance, therefore, the advantage seems to lie with those who gain from rising prices. All debtors gain and all creditors lose when the value of money is falling, the reverse being true when the value of money is rising. Thus changes in the value of money bring about an arbitrary redistribution of income.

(11) MEANINGS OF INFLATION

There is a certain ambiguity about the term *inflation*. The word has at least three meanings:

(i) Any increase in the quantity of money, however small, can be regarded as inflationary, just as any decrease in the quantity of money is deflationary. The terms *inflation* and *deflation* are used in this sense to describe the credit policy of the Central Bank. Inflation can be taken to mean conditions when the value of money is declining—that is, when prices are rising—but changes in the quantity of money, however, may or may not affect prices. If an increase in the quantity of money is accompanied by a proportionate increase in the quantity of goods and services available for purchase, then (assuming that no change takes place in the velocity of circulation) the general price level will remain unchanged.

(ii) Inflation, as understood in the post-1945 period, connotes something more than an increase in the quantity of money. In its current use the word describes an unstable situation. Inflation is present when the volume of purchasing power is *persistently* running ahead of the output of goods and services, so that there is a *continuous* tendency for prices—both of commodities and factors of production—to rise because the supply of goods and services and factors of production fails to keep pace with demand for them. This type of inflation can therefore be described as Persistent Inflation. In ordinary speech inflation is often taken to mean high prices, but high prices do not necessarily indicate the existence of inflation, for equilibrium of Supply and Demand can be established at any level of prices, and once equilibrium has been achieved inflation disappears.

(iii) The term *inflation* has acquired unpleasant associations, and in its third usage it is taken to mean a runaway inflation. At such periods the Quantity Theory seems to justify itself as an explanation of the value of money, for excessive creations of money result in huge increases in prices. This type of inflation has been variously described as "galloping," or "runaway," or as a hyperinflation.

(12) THE INFLATIONARY GAP

Inflation may be the consequence of banking policy, but a hyperinflation is almost certain to arise as a result of Government action, and is most likely to occur during a war or as a result of war. Modern wars are enormously expensive, and at such times it is impossible to cover Government expenditure from current taxation. The Government must then have recourse to borrowing, but so long as these loans come from the general public there will be no inflation, for taxation and

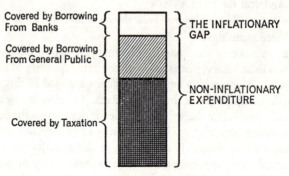

FIG. 75.—GOVERNMENT EXPENDITURE.

borrowing of this kind decrease the amount of purchasing power in the hands of the community, and so the demand for the smaller quantity of consumer goods available is reduced, and therefore there will be no tendency for prices to rise. If the Government cannot cover its expenditure by these two methods it will be compelled either to create the additional money itself or to borrow from the banks—that is, permit the banks to create the additional money required. This is known as the inflationary gap. It can occur, in times of peace if the Government is unwilling to curtail its expenditure or to increase taxation to cover it.

Both World Wars saw huge increases in the quantity of money and in prices. The increase in the quantity of money during 1945–65 was, however, a new experience for Great Britain in time of peace.

During neither of the two war periods did the increase in the quantity of money affect prices to the extent that might have been expected, the increase in the quantity of money being to some extent offset by a fall in the velocity of circulation. While a war is actually in progress people respond more readily to patriotic appeals urging them to save, and in any case hours of work are so long that opportunities for spending are reduced in this way, as well as by the curtailment of the production of consumers' goods. During a war, therefore, inflation tends to be to some extent suppressed, but after the war people's accumulations of savings formed a vast volume of potential purchasing power.

TABLE XLVII
The Quantity of Money

	1939	1945	1965
	£ million	£ million	£ million
Bank of England notes	526	1,300	2,850
Bank deposits	2,248	4,692	8,415
Total	2,774	5,992	11,265

In Great Britain rationing of consumers' goods, food subsidies, price control, control of investment, a tight system of exchange control, licensing of building and other capital projects, and restrictions on the allocation of raw materials were introduced in the Second World War and continued for some years afterwards to try to keep inflation in check. Such physical controls, however, merely suppress inflation without getting rid of it.

(13) PERSISTENT INFLATION

The Inflationary spiral. It is necessary, therefore, to consider what factors induce persistent inflation. The pressure of demand, resulting from the existence of huge amounts of purchasing power, will force up the prices of all goods and services. High prices will lead to demands for wage increases, which empoyers will generally be willing to concede, since rising prices offer the probability of increased profits. When demand is pressing it becomes possible to pass increased costs to the consumer in the form of still higher prices. Most costs of production—wages, raw material, power—rise, and as a result prices are pushed still higher, this bringing in its train a renewal of demands for wage increases. Wages force up prices; prices force up wages. This is the inflationary spiral, which if unchecked can end only with money ceasing to have any value at all.

Demand inflation. This term is used to describe an inflation which is mainly induced by excessive demand, the inflationary spiral being stimulated because supply constantly fails to keep up with demand. Thus there occurs a "demand-pull" inflation. Prices rise as a result of the high level of demand in relation to supply, the rise in wages being a consequence of the rising cost of living.

Cost inflation. If an inflation is mainly induced by rising costs of production, particularly rising wages, it can be described as a "cost-push" inflation. In this type of inflation the motivating force is mainly rising wages which push up costs of production, so that rising prices are a consequence of increased costs.

The inflations that occurred in Great Britain during both World Wars and the two post-war periods were therefore mainly demand inflations, by the early 1950s supply had caught up with demand, and since then inflation has been mainly a cost inflation.

An important cause of the persistence of inflation in Great Britain, the United States and some other countries since 1945 has been the acceptance of responsibility for full employment by the Governments of those countries. The past twenty years have also been a period of high public capital investment in Great Britain by both the State and Local Authorities in housing, schools, roads, tunnels and bridges, redevelopment of town centres, etc. As a result, for most of this period the demand for labour has been greater than the supply, and in these conditions demands for higher wages by the trade unions tend to be frequent and competitive. Indeed, one of the indications of the presence of inflation is shortage of labour, and so wages rise steeply in those occupations where the shortage is greatest, though this can do nothing to alleviate the general condition. When there is over-full employment, not only do trade unions find it easier to obtain increases in wages, but there is also a tendency for employers, who are short of labour, to bid against one another by offering higher wages than the

agreed rates—an occurrence that has come to be known as "wage drift."
It seems therefore that if full employment is to be permanently maintained persistent inflation will be difficult to avoid, though it may be
temporarily checked by brief periods of stable prices, as in 1953–54 and
1958–60 (see Table XLVIB, p. 371), although so far efforts to keep
increases in wages in line with increases in production by means of an
"incomes policy" have met with little success.

(14) HYPERINFLATION

The danger in persistent inflation is that it may become a hyperinflation. Since 1914 a number of hyperinflations have taken place, as
for example in Germany, Austria and Russia in the 1920s and in
Hungary, Roumania, China and Germany again in the 1940s. Less
disastrous, but nevertheless severe, inflations have also been experienced
by France, Italy and some South American countries. All countries of
the world have suffered some degree of inflation during the past
twenty years.

As the inflation proceeds, the velocity of circulation increases to an
even greater extent because people begin to realise that holding money
even for a single day entails considerable loss. Saving ceases, and there
is an increasing anxiety to turn all cash into real, tangible things, so
that shopkeepers' stocks are sold out as soon as replenished. Those who
try to exchange their money for foreign currency find it necessary to
offer colossal sums in exchange for a single dollar or a pound sterling.
The result is a steeper rise in prices than the increase in the quantity of
money warrants. Wages have to be adjusted each day before work
begins, and may be reckoned in terms of a foreign currency or a
commodity.

During 1922 prices in Germany were five hundred times as high as
they had been four years previously; during the final stages of the
inflation in 1923 the price even of a postage stamp reached astronomical
figures. In Hungary in 1945 prices rose to even greater heights, the
purchase of the cheapest things requiring a payment in pengö of a
number running into no less than thirty digits! Debtors found that
quite considerable debts shrank in value until they could be repaid by
the reward for a few minutes' work or dwindled away to almost
nothing. The gains of debtors were, of course, the losses of creditors.
People who had put their savings in bank deposits or Government
Stocks had them wiped out; those who had invested in real assets—
factory buildings, industrial plant, machinery, houses, land—were
more fortunate, as the value of these in terms of money appreciated
with every fall in the value of money. The business community

therefore suffered least; those who had put their savings into "safe" investments suffered most.

There is only one way to end a runaway inflation. Sooner or later currency ceases to be acceptable and transactions take place either in a foreign currency (though this may be no more than a unit of account) or in terms of some commodity. In the end a new currency has to be introduced and the old one withdrawn. In Hungary the forint replaced the pengö, in Austria the schilling took the place of the crown; in Germany the reichsmark replaced the mark, the reichsmark itself being superseded later by the deutschemark.

RECOMMENDATIONS FOR FURTHER READING

G. Crowther: *An Outline of Money*, Chapters 3 and 4 (Section 1).
D. H. Robertson: *Money*, Chapters 2 and 3.
A. Lewis: *Economic Survey, 1919–39*, Chapter 1.
J. L. Hanson: *Monetary Theory and Practice*, Chapters 10 and 11.

QUESTIONS

1. Discuss the chief factors which will cause a rise in general prices. How are such general price changes measured? (R.S.A. Inter.)

2. What are chief causes of changes in value of money? What effects are they likely to have on distribution of wealth? (I.T.)

3. How may changes in the cost of living be measured? (A.I.A.)

4. What are the defects of the Quantity Theory of Money? (I.M.T.A.)

5. Explain the difficulties involved in trying to measure the general level of prices. (B.S. Inter.)

6. Describe the quantity theory of money and discuss its validity under the present system of rationing and price control. (I.B.)

7. Describe the practical use of index numbers. How are they constructed? (I.B.)

8. What is "liquidity preference"? What are the main factors in a community which determine the degree of it? (I.H.A.)

9. How would you expect a period of rising prices to affect (a) the income of different sections of the community, (b) the revenue and expenditure of the State? (D.P.A.)

10. What are the principal causes that may bring about a change in the value of money? By what means are these changes measured? (C.C.S. Final.)

11. What factors influence the value of money? (G.C.E. Adv.)

12. Why do people hold money balances if money is only useful when it can be exchanged for goods and services? (G.C.E. Adv.)

13. "While the accuracy of the quantity equation in the theory of money is beyond dispute its usefulness is not so certain." Discuss. (G.C.E. Adv.)

14. How would you measure the average level of retail prices? What difficulties are likely to arise in doing so? (G.C.E. Adv.)

15. "A major objection to inflation is that it leads inevitably to an adverse balance of payments." Explain and discuss. (G.C.E. Adv.)

16. Discuss the rôle in monetary theory of the concept of the demand for money. (Final Degree.)

17. What do you understand by the distinction between "cost inflation" and "demand inflation," and what is the relevance to anti-inflationary policies? (Final Degree.)

CHAPTER XXII

THE ENGLISH BANKING SYSTEM:
THE COMMERCIAL BANKS

I. THE EVOLUTION OF BRITISH BANKING

(1) THE ORIGIN OF BANKING IN ENGLAND

In England banking had its origin with the London goldsmiths, who, because of the nature of their business, had facilities for storing valuables. The first banking function, therefore, was accepting deposits of cash from merchants who had no safe place in which to keep their money. The goldsmiths at first made a charge for looking after their customers' money. The second stage came when the receipts for these deposits began to be used as means of payment by merchants, and this led the early bankers to issue bank-notes of fixed denominations which were more generally acceptable. Thus the second function of banks became the issue of bank-notes. The third stage in the development of banking came when bankers began to lend money. The increasing use of bank-notes meant that fewer people wished to withdraw their deposits in cash from the bankers, who thus found it safe to lend out at interest some of the money deposited with them. This proving a profitable business, bankers began to offer the inducement of interest to encourage merchants and others to increase their deposits. Next, bankers lent their own notes, experience teaching them how much cash they ought to keep in hand to meet the demands of their customers for cash. The use of cheques made it possible for the banks to lend by allowing customers to have overdrafts—that is, to draw cheques for agreed sums above the amount standing to their credit at the bank.

(2) PRIVATE BANKS

The Bank of England was founded in 1694, primarily for the purpose of lending money to the Government, and though it undertook some ordinary commercial banking, and at an early date become the sole bank in London issuing notes, from the first it left most ordinary business to other banks. Until 1826, however, it had a monopoly of joint-stock banking in England, and in London until 1833. By the end of the eighteenth century the private bankers in London had developed the use of cheques and had established a clearing house. Outside London, private banking was more often at first a sideline to a manufacturer's or a merchant's main business—for example, Samuel Lloyd, who was in the iron and steel business in Birmingham, was the founder of Lloyds Bank. Many had sprung from "corn-merchants' offices, chandlers', tea dealers' or mercers' shops."[1] By 1821 there were 843 private banks in England, of which 62 were in London.

The large increase in the number of private banks outside London was the result of the Industrial Revolution: in 1750 there were only twelve such banks, whereas in 1821 there were 781 "country" banks. Most of these banks were small, unit banks—that is, they had no branches—and in times of crisis many of them had to close their doors. During the fifteen years 1815–30 there were no fewer than 206 bank failures.

(3) JOINT-STOCK BANKS

Banking in Scotland had developed on somewhat different lines, the Bank of Scotland (founded 1695) having no monopoly of joint-stock banking in that country. A number of joint-stock banks had therefore been established in Scotland, and it was noticed that bank failures there were rarer than in England. In the banking crisis of 1825–26, for example, not one of the joint-stock banks failed, although some Scottish banks were affected and 80 English banks had to close. Supporters of joint-stock banking, such as Joplin, pointed to the Scottish banks as proof of the greater strength of joint-stock banks as compared with private banks.

An Act of 1826 permitted the establishment of joint-stock banks in England with unlimited liability, but with power to issue bank-notes, provided that they were situated at least 65 miles from London. Joint-stock banks were opened in Bradford and Huddersfield and a number of other towns the following year, and within seven years their number had increased to 32.

An Act of 1833 permitted the establishment of joint-stock banks in London, though in their case without the right to issue notes. The first joint-stock bank to open in London was the London and Westminster, founded in 1834, and this bank had to face opposition from the Bank of England, from the London private banks and from the general public, who for some reason at first looked with suspicion upon the new joint-stock banks. By 1836, however, there were 99 joint-stock banks in England, of which 21 were in Yorkshire and two in London.

---

[1] Clapham: *Economic History of Great Britain*, I, 264.

(4) THE EXPANSION OF BANKS (i) BY OPENING BRANCHES

Small banks, whether private or joint-stock, were unable to withstand crises. The development of large-scale banking took two forms: individual banks extended their activities either by opening branches or by amalgamation with other banks. Private banks, by their very nature, tended to be local institutions, though lack of capital often hindered their expansion, and so branch banking was undertaken chiefly by joint-stock banks. Considerable progress in this direction had been made during the 50 years ending in 1890. The number of private banks fell from 321 in 1840 to 155 in 1890, but there were still over 100 joint-stock banks at the end of this period—only five fewer than at the beginning. Branch banking, however, developed only slowly. In 1865 there were only three banks with over 30 branches, the largest being the London and County, with 127 branches. By 1890 there were nine banks with over 50 branches, the largest at that date being the London and County (165 branches), the National Provincial (158) and the Capital and Counties (99), but the other 250 banks averaged only ten branches each. By 1890 branch banking had developed to such an extent that ten banks had a total of 949 branches, and by then all important Scottish banks had opened London offices, though in their case this did not deprive them of the privilege of issuing banknotes.

Advantages of branch banking. (i) When a bank has a number of branches, smaller reserves of cash can be maintained at each branch, as in case of need one branch can obtain assistance from others. (ii) The chief advantage of branch banking lies in the greater stability of such banks, for the risk of failure is reduced.

Where, as in Great Britain, industries are highly localised, a decline in the basic industry would probably result in many bank failures in that district if unit banks were customary. Though the Great Depression of 1929–35 was most severely felt in the "distressed areas," there was not a single bank failure in Great Britain, because by that time commercial banking in this country was carried on by a small number of banks, each with a network of branches, so that losses in one part of the country could be offset by gains elsewhere. The history of banking during this trade depression was, however, vastly different in the United States, where unit banking is the general rule; 7,000 banks in that country closed their doors during 1930–33, no fewer than 3,000 of them in the two months February–March 1933. In favour of unit banks it is said that, because of their better acquaintance with local conditions, they are able to provide services suitable to the local industry, but this is poor compensation for their weakness in times of crisis, and in any case branch banks generally appoint as managers men who have had previous experience in the same industrial area.

Limited liability. It was not until 1858 that the privilege of limited liability was extended to banks, though many years after that date 69 English banks and all the Scottish banks still had unlimited liability. The failure of the City of Glasgow Bank in 1878, when the demands made upon the shareholders ruined many of them, caused shareholders in other banks with unlimited liability to press for protection, and within a few years all the large banks enjoyed limited liability.

(5) THE EXPANSION OF BANKS (ii) BY AMALGAMATION

Before 1913. There were two main periods of bank amalgamation. The period down to 1913 saw the development of upwards of 40 large-stock banks. At first amalgamations took place (i) between small country banks, (ii) between London and country banks and (iii) between joint-stock and private banks. Joint-stock banks, which had previously had agents in London, were particularly anxious to join up with private banks that were members of the London Clearing House, even though to have a branch in London in the case of an English bank meant the sacrifice of the right to issue notes. For their part, the London banks, more affected than the provincial banks by the cheap-money policy of 1892–96, began to seek a country connection. Large-scale industry required large-scale banking, and this provided another motive for amalgamation. Thirdly, the earlier antipathy of the public towards joint-stock banks and its preference for private banks was reversed, many of the private banks gradually losing public confidence.

As a number of the larger banks developed they began to expand further by absorbing other smaller banks. The National Provincial came to London in 1864, the Birmingham and Midland in 1890 and Parr's in 1891. As a result of these amalgamations the total number of banks declined, so that by 1913 there were only 37 joint-stock banks (with an average of 165 branches each) and 60 private banks (with an average of fewer than seven branches each). Many private banks— for example, Lloyds and Barclays—became joint-stock banks, though Barclays did not make this change until 1896.

After 1913. In the second period of bank amalgamation large banks of equal importance began to join together, and this movement culminated in the creation of the "Big Five"—the Midland, Barclays, Lloyds, the National Provincial and the Westminster—each of these banks having between 1,000 and 2,000 branches. Few large provincial joint-stock banks still remain: Martins with over 500 branches being the largest. Some alarm, however, was caused by this development, since it was feared that in the end there would be only one large, powerful bank. In 1918, therefore, the Treasury set up a Committee of Inquiry, which recommended that no further bank amalgamation should take place without the sanction of the Treasury and the Board of Trade. Though this recommendation never became law, the approval of the Treasury has generally been sought for later amalgamations. All the "Big Five," except the Westminster, had their origin in the provinces. The amalgamation of the Westminster and Parr's in 1919 provided an example of an amalgamation that was regarded as based on sound banking principles, most of the branches of the Westminster being in the Home Counties, where deposit banking predominated, while most of the branches of Parr's were in the industrial areas of the North and the Midlands, where there was a heavy demand for loans. As a result of these amalgamations the number of joint-stock banks in England and Wales declined between 1913 and 1939 from 37 to 13, though the total number of their branches increased to over 10,000. At the present day over 85% of all the banking business in England and Wales is undertaken by the "Big Five." Scotland is still served by five banks, but except for the Bank of Scotland all of them are now associated with English banks. In 1958 the English commercial banks extended their activities by acquiring interests in Finance Companies, mainly engaged in financing hire-purchase.

II. THE PRACTICE OF BANKING

(6) FUNCTIONS OF BANKS

(i) *Accepting deposits.* This is the oldest banking function, and in the earliest days of banking a charge was made for taking care of the money. Nowadays banks pay interest on deposit accounts, the rate usually being 2% below Bank rate. This is the main type of business carried on by Savings Banks, such as the Post Office Savings Bank and the Trustee Savings Banks, which are to be found in most large towns. The Savings Banks also pay interest on deposits, and are popular with small savers. It is usual for the commercial banks to require a few days' notice of withdrawal of money from deposit accounts, though for small sums this requirement is generally waived.

(ii) *Acting as agents for payment.* Commercial banks also permit their customers to have current accounts, on which they can draw without notice by cheque. The amounts standing to the credit of customers in deposit and current accounts form over 99% of the liabilities of a commercial bank, as a glance at the balance sheet on p. 395 will show. In the United States the distinction between deposits on deposit account and deposits on current account is made clearer by the terms used in that country—time deposits (deposit accounts) and demand deposits (current accounts). The cheque has become the principal method of payment in business, and each year sees an expansion of its use by the general public. Its convenience as a means of payment, economising the carrying of cash and providing a safe means for the transmission of money through the post, explains its increasing popularity in Great Britain and the United States. Banks pay no interest on current accounts, but instead make a charge for their work in transferring sums of money from one person's account to another's.

When calculating the total volume of purchasing power that exists in the form of bank deposits it is usual to add together the amounts on deposit and current account at commercial banks, though only sums on current account are subject to withdrawal by cheque, since in practice transfers can easily be made from one type of account to the other.[1]

(iii) *Issuing bank-notes*. It has been seen above that this was the second banking function to develop, the receipts given by the early bankers in exchange for customers' deposits coming to be used as means of payment. For convenience, the receipts were replaced by bank-notes of fixed denominations, each note having printed on its face the banker's promise to pay the bearer on demand the sum stated. A bank-note is thus an acknowledgement of a bank's debt, a sort of promissory note, exempt from Stamp Duty. The issue of bank-notes was an important function of early banks, though about the middle of the eighteenth century the London banks, other than the Bank of England, ceased to issue them. In London cheques came into common use at an earlier date than in the provinces, and in the first half of the nineteenth century the provincial banks were the chief issuers of notes. Once a banker had established himself in the public's confidence, his bank-notes were accepted and circulated as money, and few people desired to exchange them for gold. This made it possible for the banker to lend his own notes, and so the issue of notes became a coveted privilege of a banker and the most profitable side of his business. Many banks, however, at times found themselves in difficulties as a result of over-issuing notes. In most countries legal restrictions have been imposed on the issue of notes by banks. Often the issue of notes is subject to tax, as in England in 1804, or Canada (the Chartered

---

[1] Deposits with the Post Office and Trustee Savings Banks are not included.

Banks), Australia (1910) and New Zealand (to 1933). In England the effect of the *Bank Charter Act* of 1844 was gradually to confine the right to issue notes in this country to the Bank of England, which since 1921 has been the sole bank of issue, but any increase in the issue must be sanctioned by Parliament.

(iv) *Lending to customers.* The most profitable business of a banker is lending, and this can be considered one of the primary functions of a commercial bank. The early bankers lent some of the cash that had been deposited with them for safe keeping. The use of bank-notes made it possible for a banker to lend his own "promise to pay" so long as he retained the confidence of the business community.

Banks nowadays make advances to customers in the following ways:

(a) *By means of a loan account.* In this case the borrower's current account will be credited by the amount of the loan, and at the same time a loan account for this sum will be opened. Thus the borrower pays interest on the full amount he has borrowed. Some banks also grant personal loans.

(b) *By means of overdraft.* When a customer obtains an overdraft from his banker this means that he is permitted to draw cheques for a sum greater by the amount of the overdraft than the balance standing to his credit. In this case, if he does not avail himself of the full amount of the overdraft, he pays interest only on the amount by which his current account is actually overdrawn. The overdraft provides the easiest and most convenient method of borrowing open to business men.

(c) *By discounting bills of exchange.* When a bank discounts a bill of exchange for a customer it is making a payment to a creditor, whose debtor has promised to pay at some future date. Thus the bank enables the creditor to be paid at once, and at the same time allows the debtor a period of credit. This therefore is really another form of bank lending, the bank collecting the debt when it is due for repayment.

(v) *Other services to customers.* Banks act as agents for their customers in the purchase or sale of stock-exchange securities, they are prepared to act as trustees or executors, they transact foreign exchange business, obtaining foreign currency for customers or exchanging foreign currency for sterling, and issue bank drafts, travellers' cheques, etc. The commercial banks also undertake acceptance business in connection with bills of exchange. During 1965-66 they began to offer credit cards guaranteeing customers' cheques up to £30.

(7) BANK LOANS CREATE BANK DEPOSITS

Whether a bank lends by overdraft or by means of a loan account, the result is the same—it increases the total volume of purchasing power, that is, the quantity of money. For example, if Dombey's account shows that he has a credit balance of £50 and he obtains an overdraft for £100 he can draw a cheque for £150, and the bank will honour it. This cheque will be paid into (say) Gradgrind's account, which will increase by £150. Dombey's account, however, cannot fall by more than £50 (although, of course, his account will show a debit of £100), so the total combined deposits at the banks of which Dombey and Gradgrind are customers will increase by £100. The loan of £100 to Dombey has increased total deposits by £100. Thus loans make deposits. Banks can also create deposits by purchasing Government Stock, which is simply a method by which banks lend to the Government. When such purchases are made the bank pays for them by cheques drawn on itself, and the payees of these cheques pay them into their own banking accounts, and so again the banks create deposits. Thus bank deposits are mainly created by the banks themselves. This power of the banks to expand credit is of enormous economic significance, for bank deposits can be used for the purchase of goods and services, irrespective of the way in which they have been created. The total quantity of money therefore depends on the credit policy of the banks.

Superficially it may appear that a bank can lend only what has been deposited with it. From the example just given, however, it is clear that cheques paid by customers are often drawn against overdrafts, though only the drawer's banker is aware of this. Whatever may be the individual bank's attitude to this, there is no doubt that the banking system as a whole is responsible for the creation of a very large proportion of the deposits of the various banks.

(8) BANK CREDIT AND TRADE CREDIT

It has been seen that when a bank grants credit it creates what it lends, and so total purchasing power is increased. If therefore a manufacturer obtains from the bank a loan of £1,000 the bank does not forgo the use of this sum in order to make the loan. In fact, as has already been seen, bank deposits will rise by £1,000, and so total purchasing power will increase. If a bank restricted its loans to the amount of cash deposited with it the bank would merely be acting as an intermediary for the transfer of a sum of money from depositors to borrowers. Banks, however, are prepared to expand their lending within the limits imposed by their liquidity rules.

It appears at first sight to be rather different when a wholesaler grants credit to a retailer, for in this case the wholesaler has to forgo for a period the use of the sum the retailer owes him. What the retailer gains the wholesaler forgoes so that there is no increase in total purchasing power. A merchant who grants credit to his customers will require more capital than one who does not, as many owners of small businesses have found to their cost, for if their customers are slow to pay they may find that they have not the means for replenishing their stock. The granting of credit by wholesalers makes it possible for people with little capital to engage in retail trade, for it enables them to sell part of their stock before paying for it. Similarly, a consumer can spend most of his wages before he receives them if retailers supply him with goods on credit.

In the case of trade credit, however, the extra purchasing power enjoyed by one person is generally balanced by an equal loss of purchasing power by another, unless, of course, the credit trading itself is financed by banks directly by loan or overdraft, or indirectly by discounting bills of exchange. Nevertheless, it was the opinion of the Radcliffe Committee (1959) that trade credit might be used to finance an expansion of production when bank credit was restricted by the monetary authorities. To some extent, therefore, trade credit appears to be similar to bank credit in its effect on total purchasing power.

(9) THE BANKERS' CLEARING HOUSES

If Dorrit has a current account at the Southern Bank and draws a cheque for £20 in favour of Copperfield, who has an account with the Northern Bank, it will then be necessary for the Northern Bank to collect £20 from the Southern Bank when Copperfield pays in this cheque. The use of cheques makes it necessary to have some means of clearing them. The London private banks were the first to allow their customers to use cheques, and by 1770 they had established a clearing house. Previous to that, bank clerks had met in the street to exchange cheques. At the present day cheques to a value of over £1,200 million pass through the Bankers' Clearing Houses every working day.

Four types of clearing may be noted:

(i) *Local branch clearings.* Suppose that Dombey receives a cheque from Nickleby, and that both of them have accounts with the Westminster branch of the Southern Bank. It is an easy matter by a book entry to credit Dombey's account with £15 and debit Nickleby's by the same amount. There is no movement of cash.

(ii) *Head office clearings.* If Pickwick's account is with the Southern Bank, Canterbury, and he sends a cheque for £8 to Weller, whose account is with the Dorking branch of the same bank, this cheque will be cleared through the Head Office of the Southern Bank, Pickwick's account being debited and Weller's credited with £8.

(iii) *Local clearing houses*. Rokesmith and Jarndyce both bank in the same town, the former at the Southern Bank, the latter at the Northern Bank. Rokesmith pays a debt to Jarndyce with a cheque drawn on the Southern Bank for £40, which Jarndyce pays into the Northern Bank. If these are the only two banks in the town a clerk will probably go from one to the other to clear the cheques. If a total of £310 has to be transferred from accounts at the Southern Bank to accounts at the Northern, and £240 from the Northern to the Southern, it will be necessary only for a cheque for the difference, £70, to be paid over to the Northern Bank by the Southern. This cheque will be cleared at the London clearing. Again no movement of cash takes place. All the larger towns have their own clearing houses, where representatives of the various banks in the town meet each day to clear cheques in this way, offsetting as far as possible indebtedness between different banks, and making a settlement by means of cheques for the differences. An exchange of cheques will then take place, the clerk from the Southern Bank, for example, collecting all cheques drawn on his bank which have been paid into the Northern Bank, so that the amounts can be deducted from the various customers. The following examples will illustrate this:

TABLE XLVIII

The Clearing of Cheques

Cheques paid into:							
Northern Bank		Southern Bank		Eastern Bank		Western Bank	
Cheques drawn on:	£	Cheques drawn on:	£	Cheques drawn on:	£	Cheques drawn on:	£
Southern	2,000	Northern	1,900	Northern	1,500	Northern	1,800
Eastern	1,700	Eastern	1,200	Southern	1,100	Southern	1,500
Western	2,100	Western	1,600	Western	1,200	Eastern	1,300

The total amounts to be credited and debited to the four banks can now be calculated:

	Northern	Southern	Eastern	Western
	£	£	£	£
Credit · · · ·	5,800	4,700	3,800	4,600
Debit · · · ·	5,200	4,600	4,200	4,900

O

The differences will be:

	£	£	£	£
Credit +, Debit — . .	+600	+100	−400	−300

It will be sufficient now for the Eastern Bank to give the Northern Bank a cheque for £400 and for the Western Bank to give cheques for £200 and £100, respectively, to the Northern and Southern Banks.

Fluctuations in the volume of clearings at provincial centres often give a good indication of the state of trade, especially where the local clearing house is situated in the main centre of a highly localised industry, as for example Manchester for the cotton industry or Bradford for wool.

(iv) *The London Bankers' Clearing House.* If Spenlow has an account with the Eastern Bank, Northampton, and draws a cheque for £25 in favour of Drood, who pays it into his account at the Western Bank, Exeter, this cheque will be cleared through the London Clearing House. All cheques originating from banks in towns other than that where they have been paid in are sent each day to the head office of the payee's bank, after which they go to the London Clearing House. The procedure there is similar to that at the provincial clearing houses, though the number of cheques and sums involved will, of course, be very much greater. The only difference is in the final settlement. Each of the commercial banks keeps a balance at the Bank of England, and so differences of indebtness are settled by cheques drawn on the Bank of England, where a series of book entries will suffice to complete the transfer of hundreds of millions of pounds between people and firms in all parts of the country, again without the movement of any actual cash. All that remains is for the cheques to be returned to the banks on which they were drawn so that the drawers' accounts can be debited, and if required the cheques can then be returned to the drawers.

There are two separate clearings at the London Bankers' Clearing Houses, the one considered in (iv) above being the Country Clearing. In addition to this, there is the Town Clearing (two per day) for the banks in the vicinity of the City.[1]

The overwhelming amount of business transacted at the London Bankers' Clearing House is seen from a comparison between the daily averages of clearings there and at the provincial clearing houses. At the present day daily average for the London clearing is approximately £1,200 million; for the combined provincial clearings the daily average is under £10 million.

---

[1] Until 1939 there were three clearings—Country, Town and Metropolitan.

(10) RESTRICTIONS ON THE CREATION OF CREDIT BY BANKS

It has been said that banks can create deposits. This is certainly true of a banking system as a whole, though it might be argued that an individual bank can lend only what has been deposited with it. In any case banks have not unlimited power to create deposits; they are restricted in a number of ways:

(i) *The Clearing House imposes a restriction on an individual bank.* A single bank cannot adopt an expansionist credit policy unless the other banks are willing to do the same. In other words, the banks in their credit policy must keep in line with one another, expanding or contracting credit together. For if one bank expands credit more than others only a fraction of the additional bank deposits thereby created will remain with it, or be paid into it by its own customers, the rest being transferred by cheque to people with accounts at other banks. If it persists in pursuing an expansionist policy it will have persistent debit balances at the Bankers' Clearing House, and in consequence a continuous depletion of its reserves at the Bank of England will occur. The banks look upon these reserves as cash, and if a serious reduction of its cash reserves takes place a bank will soon be compelled to change its policy. Similarly, if a bank adopts an over-cautious credit policy its cash reserves will increase, but its profit-earning assets will be proportionately less than those of the other banks, with the result that its competitors will show higher profits.

(ii) *The liquidity ratio.* Money consists of bank deposits and cash, the former comprising about 78% of the total. Bank deposits are largely the result of bank loans, but the banks have been able to create deposits to this extent only because most people prefer money in that form to cash. Banks lend on the assumption that their customers will wish to exchange only a small proportion of their deposits for cash. So long as a bank retains the confidence of its depositors there will be no abnormal demand for cash, and in order to retain this confidence the bank must always be able to pay cash on demand. A bank must therefore keep a sufficient reserve of cash to meet the demand of its customers for cash. Increasing confidence in banking and the greater use of cheques have reduced the demand for cash in countries which, like Great Britain, have a well-established, mature banking system.

For a long time British banks maintained a ratio of 10% between cash and deposits, as experience had taught them that this was sufficient to enable them to meet all normal calls upon them, for no bank, however efficient its management, could withstand a continuous and abnormal demand for cash. Thus the creation of credit by the banks depends on (*a*) the amount of cash there is in existence; (*b*) the amount of cash people desire to hold; and (*c*) the limitations on the creation of bank credit, and therefore on the cash reserves which the banks deem necessary. As cheques are increasingly used the demand of customers for cash falls and even before 1939 British banks found that to maintain a cash ratio of 10% gave them a greater margin of safety than they regarded as necessary. For a long time, however, the banks were unwilling to reduce their cash ratio. In 1946 the Bank of England recommended that a cash ratio of 8% should be maintained, and since then the banks have kept to this lower cash ratio.

The English commercial banks maintain two liquidity rules: (*a*) to keep a ratio of 8% between their cash reserves and deposits; and (*b*) to keep a ratio of 28% between their more liquid assets (Items 1 to 3 in the Balance Sheet on p. 395) and their total assets. At one time the cash ratio was regarded as the main limitation on the power of the banks to create credit, but the Radcliffe Report (1959) showed that if the cash ratio fell below 8% the banks could easily restore it by reducing their holding of Treasury bills, whereas such action would have no effect on the 28% liquidity ratio. It is therefore this second liquidity rule of 28% and not the 8% cash ratio that acts as a check on the commercial banks. Though there is no legal compulsion on British banks to maintain their liquidity rules, there is no doubt that the Bank of England would put pressure on them to do so if it considered such a course to be necessary.

If its liquidity ratio rises it becomes possible for a bank either to increase its liquidity or its loans; if its liquidity falls, it must reduce either investments or loans. If the banks consider changes in the ratio to be due to temporary causes no action will be taken. Shortly before Christmas and in the summer there are heavy seasonal demands for cash, but in January and early autumn the cash generally flows back to the banks. In June and early December, therefore, the ratio falls, but usually returns to normal again in early January and late August. Knowing this, the banks take no action to influence it.

(iii) *The collateral security available.* Before a bank grants a loan it will want to know the purpose and length of time for which it is required and how it is to be repaid. In addition, the borrower will probably be asked to give the bank some kind of collateral security which the bank can turn into cash if the loan is not repaid. It is, however, an important banking principle that the first consideration in such cases is the character of the borrower, for the banker prefers a loan to be repaid and for the collateral security to be at his disposal only in an emergency. The more liquid the security—that is, the greater the ease with which it can be turned into cash without loss—the more acceptable it is to the bank.

Life assurance policies form good security because they usually have a "surrender value"—that is, a present cash value. Stock-exchange securities and deeds of property are frequently given as collateral security, but the prices of Stock-exchange securities vary from day to day, and in times of trade depression the value of industrial property may fall catastrophically, as both British and American banks found to their cost in the 1930s. Documents of title, such as bills of exchange, bills of lading, warehouse warrants, etc., can be used as collateral security. Sometimes a borrower may be able to persuade someone, whose credit is approved by the bank, to act as guarantor for the loan. The amount of collateral security is not, however, a fixed quantity, for the banks can raise or lower their standards, but at any given time, and taking the bank's standard as given, the amount of security available may limit bank lending.

(iv) *The Central Bank and the State.* The final restriction on the creation of credit by the commercial banks comes from the monetary authorities, that is, in this country the Chancellor of the Exchequer, the Bank of England and the Treasury, but a consideration of monetary policy must be reserved for Chapter XXIV.

III. THE BALANCE SHEET OF A JOINT-STOCK BANK
(ii) THE THEORY OF BANKING

A bank is an institution that is prepared to accept deposits of money and repay cash on demand. The essential feature of commercial banking is lending more than the amount of cash possessed by the bank. Loans to customers form a bank's most profitable activity, but the urge to expand this side of the business is tempered by its obligation to pay cash on demand. Most borrowers do not require cash but additional bank deposits on which they can draw by cheque, but a proportion of loans will be wanted in the form of cash—for example, for the payment of wages. To expand loans will, therefore, to some extent increase the demand for cash. It has been seen that a banker knows from past experience what proportion of his assets to keep in liquid form, but he must be able to convert his other assets into cash if circumstances require it without undue delay and without loss. Thus a banker's main concern is with the liquidity of his assets. This limits the extent of his willingness to lend and the amount of investment he is prepared to undertake. We have just seen that the banker has two liquidity rules: (i) to hold an amount of cash equal to 8% of the value of his total assets (the "cash ratio"); (ii) to maintain 28% of his total assets in a fairly liquid form—cash, money at call or short notice and bills. The structure of bank assets can be seen from Table L (p. 395).

(12) THE LIABILITIES OF A COMMERCIAL BANK

The chief items on the Liabilities side of a commercial bank's balance sheet are capital, reserves, acceptances and deposits. In 1895 capital and reserves formed 12½% of liabilities, but in 1965 less than 2½%. Of the liabilities, deposits are far and away the most important, and comprise at the present day something like 95% of the total. Since 1938 deposits have risen enormously, the total for the London Clearing Banks in 1938, 1945, 1955 and 1960 and 1965 respectively being shown in Table XLIX. It will be noticed that the total in 1945 was just over double the total in 1938. During the five years 1947–51 the total was fairly stable at about £6,000 million, but since then bank deposits have again increased rapidly in times of easy credit and more slowly during periods of credit restriction.

TABLE XLIX

Bank Deposits

Date	£ million monthly averages
1938	2,277
1945	4,692
1955	6,400
1960	7,236
1965	8,415
196–	[1]

There has been a change in the distribution of bank deposits between current and deposit accounts. In the 1930s the amount on current account formed between 50 and 55% of the total; in 1965 the amount on current account was 60% of the total. This distribution, has, however, little economic significance, for transfers from one account to the other can easily be made. Deposits in both cases can therefore be regarded as purchasing power. Since 1964 the Trustee Savings Banks have been permitted to grant their customers the right to make withdrawals by cheque, thereby increasing bank deposits subject to withdrawal by cheque, and so increasing the quantity of money.

(13) THE ASSETS OF A COMMERCIAL BANK

The assets of a commercial bank are essentially claims against other people, institutions or the Government. The distribution of bank

---

[1] This space can be used for the insertion of the latest figures.

assets is the result of a compromise between (a) the necessity always to be able to pay cash on demand, and (b) the desire for profit. The more liquid the asset, the less profit it will yield to the bank. Cash—the most liquid asset—earns no profit at all, whether it be in the tills of the bank's various branches or in the bank's balance at the Bank of England. The least liquid of a bank's assets—apart from its premises—is advances to customers.

The following table shows the combined assets of the London Clearing Banks in 1938, 1945 and 1965:

TABLE L

Bank Assets (London Clearing Banks)

	1938 £ million	1938 %	1945 £ million	1945 %	1965 £ million	1965 %	196– £ million	196– %
1. Coin, notes and balances with Bank of England	241	10·2	492	10·4	720	8·2		
2. Money at call and short notice	211	8·5	347	7·5	701	7·9		
3. Bills discounted	280	11·0	188	4·0	1,260	14·0		
4. Treasury deposit receipts	—	—	1,811	38·1	—	—		
5. Special deposits	—	—	—	—	89	9·0		
6. Investments	637	28·0	1,156	24·0	1,056	10·6		
7. Advances to customers	976	42·3	768	16·0	4,726	52·6		

Source: *Monthly Digest of Statistics.*

The percentages show the relation between each asset and total deposits.

(14) THE MORE LIQUID ASSETS OF A BANK

The above table shows the maintenance of a cash ratio of 10% in 1938 and 1945 (actually 10·2% and 10·4% respectively) and of 8% in 1965 (actually 8·2%). When calculating their total cash the English Commercial banks include their balances at the Bank of England, which forms about 40% of the total. The more liquid assets comprise items 1 to 3 above—cash, money at call and short notice, and bills discounted.

Money at call and short notice. This consists chiefly of short-term loans to the money market: bill brokers, discount and acceptance houses.[1] As the term implies, such loans can be called in by the banks either

[1] See next chapter for an account of the money market.

without notice or at very short notice—one to seven days. This is a very liquid asset, and its existence makes it possible for British banks to keep a smaller cash ratio than would otherwise be prudent. In countries without a well-developed money market banks find it necessary to keep a large proportion of their total assets in the form of cash. Because of the liquidity of this asset, banks make only a small charge to the money market for loans at call or short notice.

Bills discounted. The discounting of bills is an important function of a bank. Bankers look upon bills as a most desirable asset, since they are fairly liquid and yet yield a profit. They are preferred to loans because they provide the bank with a negotiable instrument, which can be rediscounted if necessary, although it is not the practice of banks to rediscount bills which they have once acquired. Bills are said to be self-liquidating, for they arise as a result of actual trade transactions and fall due for payment at a fixed date. The use of bills of exchange to finance inland trade transactions has, however, declined during the past thirty years, and the majority of bills discounted now are Treasury bills, which yield a very small profit.

Treasury deposit receipts. During the Second World War the Government compulsorily borrowed from the banks by means of Treasury deposit receipts. This asset is therefore not to be found in the bank balance sheet of 1938, nor in those for years after 1952.

Special deposits. In 1960 the Bank of England for the first time made use of the new device of demanding from the commercial banks sums as Special deposits, as a means of reducing their liquidity.

In 1945 the more liquid assets formed 60% of deposits as against only 30% in 1938, though by 1960 the pre-1939 structure of the banks' balance sheet had been very nearly restored, the more liquid assets by that date having fallen to 31% and by 1965 to 30·1%.

(15) THE LESS LIQUID ASSETS OF A BANK

Investments and advances to customers comprise the less liquid, but the more profitable of bank assets. On account of their desire for liquidity, banks do not care for long-term investments. In this country they limit their investments to "gilt-edged" securities—mainly British Government Stocks. Advances are generally loans to provide industry with circulating capital, as it is rare for British banks to provide fixed capital. In recent years there has been an increase in personal loans. Table LI shows the distribution of bank advances in 1965.

It is usual for bank advances and investments to vary inversely, for when bank advances are not in demand the banks increase their investments. During the Great Depression of 1929–35 the banks increased their investments at the expense of advances, business men being generally unwilling to borrow during a trade slump, however low the rate of interest. With the revival of trade, banks tend to sell investments in order to increase their advances.

TABLE LI
Total Bank Advances

1965	£ million
Agriculture and fishing .	516
Industry	2,657
Retail trade .	533
Personal and professional	960
Stockbrokers	5
Other financial	713
Local Government authorities.	68
Others	45
	5,497

Source: *Monthly Digest of Statistics.*

During 1952 and again in 1955–58 and 1964–66 the banks restricted their advances to customers on the recommendation of the Bank of England, and in consequence the total for this item fell. During 1958–60 there was a huge increase in bank advances, much of this expansion being made possible by the banks selling investments.

RECOMMENDATIONS FOR FURTHER READING

J. H. Clapham: *Economic History of Great Britain*, Vol. I, Chapters 7 and 13.
R. S. Sayers: *Modern Banking*, Chapters 1, 2, 8.
G. Crowther: *An Outline of Money*, Chapter 2.

QUESTIONS

1. What are the main functions of modern banks? (Exp.)
2. Outline the advantages and the possible dangers of bank and trade credit. (I.B.)
3. Explain the working of the Bankers' Clearing Houses. (I.M.T.A.)
4. "Banks do not create money; they only lend money which has been deposited with them." Discuss. (C.I.S. Inter.)
5. To what extent are the joint-stock banks able to influence the total supply of money in circulation? (B.S. Final.)
6. Can banks create credit? If so, how? (C.I.S. Final.)

7. What are the principal investments of a British joint-stock bank and what are the general principles which tend to determine the allocation of resources amongst these investments? (I.H.A.)

8. What do you understand by the creation of credit by a bank? What limits the amount of credit which a bank may create? (C.C.S. Final.)

9. "The secret of successful banking is to distribute resources in such a way as to get a sound balance between liquidity and profitability." Discuss. (A.I.A.)

10. By what means can banks increase the total volume of bank deposits, and how will such action affect the price level? (D.P.A.)

11. Examine the limitations on the power of the commercial banks to change the quantity of money. (G.C.E. Adv.)

12. What limits the power of a joint-stock bank to increase the total amount of money loaned to its customers? (G.C.E. Adv.)

13. Describe a typical commercial bank's balance sheet. What are the chief factors determining the composition of its assets? (G.C.E. Adv.)

14. What are the liquidity principles of sound commercial banking? Why are these principles an inadequate bulwark against monetary instability? (Final Degree.)

CHAPTER XXIII

THE ENGLISH BANKING SYSTEM: THE MONEY MARKET

I. INTRODUCTORY

(1) THE FINANCIAL MARKETS

There are four important financial markets, the scope and functions of which are frequently confused. These are the money market, the discount market, the securities market (the Stock Exchange) and the capital market. Of these, the securities market is the only one that has a particular building in which its business is carried on. The business of the money market and the discount market is transacted in the neighbourhood of Lombard Street and the Bank of England, where the head offices of the commercial banks and other financial institutions are situated within easy reach of one another.

These four financial markets conveniently group themselves into two pairs. The terms *money market* and *discount market* are often used as if they were synonyms, for the connection between them is very close. The money market is essentially a market for short-term loans, just as the capital market is primarily a market for long-term loans. The second item in a commercial bank's balance sheet in order of liquidity is Money at Call and Short Notice, and this shows how much the banks are lending to the discount houses and bill brokers. These firms form the link between the money market, where the commodity dealt in is the short-term loan, and the discount market, where the commodity dealt in is the bill (trade bills and Treasury bills). Since bills are self-liquidating, and can be turned into money at a specified date, they have been called "near money." The bill brokers and discount houses borrow on short-term from the banks in order to provide themselves with funds with which to purchase (that is, discount) bills. Banks do not lend on long-term, and so firms in need of fixed capital must have recourse to the capital market. The securities market, or Stock Exchange, is the market in which existing issues of stocks and shares are bought and sold. The capital and securities markets are considered in Chapter XXV.

II. TYPES OF BILLS

(2) THE PROMISSORY NOTE

This is perhaps the simplest type of bill, being a written promise on the part of one person to pay another a certain sum of money at an agreed future date. It usually takes the following form:

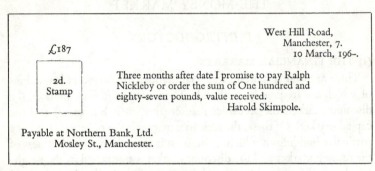

West Hill Road,
Manchester, 7.
10 March, 196-.

£187

2d.
Stamp

Three months after date I promise to pay Ralph Nickleby or order the sum of One hundred and eighty-seven pounds, value received.
Harold Skimpole.

Payable at Northern Bank, Ltd.
Mosley St., Manchester.

FIG. 76.—PROMISSORY NOTE.

In this case Ralph Nickleby has supplied Skimpole with goods to the value of £187, but Skimpole desires three months in which to pay, and with Nickleby's consent payment has been made by means of a promissory note. This falls due for payment three months and three days (these extra days being known as "days of grace") after 10th March— that is, on 13th June. On its being presented at the Mosley Street branch, Manchester, of the Northern Bank on that date, payment will be made. This particular bank has been chosen by Skimpole because he keeps his account there. Promissory notes are rarely used in business in Great Britain, though they are popular in the United States.

(3) THE BILL OF EXCHANGE

The inland bill of exchange is similar in some ways to the promissory note. Both are means by which a debtor makes acknowledgement of a debt incurred in the course of business and which he proposes to pay on demand, or, generally, at some agreed future date. Most bills are drawn for three months, but both bills of exchange and promissory notes can be drawn for payment at sight or for periods longer or shorter than three months. For both types of bill the debtor is allowed three additional days of grace in which to pay unless they are payable within three days. The Stamp Duty is now the same as for cheques. The bill of exchange differs from the promissory note in two ways: it is drawn by the creditor, and before it is of any value it has to be accepted by the debtor. An inland bill of exchange takes the following form:

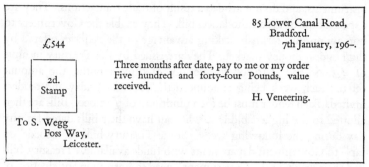

FIG. 77a.—BILL OF EXCHANGE.

After a bill has been accepted it is known as an Acceptance. Inland Bills of Exchange were quite common in 1840, though by 1870 they had been largely displaced by the cheque. They are only rarely used in Great Britain nowadays.

The foreign bill of exchange differs from the inland bill in a number of ways. It used to be made out in triplicate in case the first copy was lost in transit, but this is no longer usual. Before 1914 the import of cotton and wheat was financed by this means. The simplest form of the foreign bill is as follows:

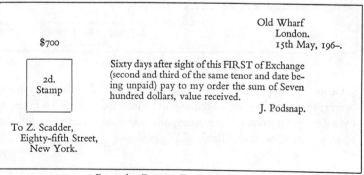

FIG. 77b.—FOREIGN BILL OF EXCHANGE.

In this example J. Podsnap of London has sold goods to Z. Scadder of New York, and has drawn a bill of exchange in payment which Z. Scadder will in due course accept and on the due date pay. In the case of a foreign bill the period before it becomes due for payment is calculated from the date of acceptance.

(4) THE TREASURY BILL

Treasury bills were created by an Act of 1877, largely on the suggestion of Walter Bagehot. Unlike trade bills, they are purely financial instruments, and do not arise as a result of trade transactions. They are a special type of accommodation bill. They enable the Government to borrow on easy terms by taking advantage of the facilities offered by the London money market. They are issued by the Treasury in units of £5,000 and £10,000 for periods of three months, the amount offered each week being announced the previous Friday and tenders invited. Each tender must be for a minimum of £50,000. Bills are then allotted to the highest bidders, who can have their bills dated for any day during the following week. Some Treasury bills are issued "on tap" to Government departments with funds available. Treasury bills had their origin in the Government's need to borrow in anticipation of revenue, and the cheapness of this method of borrowing led to a huge increase in their use, so that the value of the Treasury bill issue now greatly exceeds the outstanding revenue. The Treasury bill takes the following form:

Due 14 June 196-.

TREASURY BILL

Per Acts 40 Vict. c 2 and 52 Vict. c 6.

£10,000
London.

A
12,438

This Treasury Bill entitles   or order to payment of Ten Thousand Pounds at the Bank of England out of the Consolidated Fund of the United Kingdom on the 14th day of June 196-.

(Signed).......................................
Secretary to the Treasury.

FIG. 78.—TREASURY BILL.

Generally, no payee's name is inserted, and the bill is then payable to bearer; for safety in transit a name will be inserted if the bill is taken up by a foreign purchaser. Treasury bills are paid when they fall due upon presentation at the Bank of England.

III. THE WORK OF THE DISCOUNT MARKET

(5) DISCOUNTING BILLS

The members of the money and discount markets are the Discount Houses, the merchant bankers (or acceptance houses), the English commercial banks, a large number of foreign and overseas banks, and as lender of last resort, the Bank of England.

When Veneering, the creditor named in the bill on p. 401, agreed to Wegg's request that settlement of his debt be made by a three month bill of exchange, it was equivalent to Veneering giving Wegg three months' credit. The advantage of this type of settlement is that it gives rise to a negotiable instrument. Three courses are then open to Veneering: (i) he can hold the bill until it matures—that is, until it is due for payment; or (ii) by endorsing it he may be able to use it in settlement of one of his own debts, if some other merchant is willing to take payment in this form; or (iii) he may be able to discount it, that is, sell it to a broker. Whether the bill can be discounted will depend on Wegg's standing in the business world, for the eventual payment of the bill depends on Wegg's ability to meet it. On discounting the bill, Veneering will not receive the full amount for which it was drawn, for interest on £544 for three months will be deducted, the rate depending on the prevailing rate of interest and the risk in holding this particular bill. If Veneering discounts the bill Wegg will really be obtaining a loan, the transaction between Wegg and Veneering in effect being financed by the bill broker who discounts the bill.

Operating in the London discount market there are now nine public limited companies, of which Alexanders, the National Discount Company and the Union Discount Company of London are the largest. These nine firms are responsible for over 90% of the business of the market. In addition, there are three private firms. There are also four firms of "running brokers," but they are only agents who act on behalf of others and do not discount bills on their own account.

Many of the discount houses carry out other functions, such as lending to local authorities, acting as issuing houses or as trustees for pension funds. The discount houses enjoy the unique privilege of being able to borrow from the Bank of England when it acts in its capacity as "lender of last resort." (see p. 419).

(6) ACCEPTING BILLS

A bill of exchange has no value until it has been accepted; and unless the name of the acceptor is well known, no one will be willing to discount it. Foreign bills may be drawn on firms in all parts of the world, but few bills would qualify for discounting were it not for the existence of specialist accepting institutions. The acceptance houses are sometimes known as merchant bankers because their financial business generally developed out of their ordinary trading activities. The oldest of these firms moved into London from Europe in the late eighteenth or early nineteenth centuries during the Napoleonic War, and the most recent was founded in 1921. The names of many merchant bankers indicate their foreign origin—Schröder, Kleinwort, Lazard, Baring, Rothschild. Other merchant banks include Hambros, Hill Samuel & Co. and S. Montagu. To some extent merchant banks specialise in particular parts of the world, and, having their own agents in the chief commercial centres, they possess expert knowledge of the credit-worthiness of merchants in the areas in which they operate. For a fee, therefore, they are prepared to accept bills which would otherwise not be negotiable because the first acceptor's name was not known to the discount market. Foreign merchants can open acceptance credits with the acceptance houses, and other merchants can draw bills upon them, and such bills can be discounted in the London discount market. Thus, by guaranteeing payment, they make bills negotiable, and bill brokers and discount houses are then prepared to deal in them.

Acceptance business is not their sole activity—or few would have survived—nor, in the case of Rothschilds, is it the most important function of the merchant bankers. To offset the decline in acceptance business many of them have had to turn to ordinary banking. Thus they are prepared to accept deposits, usually paying a slightly higher rate of interest than the commercial banks, and they grant loans. They have frequently undertaken the placing of long-term loans in London on behalf of foreign firms and Governments. For example, Roths-childs assisted the purchase of a controlling interest in the Suez Canal by Disraeli's Government in 1875. The merchant bankers no longer have a monopoly of acceptance business, for only about half the total amount is now in their hands, as the commercial banks have taken an increasing share of this work during the past thirty or forty years.

When a bill has been accepted either by a commercial bank or a merchant banker it is known as a "bank bill"; when accepted by a merchant of good standing it is known as a "fine trade bill."

(7) FUNCTIONS OF THE MONEY AND DISCOUNT MARKETS

A much greater amount of discount business is transacted on the London market than on any foreign discount market. The bill brokers and discount houses borrow from the commercial banks at a very low rate of interest because the loans can be recalled at short notice. This is an advantage to the banks, as it provides them with a particularly liquid asset. It enables English banks to keep a lower cash reserve than is possible for most foreign banks. The bill brokers use these funds to discount bills which they hold for a period, usually a month, after which they rediscount them with the banks. They are able to make a profit by charging a slightly higher rate for discounting bills than that at which they borrow from the banks. The banks themselves discount bills, but prefer them to be not more than two months from maturity when they acquire them. They also like to have approximately equal amounts falling due each week. Thus they are prepared to rediscount bills for the bill brokers at lower rates than the interest they charge on their short-term loans. This loss the banks regard as a sort of fee to the bill brokers for holding bills for a period and arranging them in "parcels." Once a commercial bank has acquired a bill it usually holds it until maturity.

The existence of a well-developed money market enables the English banks to avoid borrowing from the central bank. If they ever find themselves short of cash they can call in some of their loans to the money market, and so compel members of the money market to borrow from the Bank of England. Borrowing then becomes more expensive to the members of the money market, for the Bank of England charges a higher rate than do the commercial banks both on short-term loans and for rediscounting bills. In addition the Bank of England's eligibility rule restricts the discounting of any bills to bank bills or fine trade bills. The intervention of the money market between the commercial banks and the central bank is a distinctive feature of the English banking system.

(8) RECENT CHANGES IN THE MONEY AND DISCOUNT MARKETS

During the past thirty years a number of developments have taken place affecting the London discount market. Not only has the inland bill of exchange almost gone out of existence, but even the use of foreign bills, which before 1914 were the principal means by which foreign trade was financed, has greatly declined. The main reason for this is that the foreign bill of exchange has been largely superseded by the bank draft and the telegraphic transfer of bank deposits from one country to another. If a bank draft is employed the importer obtains a draft for the required amount in the currency of his creditor and pays for it with his own cheque. A telegraphic transfer of a bank deposit from one bank to a bank in another country can be effected by a cable to a foreign bank instructing it to pay a specified sum of money to a particular merchant. Another method of payment now used in foreign trade is the documentary credit, and though this still requires the employment of a bill of exchange, it is drawn on a foreign bank and not on a merchant. The use of the documentary bill has weakened somewhat the position of the acceptance house, the services of which are no longer required in connection with such transactions, since the foreign bank is responsible for payment being made. In consequence, there is no need for the special information regarding foreign firms which only the acceptance house, with its foreign connections, could supply. Direct dealing with a foreign merchant was a risky undertaking, but commercial banks can deal safely with well-known foreign banks.

This decline in the use of trade bills has, however, coincided with a large increase in the volume of Treasury bills coming on to the market, over 90% of all bills discounted by the commercial banks now being Treasury bills. Bills discounted by the London Clearing banks in 1938 had a value of £280 million; by 1965 the total value of such bills exceeded £1,100 million. In 1910 the total issue of Treasury bills amounted to only £36 million, but by 1965 the total exceeded £6,000 million. From the point of view of both discount houses and acceptance houses the Treasury bill is not so desirable as the trade bill, since such bills do not require to be accepted. Nor is there any need for Treasury bills to be arranged in "parcels," since they are always issued in convenient amounts, and not in irregular amounts like trade bills, and a bank, too, can arrange to have them fall due daily as required. In practice, however, the commercial banks refrain from tendering directly for Treasury bills, preferring to rediscount bills offered to them by the discount houses.

Some bills are taken up by foreign banks and a few by large industrial concerns. The discount houses do not compete against one another when tendering for Treasury bills; they meet each Friday to decide the amount of their syndicated bid.

Thus the continuance of the discount market depends very largely on the willingness of the commercial banks and the Treasury to permit it to exist. However, the existence of a well-developed money market has for a long time been one of the distinctive features of the English banking system. In this country, as already pointed out, the commercial banks when short of cash never themselves borrow from the Bank of England, but instead call in some of their loans to the money market ("money at call and short notice"), and in consequence compel the discount houses and bill brokers to borrow from the central bank. In other countries commercial banks borrow directly from their central banks. In England, therefore, the money market acts as a sort of buffer between the commercial banks and the Bank of England. The discount houses, too, regard themselves as providing an important service to the Government, since they are always prepared "to cover the tender," that is, they are willing to take up whatever amount of Treasury bills the Government offers them. Thus, for a number of reasons the English commercial banks evidently prefer the London money market to remain in being, though there are, however, fewer firms in the money market than formerly and the discount houses have found it necessary to include in their activities the holding of short-dated Government stocks, the supply of which is greater than it used to be. Both they and the acceptance houses now undertake more ordinary banking business than was formerly their practice.

RECOMMENDATIONS FOR FURTHER READING

R. S. Sayers: *Modern Banking*, Chapter 3.
R. J. Truptil: *British Banks and the London Money Market*, Pt. 1, Chapters 3, 4; Pt. II, Chapters 1–3, 6.

QUESTIONS

1. Give a brief description of the organisation of the London Money Market. How has the relative importance of its several components altered in recent years? (R.S.A. Adv. Com.)

2. Explain clearly the nature of a Bill of exchange. In what ways does its "monetary character" differ from that of a Bank of England note? (Exp.)

3. Who are the chief Lenders and Borrowers in the London Money Market? (L.C. Com. & F.)

4. What are the discount houses? Explain their rôle in the London Money Market. (G.C.E. Adv.)

5. What are the functions of the contemporary discount market? What do you think of its future prospects? (Final Degree.)

6. What are the present main functions of the London Money Market? (Final Degree.)

7. The London discount market is sometimes described as a buffer between the Treasury and the Bank of England, on the one hand, and the clearing banks, on the other. Explain how the discount market does work in this way. (Final Degree.)

CHAPTER XXIV

THE ENGLISH BANKING SYSTEM:
THE BANK OF ENGLAND

I. INTRODUCTORY

(1) CENTRAL BANKING

It has become an accepted principle that a banking system requires a central bank, and few countries today are without one. This is, however, a comparatively recent development, although some of the functions of a central bank were being performed by the Bank of England before the middle of the nineteenth century. The Federal Reserve System, which undertakes central banking in the United States, was set up in 1913. Both France and Germany had central banks in the nineteenth century, but there were still many countries without this type of bank as recently as 1920. For example, central banks were not established in Canada and Argentina until 1935.

The main function of a central bank which overrides all others is to carry out a country's monetary policy. In order to be able to do this it must work closely with the State or be subject to its control, and it must have some means of influencing the credit policy of the commercial banks. In Great Britain at the present time monetary policy is the joint responsibility of the Treasury, the Chancellor of the Exchequer and the Bank of England. The aim of the central bank is not, therefore, to make maximum profit for itself. Nor should it compete against the commercial banks for ordinary banking business. The eight branches of the Bank of England are situated in the principal commercial centres— Leeds, Manchester, Birmingham, etc.—their main function being to assist the local clearing of cheques.

The necessity for a close connection between the State and the central bank led some countries to consider it desirable that the central bank should be State-owned. Both the Bank of England and the Bank of France are now nationalised institutions, but before 1946 the Bank of England was a joint-stock company, its capital being in the hands of its stockholders, as is the capital of other joint-stock companies. It makes little difference nowadays whether a country's central bank is nationalised or not, for its activities are always closely controlled by the State, and in either case it is usual for the State to take at least a share of the bank's profits. The nationalisation of the Bank of England has had little effect on its relations with the Treasury, which since 1931 has had the last word in determining monetary policy. The Nationalisation Act, however, gave the Treasury the legal right, after consulting with the Governor, to give directions to the Bank, and also gave the Bank the power to make recommendations to the commercial banks. It is generally agreed that complete independence of the central bank is undesirable because of the widespread economic effects its policy may have upon the community at large, although it might be undesirable for a central bank to be completely dependent on the State, compelled without question to carry out whatever instructions the Government of the day might issue.

It was only very slowly and by the adaptation of policy to suit particular circumstances that the practice of central banking developed in England. Not until Bagehot published his *Lombard Street* in 1877 was any attempt made to formulate the principles on which central banking should be based.

In addition to its work in connection with monetary policy the Bank of England also acts as banker both to the British Government and to the other banks. It is, too, the only bank in England with the right to issue bank-notes. When occasion demands it also acts as lender of last resort. All these can be considered to be proper functions for a central bank to undertake, but it should not compete against the commercial banks for ordinary banking business.

II. FUNCTIONS OF THE BANK OF ENGLAND

(2) THE WEEKLY RETURN

Before considering the functions of the Bank of England it will be useful to examine the Bank's Weekly Return. The *Bank Charter Act* of 1844 divided the work of the Bank of England into two departments known as (i) the Issue Department and (ii) the Banking Department, and compelled it to issue a weekly balance sheet for each department. This is known as the Bank Return and is published each Wednesday.

Consider first the Issue Department (Table LII). The liabilities of this Department consist of the notes issued by the Bank. Most of the notes (*a*) are in the hands of the banks, the general public and shop-keepers. The notes (*b*) in the Banking Department are those that have not yet been drawn into active circulation. This is the item to watch if an increase in the note issue is anticipated. It will be noticed that there was a very much larger note issue in 1965 than there was in 1937.

The following are specimen returns for the Issue Department:

TABLE LII

I. *Issue Department*

(1) Wednesday, 28th July 1937

Notes issued:	£ million		£ million
(*a*) In circulation . .	498	(*c*) Government debt . .	11
(*b*) In banking dept. . .	28	(*d*) Government securities .	185
		(*e*) Other securities . .	4
		(*f*) Coin (other than gold) .	—[1]
		Fiduciary Issue . .	200
		(*g*) Gold coin and bullion .	326
	526		526

(2) Wednesday, 18th August 1965

Notes issued:	£ million		£ million
(*a*) In circulation . .	2,785½	(*c*) Government debt . .	11
(*b*) In banking dept. . .	65	(*d*) Government securities .	2,837
		(*e*) Other securities . .	1
		(*f*) Coin (other than gold) .	1
		Fiduciary Issue . .	2,850
		(*g*) Gold coin and bullion .	⅓
	2,850⅓		2,850⅓

(3) Wednesday, [2]

Notes issued:	£ million		£ million
(*a*) In circulation . .		(*c*) Government debt . .	
(*b*) In banking dept. . .		(*d*) Government securities .	
		(*e*) Other securities . .	
		(*f*) Coin (other than gold) .	
		Fiduciary Issue . .	
		(*g*) Gold coin and bullion .	

[1] Only £14,000 of silver coin was held.
[2] This space is provided for the insertion of the latest figures.

The assets of the Issue Department are five in number. Government debt (*c*) consists of loans made to the Government by the Bank of England during the first hundred and fifty years of its existence, generally in return for a renewal of its charter. Government securities (*d*) consist of Government Bonds and Treasury Bills. Other securities (*e*) comprise other first-class securities, including bank bills and eligible trade bills. Coin other than gold (*f*) consists of silver, and in 1937 amounted to only £14,050. Items (*c*), (*d*), (*e*) and (*f*) together form the backing for the fiduciary issue. A comparison of the two Weekly Returns given above shows the big increase in the fiduciary issue between 1937 and 1965. The fifth asset of the Issue Department is gold. In 1937, 60% of the note issue was backed by gold, but after 1939 the fiduciary issue comprised more than 99% of the issue, for in 1939 most of the Bank of England's gold was transferred to the Exchange Equalisation Account.

Consider now the liabilities of the Banking Department (Table LIII). The item (*h*) is the capital subscribed by the stockholders when the Bank of England was a joint-stock company. On its nationalisation the stockholders received compensation in Government stock yielding an income equal to the dividend previously paid them by the Bank. The Rest (*i*) is the Bank's reserve, accumulated out of undistributed profits. Public Deposits (*j*) comprise the balance to the credit of the Government account. As taxes are paid in, this item will increase; when the Government makes payments it will decrease. Bankers' deposits (*ka*) are the balances of the commercial banks, forming part of their cash reserves, since they regard these balances as cash. Increased demand for cash on the part of the commercial banks will cause them to withdraw sums in cash from these balances. Payments by customers of the Commercial banks to the Government (for example, taxes) will cause public deposits to rise and bankers' deposits to fall; a payment by the Government to a customer of a commercial bank will have the reverse effect. Other accounts (*kb*) include the balances of Commonwealth and foreign banks as well as of ordinary customers of the Bank of England, and the size of this item gives an indication of the extent of ordinary business undertaken by the Bank. Special deposits (*l*) are compulsory deposits made by the commercial banks at the request of the Bank of England in pursuance of monetary policy—a new instrument of policy first employed in 1960.

The largest of the assets of the Banking Department is Government securities (*m*), and this comprises Government Stock, Treasury bills acquired directly and "Ways and Means" advances. This is the item affected when the Bank of England buys or sells securities in the open market (open-market operations). Other securities (*n*) are Dominion and foreign securities, and securities obtained by the Bank of England in the open market.

The item, Other Securities (*n*), is subdivided into (*a*) discounts and advances, and (*b*) securities. Discounts and advances (*na*) show the extent of the Bank's lending to the money market. When the commercial banks call in money at short notice the discount houses and bill brokers are compelled to borrow from the central bank, the market is

TABLE LIII

II. Banking Department

(1) Wednesday, July 28, 1937

	£ million		£ million
(h) Proprietors' capital . .	14½	(m) Government securities .	114½
(i) Rest	3½	(n) Other securities . .	20½
(j) Public deposits . . .	11	(o) Discounts and advances .	6
(ka) Bankers' deposits . .	104	(p) Notes	28
(l) Other accounts . . .	37	(q) Gold and silver coin .	1
	170		170

(2) Wednesday, August 18, 1965

	£ million		£ million
(h) Capital	14½	(m) Government securities .	300
(i) Rest	3	(n) Other securities . .	25
(j) Public deposits . . .	11	(o) Discounts and advances .	61
(k) Other deposits:		(p) Notes	81
(ka) Bankers' deposits . .	263	(q) Gold and silver coin .	1
(kb) Other accounts . .	87½		
(e) Special deposits . . .	89		
	468		468

(3) Wednesday,

	£ million		£ million
(h) Capital		(m) Government securities .	
(i) Rest		(n) Other securities . .	
(j) Public deposits . . .		(o) Discounts and advances .	
(k) Other deposits:		(p) Notes	
(ka) Bankers' deposits . .		(q) Gold and silver coin .	
(kb) Other accounts . .			
(e) Special deposits . . .			

then said to be "in the Bank." Lending by the Bank may take the form of rediscounting bills, or making loans with bills as collateral security. If the market is "in the Bank" this item will, therefore, increase. Notes (p) form the unused portion of the note issue, the reserve of notes held by the Bank of England to meet demands for cash by the commercial banks. It is the same as item (b) in the Return for the Issue Department. Gold and silver coin (q) is mostly silver, held like notes (p) for issuing when required to the commercial banks.

(3) THE GOVERNMENT'S BANK

The financing of war always severely taxed the resources and ingenuity of the kings of England from the time of William the Conqueror to that of William of Orange, and by the end of the seventeenth century the cost of waging war on the Continent had become too great to be met by expedients previously employed. It was the Government's need for money for this purpose that led to the founding of the Bank of England in 1694. In return for a charter (often renewed only in exchange for a further loan) granting the privilege of incorporation, the Bank lent the Government £1,200,000 at 8%. Thus was established the first joint-stock bank in England. An Act of 1708, by forbidding firms with more than six partners to act as bankers, ensured for the Bank of England a monopoly of joint-stock banking in England until 1826, and in London till 1833.

From its foundation, therefore, the Bank of England was the Government's bank, although it was not State-owned until 1946. As such, it receives the proceeds of taxes which are paid into the Government's account and shown in the Weekly Return under the heading of public deposits or public accounts. As agent for the Government it makes payments from this account, including the half-yearly payments, of interest on Government bonds. Thus, the National Debt came into existence at the same time as the Bank of England, and its management of the National Debt has been in the hands of the Bank ever since. Direct Government borrowing from the Bank of England is comparatively rare nowadays, but the Bank still does a little lending directly to the Government by means of "Ways and Means" advances. As the Government's bank, therefore, the Bank of England keeps the Government's account, manages the National Debt and lends to the Government.

On account of the huge increase in the National Debt its management has assumed great importance in the field of monetary policy.

(4) THE NOTE ISSUE

By the terms of its first charter, the Bank of England was given the right to issue bank-notes at least up to the value of its capital, but it was not always the sole bank of issue in England or even in London. As already noticed, the private London banks ceased to issue notes only when they developed the use of the cheque during the eighteenth century. For a long time other banks outside London continued to issue notes, and it is only since 1921 that the Bank of England has been the only bank in England with the right to issue notes. Bank of England notes were acceptable to the commercial world, and when provincial banks were established they kept their reserves in the form of Bank of England notes instead of gold. With the exception of a short period during the first two years of its existence, the Bank of England successfully maintained the convertibility of its notes into gold for a hundred years. The heavy drain on the Bank's resources during the War with Napoleon compelled it to cease payment in gold, permission to do so being granted by an Order in Council. To relieve the situation, notes in denominations of £2 and £1 were issued, the £5 note previously being the lowest denomination. The *Bank Restriction Act* of 1797, which made Bank of England notes legal tender, had been intended as a temporary measure, but it was regularly renewed until 1821, when cash payments were resumed, and Bank of England notes again became convertible.

The Act of 1826, which permitted the establishment of joint-stock banks outside a radius of 65 miles from London, also gave these new joint-stock banks the right to issue notes. This Act prohibited the Bank of England from issuing notes of denominations under £5. (In 1825 a shortage of cash had been relieved by the issue of £1 notes.) In the eighteenth and early nineteenth centuries the only Government control was over the denomination of the Bank's notes. In 1775 the Bank was forbidden to issue notes of less than £1, this minimum being raised two years later to £5, though later the issue of £1 notes was resumed.

The Bank Charter Act, 1844. The over-issue of bank-notes had been responsible for the failure of many banks between 1833 and 1843. The *Bank Charter Act* was therefore an attempt to regulate the note issue. Its chief provisions were:

(i) It separated the note-issuing function of the Bank of England from its banking business by dividing the Bank of England into two departments, (*a*) the Issue Department, and (*b*) the Banking Department.

(ii) In order to prevent an over-issue of notes it was decreed that, apart from a fiduciary issue of £14 million, all Bank of England notes were to be fully backed by an equivalent amount of gold and silver, though the amount of silver was not to exceed 20% of the value of the gold. A fiduciary issue is an issue backed by securities and not by gold. Had it not been for the fact that the Bank of England had already issued notes in excess of its holding of gold, it is probable that the Act of 1844 would have insisted on all notes being fully backed by gold. In France and some other countries a gold reserve proportional to the note issue has to be maintained, usually 35–40% of the note issue.

(iii) No new bank was to be allowed to issue notes, and existing banks having the right of note issue were not to increase their issues beyond the average circulation for the twelve weeks preceding 27th April 1844.

(iv) No bank in London, other than the Bank of England, was to have the right to issue notes, and a provincial bank on opening a London office or amalgamating with a bank with a London office was to lose its right to issue notes. Whenever another bank lost its privilege of note issue, the Bank of England was to be permitted to increase its fiduciary issue by two-thirds of the amount of the lapsed issue. As a result of this clause in the Act, the fiduciary issue had increased to £19¾ million by 1914. At the time of the passing of the *Bank Charter Act* there were seventy-two banks of issue in England; by 1914 the number had fallen to thirteen; the amalgamation of Fox, Fowler and Company with Lloyds in 1921 left the Bank of England as the sole bank of issue. Except for £4·3 million, the note issues of the banks of Scotland and Northern Ireland have to be fully backed by Bank of England notes.

(v) The Bank of England has to issue notes on demand in exchange for gold bullion at £3 17s. 9d. per standard ounce—that is, gold eleven-twelfths fine.

(vi) The Bank of England has to publish a weekly balance sheet— the Weekly Return—for both its issue and its banking departments. This publicity, it was thought, would be a safeguard against any tendency to over-issue notes.

(5) THE FIDUCIARY ISSUE

The *Bank Charter Act* of 1844 represented a triumph, it is said, for the Currency School of Thought, whose members were anxious to prevent over-expansion of the volume of money by the issue of bank-notes. Indeed, they would probably have preferred all notes to be fully backed by gold with no fiduciary issue, for the Currency School had not come to realise that the development of the cheque as an instrument by which bank deposits could be transferred from one banking account to another had resulted in bank deposits becoming money. As the Mac-millan Committee pointed out in 1931, bank deposits are of greater importance than bank-notes, for pressure to increase the note issue results from an expansive credit policy on the part of the commercial banks.

In times of crises the *Bank Charter Act* of 1844 has had to be suspended, as in 1847, 1857 and 1866, but the crisis of 1857 was the only occasion until 1914 when it was necessary to increase the note issue above the legal limit, the mere suspension of the Act being sufficient in the other cases. The clumsiness of this arrangement has evoked frequent criti-cism. The legal limit for the fiduciary issue was exceeded in 1914, but the decision of the Treasury to put out its own notes for £1 and 10s.

relieved the situation. Until 1928 Bank of England notes and Treasury Notes circulated together.

The Cunliffe Committee (1918). Although this committee favoured a more elastic currency than was possible under the provisions of the *Bank Charter Act* (1844), it considered that Act to have fulfilled its main object by preventing over-issues of notes. It recommended, therefore, that the principle laid down in this Act should be maintained, but that, with the Treasury's sanction, changes in the fiduciary issue should be made if thought necessary. It further recommended that the Bank of England should take over the Treasury issue.

The Currency and Bank-notes Act, 1928. This Act implemented the recommendations of the Cunliffe Committee. From 22nd November 1928 all Treasury Notes were to be called in and replaced by Bank of England notes, but in the meantime were to be deemed bank-notes. The fiduciary issue was raised to £260 million, backed by securities, except for £5½ million backed by silver. Changes in the fiduciary issue were to be made only with the consent of the Treasury, and notes in excess of this amount were to be fully backed by gold. Restrictions on the issue by the Bank of England of notes for amounts less than £5 were withdrawn. Pound and ten-shilling notes became legal tender in the United Kingdom for any amount, and £5 notes were legal tender for any amount in England and Wales. The profits of the Issue Department were to go to the Treasury.

The Fiduciary Issue since 1928. Between 1928 and 1939 the fiduciary issue varied between £200 and £275 million. An Act of 1939 gave the monetary authorities power to revalue the gold in the Issue Department of the Bank of England each week. Thus a rise in the price of gold would have made it possible to increase the note issue, while a fall in the price would have necessitated its contraction. War broke out, however, shortly afterwards, and most of the gold in the Issue Department was transferred to the Exchange Equalisation Account. Since 1939, therefore, most of the Bank of England's note issue has been fiduciary; in 1931 only a third of the note issue was backed by gold, but by 1939 over 60% of notes had a gold backing, whereas since 1939 less than 1% have had a gold backing. The fiduciary issue stood at £580 million in September 1939. Since then it has gradually increased, being £2,850 million in 1965.

Seasonal variations in the note issue. At certain times of the year larger demands for cash occur. The few weeks immediately before Christmas and the month of July are such occasions, and at these times there are heavy withdrawals of cash from the banks. At Christmas the cash is required for making purchases in the shops, and the shopkeepers later pay it back into the banks; in the summer the money is spent on travel, hotels, etc., and again after a short interval it returns to the banks. In December 1937 the experiment was first tried of increasing the fiduciary issue temporarily by £20 million to meet this seasonal demand for cash. In December of every year from 1948 and in every July since 1949 the fiduciary issue has been temporarily increased and usually reduced again shortly afterwards.

At the present time, therefore, this country has a fairly elastic note issue, as the frequent changes in its volume since 1939 show.

Convertibility of bank-notes. From 1821 to 1914 Bank of England notes were convertible on demand into gold sovereigns. Other note-issuing banks could exchange their own notes for Bank of England notes. During this period gold sovereigns and half-sovereigns were in general circulation. Great Britain left the gold standard on the outbreak of war in 1914 and, as already noted, Treasury notes were issued to replace the gold coinage. When this country returned to the gold standard in 1925 the gold coinage was not restored, as its maintenance is expensive, but bank-notes could be exchanged for gold, but only in the form of bars of 400 ounces. In 1931 Great Britain again left the gold standard, and since then has had an inconvertible paper currency. Pound notes, however, still have printed upon them the phrase: "I promise to pay the Bearer on Demand the sum of One Pound," and although this is supported by a facsimile of the signature of the Chief Cashier of the Bank of England, the promise now has little meaning.

Putting cash into circulation. (i) *Coin.* The Royal Mint—a Government Department—is responsible for the production of coins, buying the metal, minting the coins and then selling them to the Bank of England on demand, the Bank of England in its turn allowing the commercial banks to withdraw on demand sums in coin from their balances at the Bank—that is, from bankers' deposits. The expenses of the coinage are paid for by the Government from its account at the Bank of England (public deposits), and when coins are sold to the Bank of England the Government's account is credited by the amount of the sale. As coins are sold to the Bank of England at approximately three times their cost, the Mint makes a considerable profit.

(ii) *Notes.* The commercial banks can also withdraw sums from their accounts with the Bank of England in the form of Bank of England notes, bankers' deposits and the notes held by the Banking Department, each falling by the amount of the withdrawal. If it appears that the reserve of notes in the Banking Department is not likely to be sufficient to meet the demand of the commercial banks, then it will be necessary to increase the fiduciary issue. This, of course, requires the sanction of the Treasury, but nowadays that is a mere formality.

(6) THE BANKERS' BANK

A central bank acts as banker to the commercial banks. At first provincial banks kept only a limited amount of gold, their resources being chiefly in Bank of England notes, and so the Bank of England came to be the only bank with a large stock of gold. When cheques replaced notes as the principal means of payment, the provincial banks opened accounts with the Bank of England in order to facilitate the clearing of cheques. Some alarm was felt by the country banks when the Bank of England, taking advantage of the powers granted to it under the Act of 1826, began to open branches in the leading commercial centres. The fears of the other banks, however, proved to be groundless, for it was not the aim of the Bank of England to compete against them, but merely to provide facilities for provincial bank clearings similar to those already provided in London. Thus the Bank of England became the bankers' bank in both London and the provinces.

The development of a system of branch banking—a few large banks each with a network of branches—has simplified the clearing system. The working of the London Bankers' Clearing House was considered in Chapter XXII. The "Big Five" and the other members of the clearing house keep part of their cash reserves in the form of deposits (known as bankers' deposits) at the Bank of England. Settlements between banks at the clearing can therefore be made by transfers between the accounts of the commercial banks at the Bank of England. The final adjustment of transactions involving millions of pounds requires merely book entries at the Bank, a credit to one bank, a debit to another.

The Bank of England, as the bankers' bank, affords the commercial banks similar banking facilities to those that the commercial banks themselves render to their own customers. A man who has a current account with a bank can draw cheques on it and make payments to his creditors, and if he is short of cash he can withdraw sums in cash from his account. In exactly the same way a bank pays its debts to other banks by means of cheques drawn on its account at the Bank of England, and if it requires cash it can withdraw amounts in cash from this account. The commercial banks are therefore fully justified in regarding their balances at the Bank of England as cash. Just as a commercial bank must always be prepared to pay cash on demand to any of its customers, so must the Bank of England be prepared to pay cash on demand to the commercial banks.

The Bank of England also acts as banker to the discount houses.

(7) THE LENDER OF LAST RESORT

An essential function of a central bank is that when circumstances require it, it should act as lender of last resort. No commercial bank, however efficiently run and soundly managed, could withstand an abnormal demand for cash. In a banking crisis it becomes the duty of the central bank to allay any tendency towards panic on the part of the public by assisting the banking system to withstand the strain of excessive demands made upon it for cash. In some countries the commercial banks in times of difficulty borrow directly from the central bank. In this country the commercial banks call in their loans to the money market, and so compel the discount houses and bill brokers to seek assistance from the Bank of England. When the other banks are unwilling to lend, the central bank should be prepared to assist eligible borrowers—that is, should act as a "lender of last resort." The central bank can, of course, insist upon its own eligibility rules, and also in order to reduce such borrowing to a minimum, it can demand its own price—that is, charge as high a rate of interest as it deems the situation requires.

As with its other functions, the development of the Bank of England as lender of last resort was gradual. It was already acting in this capacity to some extent before the end of the eighteenth century, but until the Usury Laws—which prohibited more than 5% interest being charged —were modified, the Bank did not willingly assume this rôle. The Government's assistance, by the suspension of the Bank Charter Act of 1844, enabled the crises of 1847 and 1857 to be overcome. It was not, however, until the crisis of 1866 that the Bank of England fully accepted its responsibilities as lender of last resort.

(8) RESPONSIBILITY FOR MONETARY POLICY

Money has become much more than a medium of exchange. Changes in the quantity of money and in the value of money influence the level of production and the distribution of the national income. Formerly the Bank of England was responsible for monetary policy, and when Great Britain was on the gold standard its primary aim was to protect the country's gold reserves. Since 1944, when the Government for the first time accepted responsibility for the maintenance of full employment, it has had a more direct interest in monetary policy, which can now be regarded as being the joint responsibility of the Chancellor of the Exchequer, the Treasury and the Bank of England.

Monetary policy used to be regarded as mainly concerned with varying the supply of money. Changes in monetary policy, too, may be dictated by the external situation—the relation between a country's imports and its exports. If imports are considered to be excessive it may be necessary to damp down demand at home by a contraction of credit in order to reduce the demand for imported goods.

Since, however, both rising and falling prices bring about an arbitrary redistribution of income, it would seem to be more equitable to aim at stable prices, but this policy would probably make it more difficult to attain full employment. Perhaps the fairest method by which the whole community could share in the increasing prosperity of a country would be to keep all incomes stable and allow greater efficiency and higher output to bring down prices. Unfortunately, falling prices tend to check production and increase unemployment.

Two possible policies are open to the monetary authorities:

(i) *An expansionist policy.* In considering the effects of changes in the value of money we saw that one of the effects of rising prices (that is, of a fall in the value of money) was to stimulate production. If the volume of purchasing power is deemed insufficient to keep up demand to a level that will yield full employment an expansionist policy will be required. The appropriate monetary policy will then be pursued to expand credit and stimulate demand. A rise in prices will probably follow. Consequently, whenever in recent years there has been a falling away from full employment the monetary authorities have adopted an expansionist or inflationary policy.

(ii) *A restrictionist policy.* Since 1945, however, the problem has been mainly one of trying to check persistent inflation. During most of this time, therefore, there has been over-full employment—a demand for labour greater than the supply. Periodically, then, it has been found necessary to adopt a restrictionist policy, contracting credit to reduce demand, with in consequence a temporary loss of full employment—a policy popularly known as a "credit squeeze." Such a disinflationary policy has on several occasions been forced on the British monetary authorities by the external situation, excessive demand having so stimulated imports as to create a large deficit in the balances of payments and a consequent depletion of the country's reserves of gold and convertible currencies.

The main objectives of monetary policy in Great Britain at the present time can therefore be said to be:

(i) to maintain full employment;
(ii) to maintain a reasonably stable internal price level, that is, to keep inflation in check.

(iii) to stimulate economic growth and thereby increase the national income in order to raise the standard of living of the people;

(iv) to maintain stability in the external value of the currency;

(v) to keep the balance of payments in balance.

Whether all these policies can be successfully pursued at one and the same time is, indeed, doubtful, since some of these aims may conflict one with another. For example, is stability of prices compatible with the maintenance of full employment? Can economic growth be achieved without inflation? Do not full employment, economic growth and a rising standard of living all tend to stimulate imports, thereby making a balance of payments more difficult to achieve, and so endangering the external value of the currency? The consideration of questions affecting foreign exchange and international trade must be left for Chapters XXVI and XXVII.

(9) OTHER FUNCTIONS OF THE BANK OF ENGLAND

The Bank of England also performs a number of other functions:

(i) *Ordinary banking business*. From its foundation the Bank of England has had some ordinary customers, mostly now old-established businesses in the City of London, for whom it has provided the banking facilities that might be expected of a commercial bank. Since it is generally recognised that ordinary banking business is not a proper function of a central bank, no new business of this kind is likely to be undertaken by the Bank of England. The position is very different in France, where the Bank of France undertakes most kinds of banking business. Whereas the Bank of England has only eight branches, the Bank of France has over five hundred.

(ii) *Assistance to industry*. The point has been stressed both in this and preceding chapters that it is not customary for British banks to provide industry with fixed capital. During the Great Depression of 1929-35, however, the commercial banks found themselves in the paradoxical situation where their only hope of securing repayment from many of their borrowers was to continue lending to them. At that time a cessation of bank lending would have compelled many large firms to close down. It was not in the national interest to allow this to happen. and, encouraged by the Government, and supported by the commercial banks, the Bank of England began to give some assistance to industry, though only in selected cases.

Two subsidiaries, the Bankers' Industrial Development Company and the Securities Management Trust, were established respectively by the English commercial banks and the Bank of England. Aid took the

P

form of taking up debentures in the firms it was intended to help, such assistance generally being dependent on the reconstruction of a company's capital where this was considered desirable. Among firms that received assistance were the Lancashire Cotton Corporation and Shipbuilders' Security Ltd., both of which organisations concerned themselves with the rationalisation of their particular industries. The Macmillan Committee on Finance and Industry in 1931 had recommended that there should be a closer connection between the banks and industry. Since 1945 the Bank of England has indirectly assisted industry through two finance corporations in which it is an important shareholder—the Industrial and Commercial Finance Corporation Ltd. and the Finance Corporation for Industry Ltd.[1]

(iii) *External business.* The Bank of England acts as agent of the Treasury in many matters affecting Great Britain's monetary relations with the rest of the world, as for example, in the management of the Exchange Equalisation Account, exchange control, relations with other central banks and with international monetary institutions, such as the International Monetary Fund and the International Bank.

III. THE TECHNIQUE OF CENTRAL BANK CONTROL

(10) INSTRUMENTS OF CENTRAL BANK POLICY

A central bank expands or contracts the volume of purchasing power by its control over the commercial banks. This control is made possible because the commercial banks (i) think it prudent to maintain a known liquidity ratio, and (ii) keep a balance which is regarded as cash at the central bank. The maintenance of a liquidity ratio of 28% is, however, merely customary in the case of the English banks which are under no legal compulsion to maintain it, although it seems unlikely that the Bank of England would now permit them to vary it. So long as a liquidity ratio is maintained, expansion or contraction of credit by the commercial banks depends mainly on the size of their cash reserves. The English banks regard their balances at the Bank of England as cash, and are justified in doing so, since they can withdraw from these balances at any time in cash. Their cash reserves, therefore, consist partly of cash—Bank of England notes and coin—in the tills of their many branches and partly of deposits—Bankers' deposits at the Bank of England. Thus, if for any reason a bank's balance at the Bank of England falls, it regards it as a reduction of the amount of cash that it

[1] See XXV, 9.

holds. To maintain its liquidity ratio it will then have to reduce its deposits through a curtailment of its lending to a much greater extent than the amount by which its balance at the central bank has fallen.

The ultimate control over the volume of deposits of the commercial banks rests with the Bank of England. The traditional instruments of monetary policy by which the Bank of England exercises this control are Bank rate and open-market operations. Since 1951 a third instrument of policy has been used—the Directive issued by the Treasury or by the Bank of England. More recently the Bank of England has employed a new instrument of policy—Special Deposits. Nowadays monetary policy is the joint responsibility of the Treasury, the Chancellor of the Exchequer and the Bank of England. Let us now consider in turn each of the instruments of policy available to the British monetary authorities today:

(i) *Bank rate.* This is the minimum rate at which the Bank of England will discount—or more correctly, rediscount—first-class bills. The rate is fixed weekly, on Thursdays,[1] but in an emergency it can be altered at any specially convened meeting of the Court of the Bank. The importance of Bank rate lies in the fact that other rates of interest depend on it—the rate charged to discount houses, the rates charged on advances to customers and the rate offered on their deposit accounts. These rates all move up or down with Bank rate. Thus changes in Bank rate aim at influencing other rates of interest. If it is desired to check credit expansion Bank rate will be raised in order to make borrowing more expensive and so, it is hoped, reduce the demand for loans. When Bank rate is high some forms of business activity that were previously profitable may cease to be so. A high Bank rate may therefore be expected to check business activity. Curtailment of bank lending will then reduce bank deposits and so purchasing power in the hands of the community, thereby bringing about a fall in prices, which in turn will be likely to check business activity still further. By lowering Bank rate the cost of borrowing will be reduced, credit expansion will be encouraged and the reverse train of events set in motion. Such at least, is the theory of Bank-rate changes. Bank rate may also be raised for the purpose of protecting the country's gold reserve by checking an outflow of foreign funds from London. It has been suggested that Bank rate today fulfils its external function more effectively than its internal function. When bank rate is low money is said to be cheap.

(ii) *Open-market operations.* Even before 1914, when the Bank of England considered Bank rate to be its chief means of influencing the

[1] In November 1964 the change occurred on a Monday.

credit policy of the commercial banks, it was usual for the Bank to supplement it by open-market operations. It took this action, it said, in order to make Bank rate "effective." By intervening in the open market to buy or sell securities, the Bank of England can directly influence the size of bankers' deposits. If it sells securities it receives payment by cheques drawn on the commercial banks, for most of the buyers of these securities will have accounts with these banks, and upon them the cheques will be drawn. At the clearing of these cheques transfers will then have to be made from the commercial banks to the Bank of England. The balances of the commercial banks at the Bank will therefore decrease by the amount the Bank has received for the securities sold. Since the commercial banks consider their balances at the Bank as cash, if they are to maintain their 8% ratio of cash to deposits and their 28% liquidity ratio they must now reduce their deposits by calling in some of their loans to customers. By selling securities the Bank can thus bring about a reduction in the other banks' deposits and purchasing power. By buying securities it can increase the cash reserves of the other banks, and so make possible an expansion of credit. This power of the Bank is, however, dependent on the maintenance of the commercial banks of their customary cash ratio. Though the Bank used to regard open-market operations as being merely of assistance to Bank rate, it is more probable that operation in the open market was the really effective instrument and not Bank rate, as was supposed.

It is some considerable time since open-market operations of the type just described were undertaken by the Bank of England. At the present day open-market operations are undertaken for the purpose of influencing the rate of interest. The Bank of England intervenes both in the discount market and in the securities market (the stock exchange). In the discount market it employs a Special Buyer, while in the securities market operations are in the hands of the Government broker. The older weapons of the central bank, it is widely agreed, are clumsy in their operation.

(iii) *The directive.* As at first employed, this was a direct instruction from the Treasury to the commercial banks to restrict their lending. In 1951 and 1952 they were given a *quantitative* directive, that is, they were requested to restrict advances to purposes regarded as being in the national interest. In 1955 and 1957 they were told to reduce their lending whatever the purposes for which loans were required— *qualitative* directives. In 1964 and 1966 banks were told not to increase their advances by more than 5%. Since credit restriction by banks can be offset if borrowers can obtain assistance from other financial institutions, more recently the Bank of England has also made its wishes known to the merchant banks, finance companies and other financial concerns.

(iv) *Special Deposits.* In order to reduce the cash basis for their credit policy the Bank of England can ask the commercial banks for Special Deposits, usually a percentage of the banks' own deposits. This instrument of monetary policy, employed for the first time in 1960, is a somewhat similar device to that of the Special Account as employed in Australia. It is really an alternative to the older type of open-market operation and supplementary to the Directive. When the Bank of England in 1960 requested Special Deposits from the commercial banks it asked for an amount equal to 2% of their deposits from the English banks and 1% from the Scottish banks. A further request was made in 1961, but during 1962–63 these Special Deposits were released. The Bank of England again asked for Special Deposits in 1964–65.

(11) THE EFFICACY OF BANK RATE AS AN INSTRUMENT OF MONETARY POLICY

Critics point out that to raise Bank rate appears to have little effect in checking inflation in a trade boom, for in such conditions prices and profits are rising, and even a very high rate of interest is likely to be less than the rate of profit. Similarly, at the bottom of a trade depression a very low rate of interest will be insufficient to encourage business men to borrow, if they have little expectation of making a profit. Bank rate, it was conceded, is more likely to be effective in checking an expansion of credit than stimulating it. As a result, from the year 1932 when a cheap money policy was initiated Bank rate remained at 2% until November 1951, apart from a short period in September–October 1939. Thus, for nearly twenty years the Bank of England was deprived of its use of Bank rate as an instrument of monetary policy. The cheap-money policy was adopted in the first place in order to stimulate a revival of trade, and though slow to do so, eventually it had the desired effect.

The cheap-money policy was continued after 1939 to enable the Government to finance the war cheaply, and in this it was again successful, but it was pursued after 1945, again to keep down the cost of borrowing, even though conditions had completely changed and when the main problem was to check inflation.

Before the adoption of a cheap-money policy in 1932 Bank rate used to fluctuate frequently, often being changed more than a dozen times in the course of a single year—in 1875 it was altered no fewer than 24 times. Between 1860 and 1875 it was changed on the average eleven times per year. During the 50 years preceding 1914 there was only one year without a change of Bank rate. The decline in the use of Bank rate was clear even before 1914. During the 20 years 1862–81 it was changed on the average over nine times each year; during the 20 years 1894–1913 it was changed on the average four and a half times each year; during 1919–32 the average number of changes per year was two and a half. Since 1951 there has been on average little more than one change in Bank rate per year.

Though the Radcliffe Report (1959) emphasised that the liquidity position of financial institutions was of greater importance than the supply of money, it regarded variations in the structure of interest rates as an important influence on liquidity. The supply of money is of some importance, but the structure of interest rates is regarded as the vital factor in the situation.

(12) ADJUNCTS TO MONETARY POLICY

During the period when Bank rate was discredited, especially the years 1945–51, alternative instruments of policy were employed— physical controls and then fiscal policy. In 1951 the use of Bank rate was revived, and it was employed first in conjunction with physical controls (until these were withdrawn) and later alongside fiscal policy. Then variation of the hire-purchase regulations came into use. These measures are no longer regarded as alternatives to monetary policy, but rather as new instruments to supplement the old ones.

Consider now some of these adjuncts to monetary policy:

(i) *Physical controls*. As a legacy from the war there were physical controls—rationing of consumers' goods, control of prices, licensing of building, control of investment and exchange control. These were retained as a means of fighting inflation, but they succeeded only in suppressing inflation without getting rid of it.

(ii) *Fiscal policy*. The use of the budget as an alternative to monetary policy had been suggested as long ago as the 1930s. Then it was suggested that taxation should be eased at the expense of a budget deficit in order to expand demand and stimulate recovery from the slump which then prevailed. It was a simple matter, therefore, to suggest that in inflationary conditions taxation should be increased to provide a large budget surplus in order to reduce purchasing power and the pressure of demand.

(iii) *Hire purchase*. The volume of hire purchase business has increased enormously in recent years. In 1965 a sum of £1,350 million was outstanding in hire-purchase debt, two-thirds of which was owing to

Finance Houses. The regulations governing hire purchase can be varied to suit economic conditions—the initial deposit can be increased or reduced; the period of repayment can be shortened or lengthened. If it is necessary to check a recession these regulations are eased to encourage demand; in times of inflation this policy can be reversed to check an excess of demand. It was the failure of physical controls and fiscal policy to check inflation that led to the revival of Bank rate in 1951, though since then it has often been found necessary to supplement a rise in Bank rate with fiscal and financial measures, such as an increase in purchase taxes and a tightening up of hire-purchase regulations. Hire purchase has now assumed such large proportions that to expand or contract it has an important influence on the level of demand and production. The fact that a rise in Bank rate has often been accompanied by a Directive from the Treasury or the Bank of England tends to support the view still held by some people that Bank rate is ineffective, though it may only be that Bank rate is slow to take effect. In recent years until late in 1960 the banks have been more liquid than formerly, and this has often made them reluctant to curtail their lending, which is their most profitable activity. The new device of Special Deposits at the Bank of England aims to reduce the liquidity of the commercial banks and so make monetary policy more effective.

To sum up, therefore, it may be said that in order to fight either inflation or the onset of a trade recession the British monetary authorities—the Bank of England, the Chancellor of the Exchequer and the Treasury—have now available to them a variety of instruments to implement their policy, namely, Bank rate, open-market operations, fiscal policy, the Directive, the device of special deposits, control of hire purchase and, if they wished to revive them, physical controls. The employment at the same time of a number of instruments of monetary policy came to be known as a "Package Deal." It might be argued that by itself Bank rate is not always a very effective instrument of policy—or at least slow to take effect—but it may have an important part to play when used in conjunction with other instruments of monetary policy.

RECOMMENDATIONS FOR FURTHER READING

R. S. Sayers: *Modern Banking*, Chapters 4, 5 and 9.

G. Crowther: *An Outline of Money*, Chapter 6.

The Radcliffe Report on the Working of the Monetary System (H.M.S.O.).

R. G. Hawtry: *The Art of Central Banking*, Chapter 4.

J. L. Hanson: *Monetary Theory and Practice*, Chapter 14.

QUESTIONS

1. Using the Bank of England as illustration, say what are the major functions of a central bank. (I.H.A.)

2. By the Bank Act, 1844, the "fiduciary issue" of the Bank of England was then fixed at £14 million. Explain what is meant by the "fiduciary issue" of the Bank of England, and how it is backed and how its amount has varied since. Is the fiduciary issue of the Bank of England in any way limited at the present moment? If so, what is its present amount? (L.C. Com. B. & C.)

3. Does an increase in the fiduciary issue of a central bank mean that the currency is being inflated? (I.T.)

4. Why is it said that the central bank is the bankers' bank? Has it any other functions? (C.C.S. Inter.)

5. "The Bank of England, acting as lender of last resort, never refuses to create cash on demand: *but it can impose its own price.*" Explain this statement, and the particular significance of the passage in italics. (D.P.A.)

6. Explain the functions of the Bank of England (*a*) as a bank, (*b*) as a bankers' bank, (*c*) as a Central Bank. (C.C.S. Final.)

7. Describe the functions of a central bank: what powers should it possess and by what principles should their exercise be regulated? (C.I.S. Final.)

8. What is meant by the "backing of the Note issue"? Is it a necessary condition of a sound monetary system? (G.C.E. Adv.)

9. How are the activities of joint-stock banks influenced by the Bank of England? (G.C.E. Adv.)

10. What is meant by Bank rate? Explain the effects of an increase in Bank rate. (G.C.E. Adv.)

11. What are the most fundamental powers of a central bank? Give reasons for your selection, and show the relations of other conventional central banking powers to these fundamental ones. (Final Degree.)

12. "The Central Bank cannot simultaneously fulfil the rôle of lender of last resort *and* successfully control the money supply." Discuss. (Final Degree.)

CHAPTER XXV

THE CAPITAL MARKET

I. THE DEMAND FOR CAPITAL

(1) WHAT IS THE CAPITAL MARKET?

The various financial markets can be distinguished from one another by the length of the term of the loan. Thus, broadly, the money market can be defined as the market for short-term loans, and the capital market as the market for long-term loans. It would probably be more accurate, however, to describe the money market as the market for call money or very short-term loans, or even more precisely, as the market for loans to the discount market. The capital market then becomes the market for short-term, medium-term, long-term and permanent loans to the Government, industry and commerce. That part of the capital market concerned with new public issues of stocks and shares is known as the new issue market.

(2) THE FINANCING OF INDUSTRY

Industry requires both fixed and circulating capital:

(i) *Circulating capital.* In Great Britain firms generally obtain their circulating capital from the commercial banks. The item "advances to customers" in the banks' balance sheets indicates the extent to which banks supply industry with its circulating capital. For the London Clearing Banks in 1965 it amounted to approximately £4,726 million, and for all banks £5,497 million.

Another source of circulating capital is trade credit. In addition to their other functions, wholesalers act as financiers. By granting credit to retailers, they enable them to sell some of their purchases before paying for them, thereby helping them to finance their holding of stocks. The wholesalers themselves borrow from the banks, so that indirectly the banks provide circulating capital for the retail trade. Of recent years there has been a considerable increase in direct lending by the banks to retailers—especially large-scale retailers—the amount advanced to retailers reaching a total of £533 million by 1965. The bill of exchange provides another means by which a trader can obtain circulating capital, since it enables payment for goods to be postponed until they have been sold. If, as is possible, the bill is discounted by a bank the real financier of the transaction is the bank.

Thus in most cases, directly or indirectly, the provision of working capital to industry and commerce rests largely with the commercial banks. Some very large firms, however, finance themselves, providing their circulating capital from reserves.

(ii) *Fixed capital.* On account of their preoccupation with liquidity, British banks in the past have been disinclined to provide fixed capital for industry. They do not care to have their assets in the form of shares in companies, and prefer shorter-term loans, though in practice these are renewable. Many continental banks, however, used to undertake this type of business, but owing to heavy losses in trade depressions they have tended to abandon investment banking. On the other hand, the British banking system has moved slightly in the opposite direction, assistance being provided, however, through their subsidiaries, the two finance corporations.

Generally, then, British industry has to look to other sources for permanent capital. The main business of the capital market is to provide industry with permanent capital. A man setting up in business for himself as a sole proprietor usually provides most of his capital from his own past savings, supplemented perhaps by a loan from friends or relatives. One of the principal reasons for the sole trader turning his business into a partnership has generally been the need for additional capital for expansion, which the new partners provide. The development of the joint-stock company made it possible for projects requiring huge amounts of capital to be undertaken, the capital being subscribed in large or small amounts by thousands of investors. The granting of limited liability to joint-stock enterprises made it possible for the man of small means to invest some of his savings in industry without risking the loss of the rest of his savings or his personal possessions. Industry, therefore, obtains most of its permanent capital from the general public, either directly by subscription or indirectly through other institutions, such as insurance companies and investment trusts. The British insurance companies have enormous funds available for investment, and they hold large blocks of shares in the larger limited companies. The knowledge that shares in public companies can be disposed of on the Stock Exchange at their market prices makes people readier to respond to a company's appeal for subscriptions to its shares. A company may also raise fixed capital by the issue of debentures, which are loans to the company, debenture holders therefore being its creditors. Since interest on debentures is a cost to a company, the amount to be paid is deducted before net profit is calculated, thereby reducing liability to Corporation Tax. Since the imposition of this tax debentures have become a more attractive method of raising capital.

We have seen that many businesses provide themselves with circulating capital; some also finance expansion out of their profits. Instead of the whole of the profit being distributed as dividend among the shareholders, a sum is retained to provide additional fixed capital. The sole proprietor will probably look upon such a fund as his savings. The undistributed profits of the joint-stock company are similarly the company's savings. Many small businesses have grown into large firms in this way. At times tax concessions have to be made in order to encourage firms to plough back some of their profits into the business. Clearly, if a company increases its capital by using some of its profits for this purpose, its previously issued share capital does not give a true picture of the amount of capital employed by the firm. In order to correct this, firms sometimes issue bonus shares to the shareholders, the numbers received by each being proportionate to their existing holdings.

(3) THE CONTROL OF INVESTMENT

Whenever the demand for factors of production is greater than the supply, some method of apportioning them among different uses has to be employed. Under perfect competition they would be distributed among different employments according to the demand for them, equilibrium being achieved when the marginal productivity of each was the same in all occupations. As long ago as 1931 the Macmillan Committee on Finance and Industry recommended control of investment. To support his policy of full employment, Lord Beveridge suggested that since investment was easier to control than saving, the two should be brought into line by imposing control over investment.

Control over investment is necessary in time of war to ensure that investment is adequate in the industries essential to the war effort. Whenever inflation exists there will be a greater demand for factors of production than the supply, and the demand for capital will be excessive. Control of investment then becomes a method of rationing capital among the many uses competing for it. An Act of 1946 therefore made permanent the regulations for the control of investment that had been introduced during the war. The purpose in continuing this control was, in the first place, to ensure that those capital projects considered to be most important in the national interest should be able to obtain the necessary real resources; in the second place, to make possible the planning of both public and private investment.

Control was effected through a Capital Issues Committee, to which application had to be made by those desiring to raise capital by the issue of shares or other securities. Since February 1959 only Local Authorities have had to apply to the Capital Issues Committee. Control of investment can be effected by physical means. The Government can restrict its own investment by curtailing capital projects in times when there is a heavy demand for labour and other resources. It can also encourage Local Authorities to do the same. Thus, in 1965 the Government cut down its programme of road building and requested Local Authorities to postpone the erection of new civic centres.

(4) THE NEW-ISSUE MARKET

An outline of the procedure for floating a public limited company was given in Chapter VI. When the various formalities have been completed the sponsors can then issue a prospectus and appeal to the public to subscribe for the shares. The flotation can be placed in the hands of an Issuing House. These institutions act like wholesalers, purchasing the entire share issue from the new company at a price slightly below that at which the shares are to be issued to the public. Underwriting of an issue of shares in this way ensures that the full amount asked for will be forthcoming, less, of course, the payment that has to be made to the Issuing House for its services. For the sake of their own reputation in the capital market, the best Issuing Houses handle issues only after careful investigation of the new companies which seek their services. Merchant banks often act as issuing houses. A recent development is to introduce a new issue of shares through the Stock Exchange. Application is made to the Stock Exchange for a quotation for its shares, this introduction being accompanied by an arrangement with a number of insurance companies and investment trusts to take up the entire issue. In these circumstances the Stock Exchange is really acting in the capital market and not simply providing a market for existing securities, its primary function.

II. THE SUPPLY OF CAPITAL

(5) SAVINGS

The supply of capital to the capital market comes partly from individuals and partly from institutions—that is, from the savings of private individuals or firms. A private individual wishing to invest in a company's shares can instruct his banker or stockbroker to purchase them in his name. When a limited company ploughs back some of its profits into the firm it really obtains additional capital from its shareholders instead of having to go into the capital market to obtain it. The supply of capital flowing to the capital market comes from private savings, either directly, as when a man decides to buy shares, or indirectly when an institution, such as an insurance company, collects people's savings and then itself invests them.

As has already been emphasised several times, British commercial banks as a matter of policy invest only in gilt-edged securities. The Trustee Savings Banks are prohibited by law from investing in any securities other than Government or other similar stocks.

A number of other institutions collect small savings, and some of these invest part of their funds in equities—that is, in ordinary shares in public companies. Among these are investment trusts, unit trusts and insurance companies.

(6) INVESTMENT TRUSTS

The large investor is careful to avoid putting all his eggs in one basket. He safeguards himself against heavy losses by spreading his investments over as wide and varied a field as his resources will allow. If he holds shares in a dozen different companies loss in one may be offset by gain in another. The smaller investor who puts all his savings into one company runs the grave risk of losing the whole should misfortune overtake that particular company. The investment trust, however, makes it possible for the small investor to spread quite a moderate amount of savings over a large number of companies, thus lessening his risk of loss. Investment trusts are purely financial institutions which use their capital for the purchase of shares in a number of other companies, the aim being to reduce the risks of investment. A single share or unit in an investment trust may represent one-hundredth of a share in each of a hundred different companies. The management of the trust is generally free to invest in whatever enterprises it pleases and may, if it thinks it desirable, dispose of shares in some companies and re-invest in others. An investment trust derives its income from the dividends paid on the shares it holds, and after deducting expenses of management, what remains is available for distribution among its own shareholders. Some investment trusts specialise in particular fields of activity, such as bank, insurance or industrial shares.

There are in existence a number of old-established investment companies, the shares of which are bought and sold in the ordinary way on the stock-exchange. To invest in these companies, therefore, it is necessary to buy shares. At the present day the most popular form of investment trust, however, is the unit trust, which came into existence during the 1930s, although they attracted little attention from investors until the 1950s. During the 1960s many new unit trusts were established and the older ones expanded very considerably. In principle they are similar to the investment trust companies, in that they use their funds to buy shares in a large number of companies—perhaps a hundred or more. They obtain their funds, however, by the issue of units, often in quite small denominations—maybe of 5s. or even less—and units can be bought direct from the managers of the trust. In the case of a flexible trust the managers have power to vary the investments of the trust at their discretion. Most unit investment trusts are formed for limited periods of time, though generally the period can be extended. In 1964 the total assets of investment trusts exceeded £2,900 million. In the same year the combined assets of the unit trusts stood at over £400 million—an increase of £210 million in four years.

(7) INSURANCE COMPANIES

The probability of many risks can be mathematically calculated, and it is against these that insurance can be effected. Insurance is based upon the principle of the *pooling of risks*. Those who insure contribute to a common fund, out of which payments can be made to those who suffer loss. It is possible to insure against such risks as fire, theft, accident, goods in transit, employers' liability, sickness and a great many other contingencies.

Nearly 40% of the total of insurance business is in the "life" branch—that is, it is really assurance because the "risk" is certain to happen at some time. Most of this is not pure assurance, as the endowment policy is now the most popular. In this case the person whose life is assured undertakes to pay premiums for a limited period of time—ten to forty years or until he reaches a certain age. If he dies before the expiry of this term the assurance company pays an agreed sum to his dependants; if he survives he receives the agreed sum, generally with the addition of a bonus, depending on the company's profits. Thus this type of assurance is partly a method of saving. Life assurance probably dates from the seventeenth century, but other forms of insurance are much older, there being evidence of the existence of marine insurance as early as 916 B.C.! Acts of 1870 and 1909 contain provisions for the protection of policy-holders, one of these being the separation of the "life" fund from the funds of any other kind of insurance the company may transact.

Insurance companies, therefore, have huge funds at their disposal and available for investment, and during the past thirty years these funds have increased enormously. The total premium income of all British insurance companies increased from £60 million in 1900 to over

£1,800 million in 1964, of which, in the latter year, over £500 million was for life assurance. In 1920 the total funds of all these companies came to about £400 million; in 1964 the total was over £6,000 million. It is interesting to note, as set out in the table below, the chief forms of investment into which the funds of the forty British insurance companies have gone.

TABLE LIV
Investments of British Insurance Companies

Type of investment	£ million
British Government Stocks	1,267
Commonwealth Government Stocks . . .	254
Foreign Government Stocks	261
Debentures and Preference Shares	1,733
Ordinary Shares	1,620
Mortgages (on property)	891
Total	6,026

During recent years British insurance companies have invested heavily in British industry.

(8) FINANCE HOUSES

Hire purchase is a method by which medium-term credit is made available to consumers, and is sometimes known as consumer-credit or instalment credit. Generally, the consumer pays a small deposit and the balance, including interest, in equal instalments spread perhaps over two years. The credit may be provided by the retailer from his own resources or more probably nowadays by a finance house. Of the total of over £1,350 million of hire-purchase debt in 1965 (an increase of 40% in four years) £856 million was owing to finance houses. It is possible too for a manufacturing business to buy new machinery on this system.

The Radcliffe Committee in 1959 reported that there were in existence at that time seventeen large finance houses, and eighteen smaller companies calling themselves industrial bankers, these together being responsible for the financing of more than 70% of all hire-purchase business in Great Britain. The remaining business was in the hands of over a thousand smaller firms. Ten of the large finance houses are controlled by the English commercial banks.

The finance houses raise funds partly by borrowing from the commercial banks, especially when credit is easy, and partly by accepting deposits from the general public, the interest on deposits tending to be high, especially when credit is tight. Some of the larger finance houses and industrial bankers also undertake some ordinary banking business.

(9) BUILDING SOCIETIES

These institutions are registered under the *Building Societies Acts*, their main purpose being to enable people to purchase houses by instalments. Houses are too expensive for most people to buy outright, but if payment is spread over a period of twenty years house purchase is very little more onerous than the payment of rent. Building societies accumulate funds in order to be able to lend money to their members for the purchase of houses, repayment of the loan being spread over a long period, during which the society holds a mortgage on the property.

By accepting deposits, issuing subscription shares, and paid-up shares, building societies, like insurance companies, collect small savings. In most cases the societies themselves pay the income tax due on the interest paid. The actual interest received by a depositor depends therefore on the rate of tax he pays: the higher his rate of tax, the greater the gross interest he receives. The rate of interest to be paid by the borrower depends on the ease with which the Society itself can raise funds and therefore the rate of interest it has to pay to attract depositors. Building society rates of interest, however, do not change with every change in Bank rate. Nevertheless, when Bank rate is high building society rates will also be high, and vice versa. Only the reserves of building societies are available to the capital market, and these go into trustee securities. The rest of their funds are used to provide loans to borrowers. Most building societies are small, the Halifax Building Society and the Abbey National being exceptional in having branches in many parts of the country. During the past thirty years there has been a vast increase in the business of British building societies, their total assets expanding by over fourteen times and the number of members by over eight times during this period, though on account of amalgamations, the total number of societies has tended to fall.

(10) THE PROVISION OF MEDIUM-TERM CAPITAL

The banks prefer to lend for short periods; the capital market enables industry to obtain long-term or permanent capital. The need for the provision of capital for a term intermediate between these two extremes led to the establishment in 1945 of two institutions to supply medium-term loans. They are the Industrial and Commercial Finance Corporation Ltd., the capital of which came from the Bank of England, and the English and Scottish commercial banks (their contributions being proportional to their deposits), and the Finance Corporation for Industry, the capital of which was provided by the Bank of England, investment trusts and insurance companies. The former has power to grant loans of from £5,000 to £200,000, the function of the latter being to provide loans in excess of £200,000. As long ago as 1931 the Macmillan Committee had pointed out the need for institutions to give such assistance, especially to lesser-known firms that would find a public issue unduly expensive. The Industrial and Commercial Finance Corporation commenced its activities in 1945 with a capital of £45 million. Most of its customers have been private companies seeking additional capital either for expansion or to finance current production or to provide against the incidence of death duties. Before assistance is given, full details are required of a firm's history, activities and financial position. Help may be given by way of loans for ten to twenty years, secured by collateral security, as with bank loans, or by taking up debentures or preference shares in the firm, or in some cases even ordinary shares.

III. THE MARKET FOR SECURITIES

(11) THE STOCK EXCHANGE

A stock exchange is a place where dealings in stocks and shares take place, a market where those desiring to buy stocks and shares are brought into contact with those who want to sell. It is, therefore, mainly a market for old securities, and not primarily a source of new supply to the capital market.[1] There are stock exchanges in the chief financial centres of the world, such as London and New York, and in the more important provincial cities in Great Britain. A number of northern stock exchanges combined in 1965 to form the Northern Stock Exchange. The existence of stock exchanges makes it possible for an owner of stocks to dispose of them if he so desires. Stock exchanges serve the capital market by giving liquidity to permanent capital, that is, to securities that have no date for repayment. Some Government Stocks such as $2\frac{1}{2}\%$ Consols which have no date of maturity, and ordinary shares of public companies are also of this type. If there were no stock exchanges it would be difficult for owners of stocks such as Consols or ordinary shares to dispose of them, and people would therefore be less willing to invest in them. Thus stock exchanges assist the capital market by making securities more liquid, and so encourage people to invest in them.

The price at which a security can be bought or sold on the stock exchange will depend, as in other markets, on the relative strength of

[1] But see p. 432.

the demand for and the supply of that particular security at a particular time. All sorts of influences affect the prices of shares, through supply or demand. If business prospects are good the prices of shares will generally be high; if prospects are poor prices will be low. The publication of a company's balance sheet will affect the price of its shares, favourably or adversely, as the case might be. Other factors which influence stock-exchange prices are such things as changes in Bank rate, variations in hire-purchase regulations, the publication of foreign trade figures or even rumours of impending political changes. At the present day there are large institutional buyers in this market, and their activities tend to even out price fluctuations, and therefore the rate of yield. The Government deliberately influences the rate of yield on Government stocks, since some Government departments have funds to invest. If it is desired to keep up the rate of yield the Government broker will enter the market to sell; to keep down the rate of yield he will go into the market as a buyer of stock. Thus the Government itself can influence the rate of yield on its gilt-edged stocks.

Method of doing business. Only members are allowed access to the London Stock Exchange, and these consist of jobbers, of whom there are about 750, brokers, to the number of over 2,500 and their authorised clerks. The brokers act as agents for prospective investors or people with securities to sell. The actual dealers in securities are the jobbers, who tend to specialise in particular types of stocks or shares. Thus one jobber will specialise in gilt-edged securities, another in mining shares, another in the shares of commercial undertakings and so on. A broker wishing to obtain stock or shares for a client will approach a jobber who deals in the required security and ask him to state a price, but without informing him whether he wishes to buy or sell. The jobber will quote two prices, the higher being that at which he is prepared to sell, and the lower that at which he is prepared to buy. Thus, through the brokers and the jobbers buyers and sellers are brought into contact with one another. The London Stock Exchange is a highly organised market, and business is carried on according to a strict set of rules. Since there is easy telephonic communication between the London and provincial stock exchanges and those abroad, the market in stocks and shares is nearly perfect, prices tending to be the same in all parts of the market, even though, as in the case of some shares, the market may be world-wide.

(12) SPECULATION AND ITS CONTROL

There are two motives for people buying securities on the Stock Exchange. Most people or institutions buy for the sake of investment

—that is, they intend to hold the securities in order to secure an income from their capital. Generally, having once obtained certain securities they will retain them, unless a change in their financial affairs makes it necessary for them to obtain more cash. Then as the Stock Exchange assisted them to buy, so it will help them to sell their securities. So long as they derive what they consider to be a reasonable income from their investments, they may care little about fluctuations in their market prices. This is particularly the case with Government Stock that bears a fixed rate of interest. A man with an annual income of £50 a year from Consols may be quite unconcerned whether they stand at 65 or 40 in the market, since this has no effect on his income. He would be interested in the market price only if for some reason he wished to sell his stock.

There are other people, however, who pay little attention to the income to be obtained from securities, but who are keenly interested in fluctuations in their market prices. When they buy they do so because they consider the price to be low and likely to rise. Then when they believe prices are at the peak they sell, because they judge prices will fall. If the market is keen to buy it is said to be "bullish"; if it is keen to sell it is "bearish." Those who buy hoping that prices will rise are known as "bulls"; those who sell expecting prices to fall are known as "bears". These people are speculators, and their aim is to take advantage of fluctuations in the prices of stocks and shares in order to make a quick profit for themselves. Such profits are known as capital gains. Speculators are also to be found on the highly organised markets dealing in securities, foreign exchange, wheat or wool, etc.

It would be wrong to condemn all types of speculation outright. The existence of speculators in a market means that it is always possible to buy or sell at any time. The small holder of securities, suddenly finding himself in need of cash, knows that he can sell his securities at the market price at any time. If there were no speculators in the market there might be times when it would be impossible to find buyers. Speculation, therefore, makes securities more liquid. The activities of some speculators tend to steady prices, for they enter the market as buyers when most other people desire to sell, and so they prevent prices falling as much as they otherwise might; when others are wanting to buy they enter the market as sellers, and so prevent an undue rise in prices.

Speculation, however, is bad when those indulging in it attempt to influence prices by their own activities, trying to push prices down just before they buy, or to raise prices before they sell. The prices of shares are important to the economic system because these prices reflect the relative profitability of different lines of production, and high returns on investment attract new capital. Speculation of an undesirable kind may therefore result in capital not being employed to the best advantage, and so lead to the misuse of real resources. The greater the risk, the greater the possible profit, and so in times of trade boom the more risky enterprises often find it easier to obtain capital than the less risky but sounder and more socially desirable undertakings. Excessive speculation can lead to disasters such as the historic crash which occurred on Wall Street, New York, in 1929, and precipitated a trade depression.

Control of speculation. Various suggestions have been put forward for restricting the activities of speculators on the securities market:

(i) It has been suggested that once securities have been transferred to a new owner he should not be permitted to dispose of them until a certain minimum period has elapsed. The imposition of a high stamp duty on transfers, the rate decreasing with the length of time the securities have been held, might restrain some speculation.

(ii) Control of investment, that is, new issues, will prevent any serious diversion of real resources to wasteful uses. It ensures priority for those forms of production considered to be in the national interest.

(iii) Bank lending for speculative purposes might be restricted. In Great Britain only $\frac{1}{4}\%$ of total bank advances is made to stockbrokers, in contrast to the United States, where borrowing on the New York money market is primarily for stock-exchange speculation.

(iv) A capital-gains tax can be made to fall more heavily on short-term capital gains, as with the American Capital Gains Tax and the British Capital Gains Tax of 1962.

The main thing that stands in the way of controlling undesirable speculation is the difficulty of distinguishing between speculative dealings and genuine investment. Care must be taken lest any restriction of speculation should hamper the raising of capital on the capital market for legitimate purposes.

RECOMMENDATIONS FOR FURTHER READING

B. Ellinger: *The City.*
E. Lavington: *The English Capital Market.*

QUESTIONS

1. The London Stock Exchange is often described as a "perfect market." Give a sufficient description of its work to justify this attribute; and point out how the division of its members into brokers and jobbers may be considered to help towards the attaining of this perfection. (R.S.A. Adv. Com.)

2. What do you understand by the capital market? To what extent is it, in ordinary times, an organised market in this country? (R.S.A. Adv. Com.)

3. What is a Bonus Issue?

Discuss the desirability or otherwise of such an issue from the point of view of (a) the company; (b) the shareholder; (c) the National Economy. (L.C. Com. C. & F.)

4. What do you understand by share capital and loan capital? What factors might cause a firm to decide to finance expansion by one form rather than the other? (C.I.S. Inter.)

5. What do you understand by the market for new capital? (G.C.E. Adv.)

6. What part does the Stock Exchange play in the Capital Market in the United Kingdom? (G.C.E. Adv.)

7. What factors determine the market value of a joint-stock company's shares on the Stock Exchange? (G.C.E. Adv.)

8. Outline briefly the history and present position of British building societies. (Final Degree.)

9. Discuss the position of life assurance offices as providers of capital. (Final Degree.)

INTERNATIONAL ECONOMICS

PART SEVEN

INTERNATIONAL ECONOMICS

CHAPTER XXVI

INTERNATIONAL TRADE

I. THE THEORY OF COMPARATIVE COST

(1) THE ORIGIN OF INTERNATIONAL TRADE

Trade between different countries developed first where one could produce something desirable which others could not. The Phoenicians became famous in the ancient world for their purple-dyed cloths, which they bartered for other goods with the people of the countries bordering on the Mediterranean Sea. International trade therefore owes its origin to the varying resources of different regions:

(i) Mineral resources can obviously be worked only where they are found. Coal nowadays is mined chiefly in the United States, Great Britain, Germany and Russia; iron chiefly in the United States, France, Sweden and Russia; copper in the United States and Chile. Most nickel comes from Canada; most gold from South Africa, and most silver from Mexico.

(ii) Many commodities can be grown only under particular climatic conditions or in certain soils. As a result, most rubber is produced in Malaya and the East Indies; almost the entire world supply of jute comes from the Ganges delta in East Pakistan; most of the world's coffee comes from Brazil, and most cocoa from West Africa and Brazil; and Italy stands first for the production of lemons.

(iii) The inhabitants of a region may develop special skill in the production of a commodity, which in time, may acquire a special reputation for its quality. Wines such as champagne, sherry, port, chianti owe their distinctive qualities partly to the special flavour of locally grown grapes and partly to the local method of manufacture. Scotch and Irish whisky have similarly acquired distinction.

By exchanging some of its own products for those of other regions, a country can enjoy a much wider range of commodities than would otherwise be open to it.

(2) INTERNATIONAL DIVISION OF LABOUR

If international trade took place only in cases where countries could produce what others could not, the total volume of world trade would not have reached its present-day proportions. A glance through the list of commodities entering into any country's trade will show that it imports many things that it could, if it wished, produce for itself—for example, Great Britain imports wheat, dairy produce, meat and wool, all of which it is itself capable of producing. Similarly, the United States imports motor cars, motor cycles, china ware, wool, cotton and linen goods. This is not merely because a country by its own efforts cannot completely satisfy its demands for these commodities. Early in this book it was seen that division of labour within a country enables it to increase the output of everything it produces, even though specialisation entails an increase in the work of distribution. Just as division of labour within the firm can be extended to division of labour within the industry, so division of labour within a country can be extended to the international field, each country specialising in the production of a few only of the things that it is capable of producing, and leaving to others the production of some of the things that it could have produced itself had it so desired. International division of labour or specialisation results in a vast increase in the total world output of all kinds of goods.

A country's choice of the forms of production in which to specialise will be determined according to its advantages over others in the production of these things. If one country has the greatest advantage over others in the production of woollen goods, then it will tend to specialise in the production of that commodity. Another country may specialise in the production of raw wool. Such advantages will accrue to a country if it can produce particular goods of a certain quality more cheaply than other countries. This is known as the *Principle of Comparative Cost*, which is really an extension of the *Principle of Comparative Advantage* considered earlier in this book. This theory of international trade was first developed by Ricardo. Comparative cost is considered in terms of what can be produced by a given quantity of productive resources (factors of production)—that is, it is real or opportunity-cost that is involved. For example, in one country it may take 100 units of productive resources to produce 150 units of milk, or 80 units of wheat. In a second country 100 units of productive resources may produce 100 units of milk, or 60 units of wheat. The first country clearly has the greater comparative advantage over the second in milk production.

Consider again the Principle of Comparative Advantage as applied to individuals. A successful barrister would find it to his advantage to pay a man to attend to his gardening than to do this work himself, for during the time he would have to spend at work in his garden he could earn more in his professional capacity than the amount necessary to pay the wages of a hired gardener. The barrister may be both a better lawyer and a better gardener than the man whom he employs, but it will be to his advantage to specialise in that pursuit for which he has the greater comparative advantage over the other. By undertaking legal work and using part of his earnings to pay his gardener's wages, the barrister is indirectly cultivating his garden. Similarly, it is to the advantage of a nation to specialise in the production of those things for which it has the greatest comparative advantage over others. By specialising in the production of a few things and engaging in international trade, a country produces its imports indirectly.

Just as division of labour within a country increases the work of distribution, so international division of labour makes necessary a vast increase in the exchange of commodities between countries. The greater the amount of specialisation, the greater, therefore, will be the volume of international trade, and the greater will be the output of all kinds of goods by the world as a whole.

(3) ADVANTAGES OF INTERNATIONAL TRADE

In order to simplify discussion of the advantages of international trade, it is usual to assume that there are only two countries in the world and that only two commodities enter into trade. Let the two countries be Atlantis and Erewhon, and let the two commodities be cloth (typifying manufactured goods) and wheat (typifying agricultural products). There are then three separate cases to consider.

Case I. Where each country can produce one commodity, but not the other. Assume that Atlantis can produce cloth but not wheat, and that Erewhon can produce wheat but not cloth. The earliest trade between regions took place on this basis. Without exchange each country will obviously be poorer. If Atlantis can make a bargain for the exchange of some of its cloth for some of Erewhon's wheat the people of both Atlantis and Erewhon will be better off as a result of this trade, for each will then have both cloth and wheat.

Case II. Where each country can produce one commodity more cheaply than the other. Assume next that the employment (say) for a year of 100 units of resources (factors of production) in Atlantis will produce either 100 units (yards) of cloth or 50 units (bushels) of wheat, and that 100 units of resources in Erewhon will produce either 50 units of cloth or 100 units of wheat. Assume further that Atlantis possesses 2,000 units of resources or factors and Erewhon 3,000 units. If each country employs half its resources for the production of cloth and half for the production of wheat, and no exchange takes place, the total output and consumption for these countries will be as follows:

TABLE LV*a*

Country	Units of resources	Units of output	
		Cloth	Wheat
Atlantis	2,000	1,000 +	500
Erewhon	3,000	750 +	1,500
World Total . .	5,000	1,750 +	2,000

If now Atlantis and Erewhon specialise in the production of the commodity for which each has a comparative advantage over the other, Atlantis devoting its production entirely to cloth, and Erewhon producing only wheat, their total output will be as follows:

TABLE LV*b*

Country	Units of resources	Units of output	
		Cloth	Wheat
Atlantis	2,000	2,000 +	0
Erewhon	3,000	0 +	3,000
World Total . .	5,000	2,000 +	3,000

As a result of this specialisation the total output of cloth has increased from 1,750 to 2,000 units, and the total output of wheat from 2,000 to 3,000 units. If the rate of exchange is taken to be 900 units of wheat for 900 of cloth, then the consumption of each commodity by the two countries will be as follows:

TABLE LV*c*

Country	Units of resources	Units consumed	
		Cloth	Wheat
Atlantis	2,000	1,100 +	900
Erewhon	3,000	900 +	2,100
World Total . .	5,000	2,000 +	3,000

As a result of specialisation and exchange, Atlantis has increased its consumption of cloth from 1,000 to 1,100 units and its consumption of wheat from 500 to 900. At the same time Erewhon has increased its consumption of cloth from 750 to 900, and of wheat from 1,500 to 2,100. The gain of the two countries is clear:

TABLE LV*d*

Country	Units of resources	Units consumed	
		Cloth	Wheat
Atlantis	2,000	100 +	400
Erewhon	3,000	150 +	600
World Total . .	5,000	250 +	1,000

Both countries, therefore, benefit from international trade.

Case III. Where one country can produce both commodities more cheaply than the other. Assume now that the employment for (say) a year of 100 units of resources in Atlantis will produce either 100 units of cloth or 100 units of wheat, and that the employment of 100 units of resources in Erewhon will produce either 40 units of cloth or 80 units of wheat. As before, assume also that Atlantis possesses 2,000 units of productive resources and Erewhon 3,000 units. If each country devotes half its resources to the production of each commodity, and if no specialisation and exchange take place, the respective outputs (and consumption) in the two countries will be as follows:

TABLE LVI*a*

Country	Units of resources	Units of output	
		Cloth	Wheat
Atlantis	2,000	1,000 +	1,000
Erewhon	3,000	600 +	1,200
World Total . .	5,000	1,600 +	2,200

In this case Atlantis can produce both commodities more cheaply than Erewhon, but it has a greater comparative advantage in the production of cloth than of wheat. Specialisation and exchange will still be of advantage to both countries. Atlantis will specialise in the production of cloth, because it has a greater comparative advantage in the production of that commodity; Erewhon will specialise in the production of wheat. In this case it is unlikely that Atlantis will give up entirely the production of wheat, for Erewhon can produce only 2,400 units of wheat, even if it devotes all its resources to the production of this commodity. Assume that Atlantis continued to use 10% of its resources for wheat production. Then, as a result of this specialisation, but before exchange takes place, output will be as follows:

TABLE LVI*b*

Country	Units of resources	Units of output	
		Cloth	Wheat
Atlantis	2,000	1,800 +	200
Erewhon	3,000	0 +	2,400
World Total . .	5,000	1,800 +	2,600

The total world output of each commodity is greater than it was before, the production of cloth having been increased from 1,600 to 1,800 units and wheat from 2,200 to 2,600 units. If an exchange is effected of (say) 700 units of cloth for 1,000 units of wheat each country will be able to consume more of each commodity than was possible without specialisation. As a result of international trade each country, therefore, is richer:

TABLE LVI*c*

Country	Units of resources	Units consumed					
		Cloth			Wheat		
		Output	Import or export	Total	Output	Import or export	Total
Atlantis . .	2,000	1,800 −	700 = 1,100		200 + 1,000 = 1,200		
Erewhon . .	3,000	0 +	700 = 700		2,400 − 1,000 = 1,400		
World Total .	5,000		1,800			2,600	

Thus, it is *comparative* and not *absolute* differences in cost that are important. This case also provides an illustration of a country (Atlantis is this example) importing a further quantity of a commodity (wheat) which it produces itself. Some people in Atlantis might urge that more wheat should be grown and less imported. It can, however, be clearly seen from this example that there would be no *economic* justification for this. Atlantis, like any other country, has only a limited supply of productive resources, and more wheat can be grown there only if resources are withdrawn from the production of cloth or some other commodity. If Atlantis diverts 100 units of resources from the production of cloth to the production of wheat the country will be poorer, for 100 units of resources will produce in that country either 100 units of cloth or 100 units of wheat, but in the above example 70 units of cloth can be exchanged for 100 units of wheat.

(4) THE TERMS OF TRADE

By terms of trade we mean the rate at which one country's products exchange for those of another. How much wheat Erewhon will have to give Atlantis for a quantity of cloth will depend, as J. S. Mill pointed out, on the strength of the demand of Erewhon for cloth relative to the demand of Atlantis for wheat.

In Case III above it was assumed that these relative demands were such that 100 units of wheat were exchanged for 70 units of cloth. However great is the demand of Atlantis for wheat, not more than 100 units of cloth will be given for 100 units of wheat. If the price were higher it would be more profitable for Atlantis to increase its own production of wheat by curtailing its production of cloth, for the opportunity cost of 100 units of wheat in Atlantis is 100 units of cloth. Similarly, however great is Erewhon's demand for cloth, the highest price that it will pay for 100 units of it will be 200 units of wheat, for the opportunity cost of producing 100 units of cloth in Erewhon is 200 units of wheat. The price of 100 units of cloth, therefore, will be at some point between 100 and 200 units of wheat.

The terms of trade depend, therefore, on the prices of commodities entering into international trade. The terms of trade are said to be favourable to a country when the prices of its exports are high relatively to the prices of its imports. In the period between the two World Wars the terms of trade became more favourable to Great Britain because the world prices of primary products—raw materials and foodstuffs—fell more than the world prices of manufactured goods. On the other hand, after 1945 the demand for primary products was so great that the terms of trade turned sharply against Great Britain and continued to do so until 1953. During 1956–60 the terms of trade again became more favourable to Great Britain, as also during 1961–65, as the following table shows:

Export Index as a Percentage of Import Index

1954	.	.	.	87	1960	.	.	.	97
1955	.	.	.	86	1961	.	.	.	100
1956	.	.	.	87	1962	.	.	.	102
1957	.	.	.	89	1963	.	.	.	101
1958	.	.	.	96	1964	.	.	.	99
1959	.	.	.	96	1965	.	.	.	101

N.B. The larger the number, the more "favourable" the terms of trade.

(5) ASSUMPTIONS OF THE THEORY OF INTERNATIONAL TRADE

The Theory of Comparative Costs shows quite clearly that international trade is to the advantage of all countries taking part in it. It is, however, based on a number of assumptions:

(i) the existence of perfect competition;
(ii) that there is full employment in all countries;
(iii) the absence of currency restrictions; and
(iv) that trade is free from artificial restrictions, such as tariffs or quotas.

The effects of interference with the freedom of international trade are considered below.

In addition to these important assumptions a number of others are made in order to simplify demonstration of the theory:

(v) that there are only two countries in the world, and only two commodities entering into international trade;

(vi) that there are no costs of transport, since to take account of such costs will merely reduce the range by the cost of transport within which the world price of a commodity will fluctuate;

(vii) that expansion or contraction of production in the two countries Atlantis and Erewhon is possible without either diminishing or increasing returns coming into operation. To allow for the possible effects of the Laws of Returns would unnecessarily complicate the exposition.

II. RESTRICTIONS ON FREEDOM OF TRADE

(6) FREE TRADE AND ITS DECLINE

Effects of restrictions on trade. Import duties aim at checking imports by making them dearer; import quotas more directly limit imports to certain pre-determined amounts; both therefore reduce the total volume of international trade. Preferential duties (that is, the imposition of lower rates of duty to certain privileged countries) and exchange control (limiting the amounts of foreign currency people can acquire) both divert trade from its normal channels. Whatever forms the inteference with free trade takes, the results are the same—the production of goods in regions that do not possess the greatest comparative advantages for their production, and in consequence a reduction of the total world supply, thereby making the world as a whole so much the poorer economically.

Decline of free trade. Never, however, since the nation-state came into being has any country completely carried out a policy of free trade. The nearest approach to free trade in Europe occurred during the decade 1860–70, when, largely as a result of the influence of Napoleon III, there was an all-round lowering of import duties. In the late nineteenth century there was a reaction against free trade, and both Germany and the United States built up their industries behind tariff barriers. British prosperity under free trade made this country cling to the doctrine longer than other countries, but the Great Depression (1929–35) caused all countries to seek the protection of high tariffs, and in 1932 Great Britain forsook free trade.

Efforts to secure a general reduction of tariffs have usually had only a limited success. The World Economic Conference of 1933 was a complete failure, but the conferences of recent years, held under the auspices of GATT (the General Agreement on Tariffs and Trade), have had a greater measure of success, and some slight reductions in tariffs were agreed upon. The establishment of the European Common Market was a reaction in favour of free trade on a regional basis.[1]

(7) THE CASE FOR PROTECTION

(i) *Some non-economic arguments.* If the advantages of international division of labour and trade are as strong and irrefutable as economists assert, the student of international trade may well be puzzled by the extent to which Governments impose restrictions on their foreign trade. The actions of Governments, however, are not swayed entirely by economic considerations. A re-armament programme, for example, by diverting resources from the production of consumers' goods to the forging of weapons of war, will make a nation poorer, but its people may be willing to pay this price if they value freedom more than material wealth. Similarly, some of the arguments for protection are based on non-economic grounds. A country may desire to protect its farming industry in order to be able to feed itself in case of blockade in time of war; or it may desire to build up an iron and steel industry for war purposes. When, too, a country aims at economic self-sufficiency the reasons are generally political.

If a conference is called to consider a reduction of tariffs a country that had imposed no restrictions on imports would find itself at a disadvantage, since it would have no concessions to offer. It has been suggested, therefore, that a country believing in free trade should impose import duties for use as a means of bargaining with others for a reduction of tariffs.

(ii) *To assist new industries.* One of the few economically sound arguments in favour of protection is in the case of "infant" industries—

---

[1] See p. 457 below.

Q

that is, newly established industries. If heavy initial fixed costs have to be incurred by a new industry the cost of producing a small output will be very heavy, but expansion of output may be accompanied by decreasing costs. In the early stages of its development the industry may be unable to stand up to its foreign competitors. Unless protected while "young," the industry will never be able to establish itself. A protective tariff for infant industries, however, can be justified only if it is removed once the industry has become firmly established. The difficulty is to decide when protection is no longer needed, for once tariffs have been imposed it is not easy to secure their removal. There is the danger, too, that protection will be given to industries that have no chance of survival without it, so that resources are diverted from more to less advantageous use.

(iii) *To protect a country's standard of living.* In countries where the people enjoy high real wages, it is often felt that their standard of living will be undermined if cheap goods are imported from countries where wages are low. The development of manufacturing industry in the Far East has given special point to this argument. A people's standard of living, however, depends on the quantity and quality of their country's factors of production, and high wages are therefore the *result*, and not the *cause*, of favourable conditions of production. To boycott goods produced in a country where wages are low will therefore depress wages still further there, whereas an increased demand for labour, arising from increased demand for that country's products, will raise wages there. Indeed, the basic principle underlying international trade is that costs of production are not the same everywhere. A serious difficulty arises, however, when areas with the greatest comparative advantages develop after a vast amount of highly specific fixed capital has been laid down elsewhere. Great Britain obtained a long start over other countries in most branches of manufacture as a result of being the first country to experience an industrial revolution, and cotton goods could be made most cheaply in Lancashire at the time when the industry developed there. If some other countries can now produce cotton goods more cheaply than Lancashire it might be argued on economic grounds that advantage should be taken of this, and cheap cotton goods be imported by Great Britain. Factors of production could then be released from cotton manufacture in Great Britain and devoted to the production of other commodities, most of which could be retained here, because the cheapness of imported cotton goods would require only a small quantity of other goods in exchange for them. Unfortunately, such a course would mean scrapping a large amount of fixed capital, and in the short period would cause structural unemployment. Hence the demand for protection. To accede to this demand would help the industry only in the home market, since protection cannot assist the export trade.

(iv) *Other arguments for protection.* When the production of a commodity abroad is carried on by a foreign monopolist a high tariff may be demanded in order to protect home producers against dumping of foreign goods on the home market at a much lower price than that at which the monopolist is selling them in his own country. This form of price discrimination was considered in Chapter XIV.

Sometimes a tariff is advocated in order to correct an adverse balance of payments. If imports exceed exports duties on imports will make them dearer, and so reduce their volume. If this policy also checks exports, as it may well do if other countries retaliate for their loss of exports by themselves restricting imports, the eventual result will be to reduce the total volume of trade. An excessive demand for imports is symptomatic of an inflationary condition in a country's economy, a situation that can be remedied in the long run only by internal monetary policy and not by the imposition of a tariff or other measure to restrict imports. In a trade depression, however, a tariff may be imposed as an emergency measure, for, as has been seen, the Theory of International Trade is based on the assumption that there is full employment, and if heavy unemployment exists, a Government may pursue any policy it thinks will alleviate it, regardless of any ill effects it may have. During the Great Depression most countries increased their tariffs, but this did not rid them of unemployment. As a short-term measure in 1964 the British Government imposed a surcharge on imports.

(8) IMPORT QUOTAS

An an alternative to the tariff, restriction of imports can be brought about by means of quotas. These fix the maximum amount of a commodity that can be imported during a particular period. The amount of a commodity having been determined, licences are then issued to supplying countries, stating the maximum amount each is permitted to supply.

A tariff or an import surcharge restricts imports by increasing their prices; import quotas enable a Government to restrict imports to definite quantities of what it regards as essentials. Unless the prices of these goods are also controlled, restriction of imports by quota will tend to raise their prices. When the amount of a quota is determined by a trade agreement with a foreign Government this may be for a period of years. In such cases a fall in world prices is of no benefit to home consumers. In the case of tariffs it is the Government which gains from the higher prices resulting from the import duties, but when imports are restricted by quotas (unless the Government undertakes the buying) the higher price benefits the importers of the commodity.

(9) MULTILATERAL *v.* BILATERAL TRADE

By multilateral trade is meant freedom of countries to trade with whatever other countries they please. Bilateral trade occurs when two countries try to balance their trade with one another, and this may be brought about by a trade agreement between them. A diagrammatic illustration of the advantages of multilateral over bilateral trade is given in Figs. 79a and 79b below.

(i) *Multilateral trade.* Assume that there are three countries—Atlantis, Erewhon and Utopia—taking part in world trade, and that there are no restrictions of any kind on freedom of trade, and that all three currencies are freely convertible. In the following table the arrows indicate the direction of a country's exports, the arrow pointing to the importing country. The sign − denotes exports and the sign + imports. The figures denote units of imports or exports. Transport costs are ignored.

Atlantis	Erewhon	Utopia
+ 20 ←———————— − 20		
− 30 ——→ + 30		
	− 50 ——→ + 50	− 40
	+ 40 ←————————	
− 25———————————→ + 25		
+ 35 ←————————————		− 35
+ 55 − 55	+ 70 − 70	+ 75 − 75

FIG. 79a.—ADVANTAGES OF MULTILATERAL TRADE

When multilateral trade is in operation it is not necessary for each country to balance its exports and imports individually with each other country. For example, Atlantis imports 35 from Utopia, although itself exporting only 25 to that country, but this is balanced by an export of 30 to Erewhon, with an import from that country of only 20. The trade of Erewhon and Utopia shows the same features, so that each country exactly balances its trade.

(ii) *Bilateral trade.* Assume now that for some reason multilateral trade breaks down and that each pair of countries enters into a trade agreement. Atlantis desires only 20 from Erewhon, and so Erewhon can have only 20 from Atlantis; Erewhon can make an exchange with Utopia of only 40; and Utopia and Atlantis will exchange only 25. In the case of bilateral trade each pair of countries must balance their trade with one another, with the result that the volume of trade between them is determined by the lesser of the two demands for imports. The total trade of the three countries, therefore, will now be as follows:

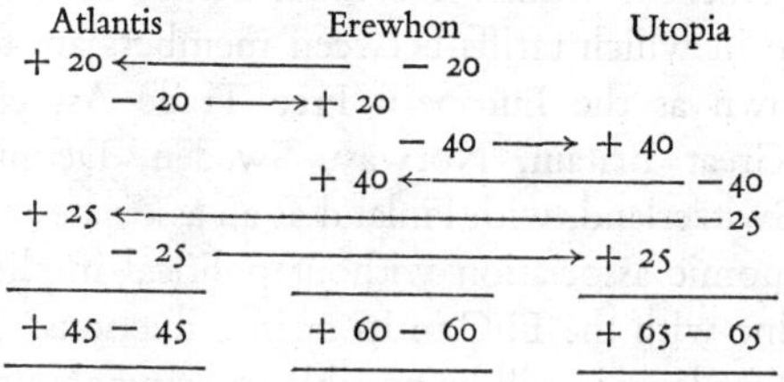

```
        Atlantis         Erewhon          Utopia
      + 20 ←────────────   − 20
        − 20 ────────→+ 20
                         − 40 ────→ + 40
                         + 40 ←──────────── −40
      + 25 ←──────────────────────────────  −25
        − 25 ─────────────────────→ + 25
      ─────────         ─────────        ─────────
      + 45 − 45         + 60 − 60        + 65 − 65
```

FIG. 79b.—BILATERAL TRADE

Each country has suffered a reduction in its trade, Atlantis by ten units, Erewhon by ten and Utopia by ten, the total for the three having fallen by thirty. Multilateral trade is clearly advantageous to them all.

(10) REGIONAL FREE TRADE

In recent years several groups of countries have formed areas in which free trade between the members will gradually be introduced.

First among these was the European Economic Community (E.E.C.), better known as the European Common Market. As long ago as 1947 the Netherlands, Belgium and Luxembourg formed themselves into a single customs union, known as Benelux, to encourage trade with one another. Then in 1952 these three states joined with France, West Germany and Italy to establish the European Coal and Steel Community. It was the success of these two efforts that led to the establishment in 1957 of a European Common Market, the members of which would eventually trade with one another unhindered by tariff barriers. The aim was not entirely economic, as it was hoped that economic co-operation would lead in time to political union. They agreed to reduce their tariffs against one another year by year, beginning with a reduction of 10% in January 1959, the aim being to establish by 1969 a common market with free trade between members but with a common tariff against the rest of the world. Other European countries are eligible for membership.[1]

Great Britain's attitude to the Common Market is affected by its relationship to the members of the Commonwealth, which all enjoy preferential tariffs in one another's markets. It was on this account that Great Britain did not become a founder-member of the European

[1] Greece, Iceland, Ireland, Spain and Turkey have been admitted as associate members.

Economic Community. Since, however, Great Britain's trade with countries of the EEC is increasing, this country is anxious not to suffer from being outside this organisation, but in spite of protracted negotiations during 1962–63 between Great Britain and the EEC, agreement could not be reached. Meanwhile Great Britain has helped to form a second region in which tariffs between members are to be gradually reduced, known as the European Free Trade Association (EFTA), comprising Great Britain, Norway, Sweden, Denmark, Portugal, Austria and Switzerland, with Finland as an associate member. This is a purely economic association without political implications. EFTA has kept in line with the EEC in its tariff reductions. Most members hope that before long it will be possible to bring about a union of the two organisations.

A third area of regional free trade with seven members was established in 1960, known as the Latin American Free Trade Association (LAFTA).

The Theory of International Trade supports the view that a lowering of tariffs between countries will have the effect of increasing their trade with one another. This appears to have been proved in the case of both the EEC and EFTA. Since 1958 not only has trade within each group increased but so also has trade between the two groups. Within the EEC trade expanded in value by over 160% during 1958–65 and within EFTA by over 80%, demonstrating that an increase in international trade is to the advantage of all countries taking part in it.

III. THE BALANCE OF PAYMENTS

(11) THE VISIBLE BALANCE OF TRADE

International trade gives rise to indebtedness between countries. The balance of payments shows the relation between a country's payments to other countries and its receipts from them, and is thus a statement of income and expenditure on international account. Payments and receipts on international account fall into three groups: (i) the visible balance of trade; (ii) invisible items; and (iii) capital movements.

The chief payments and receipts are, of course, for goods—imports and exports respectively. Great Britain's imports are mainly foodstuffs and raw materials, its exports being mostly manufactured goods. Great Britain, therefore, has to pay those countries which supply it with food and raw materials, and receives payment from those countries which buy its manufactured goods. Items in the balance of payments which relate to goods are known as *visible* items, and the relation between imports and exports is known as the balance of trade. With the surprising exception of 1956 and 1958, Great Britain has consistently had an adverse (or passive) trade balance—that is, an excess of imports over exports—every year since 1890. In the nineteenth century, when Great Britain was the workshop of the world, this country had a favourable balance of trade.

(12) INVISIBLE ITEMS IN THE BALANCE OF PAYMENTS

There are, however, many other payments and receipts which enter into a country's balance of payments, and these are known as *invisible* items, often being called invisible exports in the case of receipts. They arise chiefly as a result of services provided by one country for another and include the following:

(i) *Shipping and civil aviation*. Payment has to be made to shipping and aircraft companies for the carriage of goods and passengers from one port to another.

TABLE LVII
Shipping and Civil Aviation

	Shipping			Civil Aviation			
	Receipts	Payments	Net	Receipts	Payments	Net	Overall Balance
	£ million	£ million	£ million	£ million	£ million	£ million	£ million
1938	100	80	+ 20				
1948	255	178	+ 77				
1952	401	296	+ 105				
1958	637	615	+ 22	68	60	+ 8	+ 30
1960	644	669	− 25	96	78	+ 18	− 7
1962	647	659	− 12	115	94	+ 21	+ 9
1964	703	728	− 25	135	108	+ 27	+ 2

At one time Great Britain enjoyed almost a monopoly of the world's carrying trade, and as recently as 1913 was responsible for carrying 70% of the goods entering into world trade. In spite of the appearance of rivals after the First World War Great Britain still retained over 50% of the carrying trade. The Second World War was a further setback for this country, but by 1965 Great Britain's merchant tonnage, though at that date forming only 25% of the world's total, exceeded that of 1939,[1] but for some years shipping has been a debit item in the British

[1] Tonnage of British merchant shipping:

1939	.	.	.	.	.	18·7 million
1945	.	.	.	.	.	16·4 „
1965	.	.	.	.	.	21·6 „

balance of payments (see Table LVII). An increasing amount of freight is now carried by air. Even however when civil aviation is taken into account transport is no more than a self-balancing item.

(ii) *Financial services.* During the greater part of the nineteenth century London was the financial centre of the world, providing banking and insurance services for many countries. As with shipping, the two World Wars seriously affected Great Britain's position, but income from this source is still an important credit item to the British balance of payments.

(iii) *Investments abroad.* At one time the capital for a considerable amount of industrial development in foreign countries came from British investors. This was supplied in a number of ways. Sometimes British companies with British capital established themselves abroad to build railways (as in South America) or to develop oil-mining (as in Mexico, Iraq and Iran); sometimes British investors put their money into foreign companies; sometimes foreign governments raised loans in Great Britain; sometimes the British Government itself lent to foreign governments. In all cases the effect was the same: dividends or interest had to be paid from other countries to Great Britain, and this income became another invisible receipt. In the thirty years before the First World War Great Britain's income from foreign investments quadrupled:

TABLE LVIII

Income from Foreign Investment

	Receipts	Payments	Net
	£ million	£ million	£ million
1870	—	—	+ 50
1891	—	—	+ 100
1907	—	—	+ 140
1913	—	—	+ 200
1938	205	30	+ 175
1950	271	117	+ 154
1960	634	455	+ 179
1964	866	461	+ 405

During the early years of the Second World War many foreign investments held by British people were purchased by the Government and sold to pay for imports required for the prosecution of the war. Income from foreign investments has to be offset by the payment of interest and dividends on the investments of foreigners in Great

Britain. There has been a great increase in foreign investment in this country in recent years. Since 1952 there have, too, been repayments of the American loan. British investment abroad, however, has again increased, but in 1965 owing to its adverse effect on the balance of payments, the Government had to restrict it.

(iv) *Other invisible items.* One or two other invisible items may be briefly mentioned. Expenditure by British tourists abroad is a payment; expenditure by foreign tourists in Great Britain is a receipt, this item nowadays showing only a small net debit in the balance of payments. The renting of American films by British cinemas is another payment, while the hiring of British films by American cinemas is a receipt. Expenditure of the British Government abroad is now a serious debit item, having risen from only £16 million in 1938 to over £483 million in 1964.

The following table shows the chief items in the British balance of payments:

TABLE LIX

The British Balance of Payments.[1] *Current Account*

Payments	£ million			
	1938	1963	1964	19–[2]
I. Imports (Visible Items) . .	835	4,366	5,005	
II. Invisible Items:				
(i) Government expenditure abroad . .	16 ⎫	422 ⎫	483 ⎫	
(ii) Shipping and Aviation .	80 ⎪	775 ⎪	836 ⎪	
(iii) Interest, profits and dividends . . .	30 ⎬ 173	441 ⎬ 2,280	461 ⎬ 2,494	
(iv) Travel (tourists) . .	40 ⎪	241 ⎪	261 ⎪	
(v) Other items . . .	7 ⎭	401 ⎭	453 ⎭	
Total payments .	1,008	6,646	7,499	
Receipts				
I. Exports and re-exports (visible):	533	4,287	4,471	
II. Invisible Items:				
(i) Shipping and Aviation .	100 ⎫	788 ⎫	838 ⎫	
(ii) Interest, profits and dividends . . .	205 ⎬ 405	828 ⎬ 2,464	866 ⎬ 2,616	
(iii) Travel (tourists) . .	28 ⎪	188 ⎪	190 ⎪	
(iv) Other items (net) . .	72 ⎭	660 ⎭	722 ⎭	
Total receipts .	938	6,751	7,087	
Balance . .	−70	+105	−412	

[1] The figures have been taken from The White Papers on the United Kingdom Balance of Payments (H.M.S.O.).
[2] This column can be completed with the latest figures.

(13) EFFECTS OF CAPITAL MOVEMENTS

All the above items in the balance of payments, visible and invisible, affect the current income and expenditure of a country with the rest of the world. The balance of payments is also affected by capital movements. The income from foreign investments is a receipt, but when the investment was originally made, it is a payment. For a long time sterling has been regarded as an international currency. Nowadays it shares this function with the U.S. dollar. Other countries hold balances in these currencies to cover their international transactions. Fear for the safety of these balances, however, may cause holders to convert them for gold, thereby causing an outflow of capital from this country. Capital movements have a disturbing effect on the balance of payments of the countries concerned, as Great Britain has found to its cost on a number of occasions. This danger has been rendered more serious by the increase in the size of these balances, the sterling balances by 1965 having increased in value by seven times compared with 1939. Since 1953 however dollar balances have been greater in total than those held in sterling. A favourable balance on current account can be turned into adverse balance by capital movements, as indeed occurred in 1954, 1959 and 1963. In 1955, 1960 and 1964, when Great Britain had large deficits in its balance of payments on current account, the situation was aggravated by large deficits also on capital account (see Table LX).

(14) THE BRITISH BALANCE OF PAYMENTS

A debit balance on visible trade can be offset by a credit balance on invisible items, or vice versa, so that an overall balance can be achieved. During the early nineteenth century Great Britain generally had a credit balance in its balance of trade, which was mainly devoted to investment abroad, thereby increasing still further its income from foreign investment. As a result, by the second half of the nineteenth century Great Britain was able to import considerably more goods than it exported, the adverse balance in the balance of trade being easily covered by the favourable balance in invisible items.

Two World Wars weakened Great Britain's position as a trading nation. Not surprisingly the years immediately following the Second World War found Great Britain in serious difficulties with its balance of payments. Not only had Great Britain's income from foreign investment declined but huge debts had been created by purchase from abroad on credit. The loss of foreign investments and the reduced net income from shipping made it imperative for Great Britain to export more than before the war, especially if assistance was to be given to developing nations in Africa and Asia. The following table shows the British balance of payments in recent years:

TABLE LX

The British Balance of Payments

Date	Balance of Trade (Visible items)	Invisible Items	Current Balance of Payments	Long-term Capital Movements
	£ million	£ million	£ million	£ million
1928	− 352	+ 475	+ 123	
1938	− 302	+ 232	− 70	
1947	− 415	− 28	− 443	
1950	− 133	+ 433	+ 300	
1951	− 743	+ 336	− 407	
1952	− 120	+ 258	+ 138	
1953	− 218	+ 333	+ 115	
1954	− 204	+ 325	+ 121	− 191
1955	− 313	+ 156	− 157	− 122
1956	+ 53	+ 156	+ 209	− 187
1957	− 29	+ 245	+ 216	− 106
1958	+ 32	+ 298	+ 330	− 193
1959	− 116	+ 248	+ 132	− 251
1960	− 404	+ 131	− 273	− 185
1961	− 149	+ 135	− 14	+ 77
1962	− 98	+ 191	+ 93	− 93
1963	− 79	+ 184	+ 105	− 162
1964	− 534	+ 122	− 412	− 344
1965	..	..	− 136	− 218

+ = credit. − = debit balance.

As Table LX shows, Great Britain has had difficult years, but has achieved a credit balance on current account in the majority of the years shown to 1965, giving an overall balance for that period of over £900 million. Difficulties have arisen mainly on capital account, due partly to excessive investment abroad, assistance to developing nations and the fact that Great Britain acts as banker to the whole Sterling Area, and partly to a temporary loss of confidence in sterling as an international currency, resulting in withdrawals of sterling by foreign holders. Sterling crises have tended to occur in those years when Great Britain has had an adverse balance of payments on current account, for its reserves of gold and convertible currencies have been inadequate to meet severe strains. Table LXI shows how these reserves have fluctuated in recent years.

(15) THE PROBLEM OF BALANCE

When a country has an adverse or debit balance in its balance of payments it regards it with serious concern; when it has a favourable or credit balance there is satisfaction. Yet for all countries of the world total payments must be exactly equal to total receipts, since every

TABLE LXI

Great Britain's Reserves of Gold and Convertible Currencies

End of year	£ million	End of year	£ million
1951	834	1959	977
1952	659	1960	1,154
1953	899	1961	1,037
1954	986	1962	1,002
1955	757	1963	949
1956	799	1964	827
1957	821	1965	940
1958	1,096	1966	

payment is at the same time a receipt. Since, then, all countries cannot achieve favourable balances in the same year, the aim should be a balance, neither more nor less, over a period of time.

In one sense each individual country's balance of payments must balance each year. When all items, both visible and invisible, have been taken into account a balance is achieved by showing how the deficit (if there is an adverse balance) or the amount of the credit (if the balance was favourable) has been covered.

If there has been a deficit it must have been covered in one of the following ways: (i) by borrowing from another country; (ii) by obtaining assistance from the I.M.F. (the International Monetary Fund) or an international body such as the Group of Ten—the leading central banks; (iii) by imports on credit; (iv) by receiving gifts from another country; (v) by selling foreign investments; (vi) by exporting gold. Most of these methods of covering a deficit in the balance of payments make things more difficult for a country afterwards—loans have to be repaid, goods bought on credit have to be paid for later, the sale of foreign investments reduces future income. Such measures are therefore to be taken only in exceptional circumstances. When the deficit is small it can be covered by an export of gold.

When a country earns a credit balance it can use it to increase its foreign investment or to add to its gold reserves.

RECOMMENDATIONS FOR FURTHER READING

G. Crowther: *An Outline of Money*, Chapter 10.
P. B. Whale: *International Trade*.
R. F. Harrod: *International Economics*.

QUESTIONS

1. Explain what is meant by the "infant industry" argument in support of protective tariffs. (L.C. Com. Econ.)

2. What do you understand by the "Theory of Comparative Costs"? Can it be applied to home trade? (A.I.A.)

3. How does inflation affect our export and import trade? (Exp.)

4. Carefully distinguish between the "balance of trade" and the "balance of payments." Outline the outstanding changes that have taken place in the balance of payments of the United Kingdom since 1938 and comment upon the significance of these changes. (I.B.)

5. What is meant by an adverse balance (*a*) of trade, (*b*) of payments? How can an adverse balance of trade be remedied? (L.G.B.)

6. How are the terms of trade of a country measured? Is an improvement in the terms of trade bound to lead to an improvement in the balance of trade? (C.C.S. Inter.)

7. Distinguish between the Balance of Trade and the Balance of Payments and explain the meaning of (*a*) unrequited exports, and (*b*) invisible exports. (I.M.T.A.)

8. What is meant by "deterioration in the terms of trade," and for what reasons may this occur? Can such a deterioration ever be to the advantage of the country suffering it? (D.P.A.)

9. "It is comparative advantage, not absolute advantage, which determines the pattern of trade between countries." Elucidate and discuss. (C.I.S. Inter.)

10. How is a country affected by a change in its favour of the terms of trade? (C.I.S. Final.)

11. Import controls are a way of correcting an unsatisfactory balance of payments. Discuss the objections to their use. (I.B.)

12. What part do capital movements play in the United Kingdom Balance of Payments? (G.C.E. Adv.)

13. In Malanesia a unit of resources will produce either 100 yards of cloth or 20 units of steel. In Indolaysia a unit of resources will produce 90 yards of cloth or 15 units of steel. Explain the effects of international trade on production of each of the commodities in each country. (G.C.E. Adv.)

14. What are invisible exports and invisible imports? Give examples of both and discuss their relative importance for the United Kingdom. (G.C.E. Adv.)

15. Can a deterioration in a country's international terms of trade cause an improvement in that country's balance of trade? (C.C.S. Final.)

16. "The main justification of tariffs is to protect the industries of advanced nations from the unfair competition of backward ones." Discuss. (G.C.E. Adv.)

CHAPTER XXVII

FOREIGN EXCHANGE

I. THE FULL GOLD STANDARD (TO 1914)

(1) MONEY IN THE INTERNATIONAL SPHERE

We have seen that money first came to be used as a medium of exchange to obviate the clumsiness of barter, the early forms of money all being commodities that were wanted for their own sake. By the beginning of the nineteenth century money consisted of gold or silver coins; at the end of that century most countries had currency systems linked to gold; at the present day when bank deposits are the most important sort of money in many countries, inconvertible paper is the principal kind of cash in circulation. When commodity money was in use the settlement of international debts presented no special difficulty. Cattle were generally acceptable to different peoples, and so were capable of being used for the settlement of international transactions; nor was there any difficulty about the international use of the precious metals, for even after the invention of coinage the coins could be weighed, so that it was of little importance whether they were sovereigns, francs or dollars. No one, however, wants inconvertible paper for its own sake.

International dealings in recent times have been complicated by the fact that each country has its own currency, and a balance of payments can be compiled only after prices, expressed in many different currencies, have been converted to a common denominator—the currency of the country concerned. The consequences of an unfavourable balance of payments and the methods of correcting it vary according to the system of foreign exchange in operation. It is the purpose of this chapter therefore to give a brief survey of foreign exchange over the past 50 years or so, and therefore the gold standard, as it operated down to 1914, will first be considered.

(2) FEATURES OF THE GOLD STANDARD

On the full gold standard the monetary unit consists of a fixed weight of gold of a definite fineness; the price of gold is fixed by law; and there is complete freedom to buy or sell gold, to import it or to export it. When Great Britain was on the gold standard the Bank of England was legally obliged to buy gold at £3 17s. 9d. and to sell it at £3 17s. 10½d. per standard ounce, that is, gold eleven-twelfths fine. Changes in the supply of gold or in the demand for it could therefore have no effect on its price in terms of money. A change in the price of gold could be seen only indirectly through the prices of other things: a fall in the price of gold meant that fewer other things could be obtained in exchange for a given amount of it; a rise in its price meant that more of other things could be obtained for the same amount of gold. There was thus a close relation between the supply of gold and the prices of other things.

The mint par of exchange. The rate of exchange between two currencies both on the gold standard depends therefore on the quantity of gold in a unit of each. If an Erewhon dollar contains five times as much gold as an Atlantis franc, than the rate of exchange between the two currencies will be five francs to one dollar. This is known as the mint par of exchange.

Gold points. A heavy demand for Atlantis francs in Erewhon will, however, raise their price there. So long as Atlantis is on the gold standard and its paper francs are convertible into gold, the price of francs in Erewhon cannot rise above the cost of transporting gold between the two countries. Similarly, the price cannot fall by more than this amount, for if it did, paper money could be purchased and exchanged at a profit for imported gold. Thus, when countries are on the gold standard the rate of exchange between their currencies can fluctuate only within these narrow limits—that is, between the specie or gold imports and export points. The extent of fluctuations will depend in each case on the cost of transport and insurance, so that on the full gold standard before 1914 the rate of exchange between sterling and American dollars would be liable to slightly wider fluctuations than the rate of exchange between sterling and French francs.

(3) THE DUAL FUNCTIONS OF THE GOLD STANDARD

The gold standard really performs two functions, to a certain extent separate and distinct. There is, firstly, the internal gold standard, some of the features of which have just been considered, and secondly, the external gold standard, which regulates the rate of exchange between different currencies.

The internal gold standard. On the full gold standard, gold coins are in circulation and on demand bank-notes can be exchanged for gold. This means that an adequate reserve of gold must be kept to meet this demand. In some countries the law insists upon the maintenance of a gold reserve proportionate to the note issue. In Great Britain the *Bank*

Charter Act of 1844 permitted a small fiduciary issue, but the rest of the issue required a full gold backing. The amount of cash in the country then depended on its stock of gold. If this stock increased the quantity of cash could be expanded; if it declined the amount of cash had to be reduced. On the gold standard the volume of cash is then directly and rigidly controlled; the volume of bank deposits is dependent on the amount of cash held by the commercial banks, and so this kind of money also is indirectly controlled.

The external gold standard. In the international field the gold standard provides stability of exchange rates between different currencies, for the rate cannot fluctuate beyond the limits of the gold points. Fluctuating exchange rates handicap international trade, for traders will be reluctant to make forward contracts if a change in the rate of exchange is feared. On the gold standard, a country with an adverse balance of payment will have to make up its excess of payments over receipts by the export of gold; a country having a favourable balance will import gold.

The interaction of the functions of the gold standard. Since a single gold reserve had to serve both internal and external needs, the export or import of gold to meet the needs of the balance of payments will affect the internal situation. An export of gold reduces the gold basis for the internal currency, the volume of which must then be reduced. To accomplish this the banking system must adopt a policy of *deflation*. Bank rate will be raised, and by open-market operations the central bank will reduce the cash reserves of the commercial banks, which in their turn, in order to maintain their cash ratio, will reduce deposits by restricting their loans. As a result internal prices—including wages—will fall. This will make foreign goods relatively dearer, and so imports will be checked, while the export of home-produced goods will be stimulated because they will now be cheaper on the world market. In this way an adverse balance of payments will be rectified.

If, on the other hand, a country on the gold standard has a favourable balance of payments it will receive gold. This will increase the cash basis for the internal currency, and the banking system should then adopt a policy of credit expansion—that is, of *inflation* in order to increase the quantity of money. This will raise prices and wages, increase the demand for imports, while exports, now being dearer, will be discouraged. In this way a favourable balance will tend to disappear.

The following diagram illustrates the self-regulating character of the gold standard, a deficit or surplus in the balance of payments being corrected "automatically":

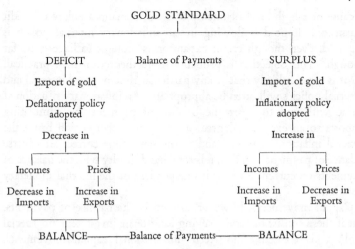

Thus, the "rules" of the gold standard compel a country to deflate when it is losing gold, and to inflate when gold is flowing in. Provided that these two rules are obeyed the balance of payments is "automatically" brought into balance. The report of the Cunliffe Committee (1918) describes the working of the gold standard before 1914 on these lines. It is extremely doubtful, however, whether the gold standard ever worked quite so smoothly as the Cunliffe Committee believed.

(4) THE ADVANTAGES AND DISADVANTAGES OF THE GOLD STANDARD

Advantages. Provided that the fiduciary issue (if any) is fixed, the volume of a country's currency depends on its stock of gold, and so it is impossible for an over-issue of bank-notes to occur. There can be no hyperinflation on the gold standard. In international dealings the gold standard provides fixed rates of exchange, and if a country keeps to the rules its balance of payments can be left to take care of itself.

Disadvantages. Internal purchasing power can be increased only if more gold is acquired. An expanding economy requires the volume of purchasing power to be more elastic than this, for it is foolish to make industrial development dependent on a country's stock of gold. The principal drawback to the gold standard is that it links internal monetary policy too closely with the requirements of the balance of payments, making it impossible for a country to pursue an independent monetary policy. If gold is flowing out, an internal policy of deflation has to be followed, even though the internal economic situation may, because of a high level of unemployment, demand a policy of credit expansion. If gold is flowing in, an inflationary internal policy is required, even though credit expansion is thought to have gone far enough. This objection is probably more theoretical than practical, for it is most unlikely that at any particular time opposed internal and external policies will often be appropriate. An inflationary situation at home will tend to upset the balance of payments by stimulating imports to an excessive degree: a policy of deflation will bring the internal inflation to an end and at the same time correct an adverse balance of payments. In fact, it is rare that difficulty with the balance of payments on current account is independent of the internal monetary situation.

Capital movements, however, also affect the balance of payments, but if these consist of funds seeking long-term investment no special problem is created. Short-term international capital movements, however, can have a disturbing effect on the balance of payments. A further disadvantage of the gold standard is the necessity of maintaining an additional gold reserve to support the internal note issue.

II. OFF THE GOLD STANDARD: FREE EXCHANGE RATES (1919-25)

(5) THE DETERMINATION OF THE RATE OF EXCHANGE

The outbreak of war in 1914 brought about the suspension of the gold standard. During the war, fixed rates of exchange were in operation, but for some years after the war—the actual period varied for different countries—the rates of exchange between many currencies were free to fluctuate, like other prices, according to the conditions of the market. Thus the value of the pound in dollars fell from 4·76½, the rate at which it had been fixed during the war, to 3·40 in 1919. The price of one currency in terms of another depended therefore on the relation between the supply of, and the demand for, it on the foreign-exchange market. The supply of Erewhon dollars will increase in Atlantis if Erewhon has been importing goods from Atlantis; the demand for Erewhon dollars in Atlantis will depend on the demand for Erewhon's export by Atlantis. A series of different exchange rates would emerge between each pair of countries, depending on the demand of each for the other's products, if traders were the only people to enter the foreign-exchange market. If, however, Erewhon dollars could be bought in Atlantis and sold at a profit in Utopia, speculators would intervene in the market, with the result that the same rate of

exchange would eventually prevail in all centres. This type of speculation is known as *arbitrage*.

The Purchasing Power Parity Theory, as refined by Cassel, attempted
to show that under a system of free exchange rates the rate of exchange
between two currencies depended on the relative price levels in the two
countries. If, for example, the rate of exchange between Erewhon
dollars and Atlantis francs moved from 150 to 200 francs to the dollar
it was thought to be due to a rise in prices of $33\frac{1}{3}\%$ in Atlantis. This
is an interesting theory, but though it contains an element of truth, it is
open to serious criticism.

(i) *The difficulty of comparing purchasing power in different countries.*
The construction of a cost-of-living index number is difficult because
different groups of people even in the same country buy different
assortments of goods. How much more difficult is it, then, to compare
price levels in different countries when perhaps in one the people drink
tea, and in the other coffee or wine?

(ii) *Effect of changes in demand.* If the Erewhon demand for Atlantis
perfume increases, it will increase the Erewhon demand for Atlantis
francs on the foreign-exchange market, and so raise the price of francs
in terms of dollars. As a result, all Atlantis goods will be slightly dearer
to the people of Erewhon, and all Erewhon goods will be slightly
cheaper to the people of Atlantis. Apart from imports, however, the
relative cost of living in the two countries will remain unchanged.

(iii) *Other influences in the rate of exchange* include any payments that
enter into the balance of payments. Where exchange rates are free to
fluctuate they are responsive also to speculative, political and psychological influences.

(6) FREE EXCHANGE RATES AND THE BALANCE OF PAYMENTS

As on the gold standard, the balance of payments can again be left
to take care of itself. An adverse balance means an excess of imports,
and this will cause the supply of the country's currency on the foreign-
exchange market to increase relatively to the demand for it. As a
result, the price of its currency in terms of others will fall. Thus imports, being dearer, will be discouraged, and exports, being cheaper,
will be stimulated, and a balance automatically achieved. Suppose
the rate of exchange between Erewhon dollars and Atlantis francs to be
120 francs to the dollar. An increase of Atlantis imports from Erewhon
increases the supply of francs in the market, and causes the franc to
depreciate to 180 francs to the dollar. As a result, the people of Erewhon
can now buy Atlantis goods previously costing one dollar for two-
thirds of a dollar, and so Atlantis exports to Erewhon will increase; to

the people of Atlantis, however, goods formerly costing 120 francs will now cost 50% more, and so they will tend to import fewer goods from Erewhon. Thus on a system where exchange rates are free to fluctuate *depreciation* of the currency corrects an adverse balance of payments.

(7) ADVANTAGES AND DISADVANTAGES OF FREE EXCHANGE RATES

Advantages. On this system of foreign exchange a country can pursue at any time whatever monetary policy suits the needs of its own internal situation. If it considers that a permanent policy of mild inflation is desirable in order to stimulate business activity this can be adopted. In fact, when free exchange rates are in operation a country need never adopt a policy of deflation. On the gold standard the needs of the balance of payments dictate the internal monetary policy, but with free exchange rates the balance of payments is brought into equilibrium by the rate of exchange, and this is influenced by internal policy. On or off the gold standard, however, the internal and external situations affect one another. Inflation at home will increase imports and discourage exports, and so lead to depreciation of the currency.

Disadvantages. The chief drawback to free exchange rates is the harmful effects of fluctuating exchange rates on international trade. There is, too, greater danger of a runaway inflation. The gold standard does not prevent inflation, for it is possible for all countries on the gold standard to inflate together, but it does put an effective brake on inflation in a single country. Shirking unpopular policies—increased taxation or retrenchment—a Government may take the easy way of financing its activities through inflation. During the period when free exchange rates were in operation there were many severe inflations and several runaway inflations.

III. THE RESTORED GOLD STANDARD (1925–31)

(8) NEW FORMS OF THE GOLD STANDARD

(i) *The gold bullion standard.* It was the chaos of the monetary systems in the years following the First World War that made the authorities in many countries believe that recovery could be achieved only by a return to the gold standard. The Cunliffe Committee recommended that Great Britain should follow this course. In 1922 the gold standard was restored in Austria, in 1924 in Germany, in 1925 in Britain and in 1928 in France. Great Britain did not, however, return to the full gold standard, for under the restored standard there was no gold coinage. Paper money was convertible, but only into gold bars, each weighing 400 ounces and worth about £1,560. The gold bullion standard had two advantages over the full gold standard: (a) it was not necessary to incur the expense of replacing worn coins, nor (b) was there any need to maintain a gold reserve against the internal note issue, although, of course, a gold reserve was still required for international settlements.

(ii) *The gold exchange standard.* Some countries sought to obtain the advantages of the gold standard even more cheaply than was possible on the gold bullion standard. On the gold exchange standard a country keeps its reserves in a currency based on the gold standard. The Scandinavian countries adopted this form of gold standard and chose to keep their reserves in sterling—mainly in Treasury bills. The advantage of this system is that a country's reserves can earn interest, whereas the guarding of a stock of gold involves considerable expense. The disadvantage is that countries on the gold exchange standard become dependent on the "parent" country, for if the "parent" country leaves the gold standard the value of the reserves of all countries on the gold exchange standard will depreciate. When Great Britain left the gold standard in 1931 many countries on the gold exchange standard suffered in this way.

(9) THE BREAKDOWN OF THE GOLD STANDARD

A number of causes contributed to the breakdown of the gold standard:

(i) *Not obeying the 'rules.'* The successful working of the gold standard before 1914 depended on the rules being obeyed. The first rule was that if there was an outflow of gold a policy of deflation must be adopted. The second rule was that in case of an inflow of gold a policy of inflation was required. During the period of the restored gold standard, however, countries did not always adhere to these rules. Deflation was both unpopular and difficult to carry out, for a contraction of credit requires a reduction in prices and wages, and trade unions were stronger in 1925 than in 1910 in resisting cuts in wages. It was not possible to deflate to the required extent because wages were difficult to adjust. Deflation also checks business activity, because falling prices reduce profit margins. Similarly, a country receiving gold was often unwilling to inflate for fear that a rise in prices might check its export trade. The United States imported a huge amount of gold, but it was not allowed to influence the cash basis for credit expansion—that is, it was "sterilised." After 1928, France acted in a similar fashion. It must be emphasised, however, that the rules were easier to carry out before 1914 than after 1925, as in the period of the restored gold standard the necessary adjustments—that is, the extent of inflation or deflation—were much greater than had been previously required. To obey the rules during 1929–30 required Great Britain to deflate in a time of depression and the United States to inflate when already experiencing a trade boom and inflation.

(ii) *Capital movements.* In the pre-1914 period, most big movements of capital were for long-term investment. During the years following the First World War a mass of short-term funds came into existence, and this "refugee capital" or "hot money" moved from one centre to another. Safety rather than the rate of interest was the prime considera-tion, and often a high Bank rate, instead of attracting foreign invest-ment, came to be looked upon as a sign of weakness and actually caused a withdrawal of funds. The repayment of war debts and reparations payments also added to post-war difficulties.

(iii) *The over-valuation of sterling.* When Great Britain returned to the gold standard in 1925 the pound sterling was given the same value in terms of U.S. dollars as it had in 1914, the price of gold being fixed as before at £3 17s. 9d./£3 17s. 10½d. per standard ounce. Great Britain was still the leading financial centre of the world and sterling an international currency, and the reason for selecting this rate was chiefly a matter of prestige. It was, however, fairly generally acknowledged at the time that this rate greatly over-valued sterling, making imports relatively cheap and exports dear.

The rules of the gold standard required Great Britain to deflate, but because of the over-valuation of the pound, the amount of deflation needed was too great, and prices and wages could not be reduced to the extent required. Every fall in prices also increased the burden of the National Debt, for though incomes fell, the taxation necessary to pay the interest remained the same. Deflation could not go nearly far enough, and so prices were not sufficiently reduced, with the result that the main consequence was a reduction of output and an increase in unemploy-ment. The effect of the deflation consequent on the over-valuation of sterling was that a trade depression beset Great Britain fully two years ahead of the world trade depression.

In contrast, the French franc at one-fifth of its pre-1914 parity was under-valued and for a time France enjoyed a favourable balance of payments and an inflow of gold.

Devaluation. In exceptional circumstances, when it is clear that a currency is over-valued by the rate of exchange, a country may decide to devalue its currency in order to remain on the gold standard. Great Britain, for example, would have been perfectly justified in devaluing at any time during 1925–31. On the other hand, there was really no justification whatever in 1933 for the devaluation by the United States of the dollar to 60% of its previous value in gold. This gave a rate of over $5 to £1 sterling. In 1935 Belgium also devalued its currency. France devalued the franc on several occasions.

When there is a fundamental disequilibrium in a country's balance of payments, and the amount of deflation required to correct it is very great, devaluation is justified. Like deflation, it will cheapen exports and make imports dearer (in terms of other currencies), but unlike deflation, there will be no need to reduce *money* wages. It is, however, a remedy to be applied only in times of extreme crisis, for stability of exchange rates is the principal advantage of the gold standard, and fear of further devaluation may destroy confidence in a currency.

(10) IMMEDIATE CAUSES OF GREAT BRITAIN LEAVING THE GOLD STANDARD

After the collapse of the mark in the great German inflation in 1923, Germany, not unnaturally, found it difficult to borrow, and in consequence had to pay a high rate of interest on loans. Germany, however, would have been unable to buy from abroad at all unless given credit, and both Great Britain and the United States lent considerable sums to that country. During 1928–31, Great Britain's *net* lending abroad averaged over £123 million per annum, and a favourable balance of payments on current account during those years was offset by these heavy capital movements, which turned a favourable balance into an average annual deficit of £65 million, which had been largely recovered by short-term borrowing.

The trade depression, which had already hit Great Britain, began to spread to the United States and Germany in 1930, and American financial assistance to Germany abruptly came to an end. Fear of the consequences of this led those of Germany's creditors who could do so to withdraw funds from that country. This, and the general collapse of world prices, brought on a financial crisis in Germany in 1931, one bank failing and others temporarily having to close their doors. It was well known too that Great Britain was heavily involved in Germany, and so both its creditors and countries on the gold exchange standard, as well as others with sterling balances, began to withdraw their short-term loans from London. There had been over-lending, and the moratorium in Germany and some other countries laid bare the weakness of the British position. Confidence in Great Britain's ability to remain on the gold standard was further shaken by forecasts of a large budget deficit. In 1931 Great Britain had a deficit of over £100 million in its current balance of payments, the shrinkage of world trade causing a sharp decline in its invisible exports. Although both the United States and France came to Great Britain's assistance with loans, it proved to be impossible to withstand the heavy drain of gold, and therefore, in September 1931, Great Britain had to leave the gold standard.

During the years 1931–36 one country after another left the gold standard.

IV. EXCHANGE CONTROL

(11) THE ORIGIN OF EXCHANGE CONTROL

When countries left the gold standard in the 1930s there was no desire to return to free exchange rates, for too many people, especially in Central Europe, remembered the severe inflations suffered in the previous decade. In most cases, therefore, some form of exchange control was introduced. This might merely aim at keeping exchange rates stable, or it might take the form of maintaining a rate of exchange either higher or lower than the equilibrium rate of a free market. A country "pegging" the rate at a low level—that is, under-valuing its currency—did so to stimulate its export trade. New Zealand followed such a policy after 1933. A policy of over-valuation might be pursued in order to bolster up confidence in the currency at home, to cheapen imports during time of war or to lessen the burden of an external debt payable in a foreign currency. Thus the German reichsmark was over-valued in 1931. Consequently, strict measures of exchange control were necessary to maintain the exchange rate, for over-valuation encourages imports, and checks exports, thereby increasing the country's difficulties with its balance of payments.

(12) THE GERMAN SYSTEM OF EXCHANGE CONTROL (1931–39)

Germany over-valued its currency by pegging the mark at a rate above the equilibrium. The high value of the mark encouraged imports and checked exports, so that it became necessary to restrict the amounts of foreign currency available to the German people. It is probable that if this had not been done, the Germans, remembering the great inflation of 1923, would have rushed to change marks for other currencies, and the mark would have been rendered worthless for the second time in eight years.

A most rigid system of exchange control was built up. If any German desired foreign currency he had to apply to the Reichsbank for it. If a German required it for personal reasons—a holiday in Switzerland, for example—his application would almost certainly be refused, as also would be that of a person desiring to import luxury goods. On the other hand, importers of things such as tin, rubber, oil would have little difficulty in obtaining the necessary foreign currency. The foreign trade of Germany came under the control of the Reichsbank, and it thus became possible for imports to be restricted to "essentials," these soon being interpreted as things required for war purposes. At the same time a German acquiring foreign currency was compelled to sell it to the Reichsbank. Even foreigners who had acquired German marks in Germany were forbidden to exchange them for other currencies, and had to accept credits in *blocked accounts*, on which they could draw only for expenditure in Germany itself. Instead of one rate of exchange for marks, there were multiple rates, each depending on the purpose for which the foreign currency was required, and varying with the urgency of Germany's desire for imports or reluctance to part with exports. Such a policy could not be pursued for long without causing reprisals. Eventually trade with Germany was reduced almost to barter.

(13) BRITISH SYSTEMS OF EXCHANGE CONTROL

(i) *Before 1939*. After Great Britain left the gold standard sterling was at first left free to fluctuate, and by March 1932 it had steadied itself at about 70% of its value on the gold standard. The aim of British policy at that time was to stabilise the exchange rate for sterling. In June 1932, therefore, the British Treasury established an *Exchange Equalisation Account*, for which the Bank of England was to act as agent. The sterling resources of the Account were in Treasury bills, and these funds were to be used for intervention in the foreign-exchange market. At the time when the British Exchange Equalisation Account was set up, confidence in sterling was returning, and as a result, the Account was able to acquire a considerable amount of foreign currency. The aim was to use these resources of sterling and foreign currency to counteract those fluctuations in the value of sterling on the foreign-exchange market which were due to causes other than changes in the demand for imports and exports—for instance, to cut out, if possible, the effect of movements of refugee capital. If foreigners were selling sterling, the Account bought sterling; if foreigners were buying sterling, the Account sold sterling for other currencies. In face of an increased demand for imports from abroad, the Account would have been ineffective, but its resources were sufficient to enable it to offset purely temporary fluctuations. Thus, the system adopted by Great Britain before 1939 was the mildest possible form of exchange control, since it was simply intervention in the foreign-exchange market by the Bank of England, acting on behalf of the Treasury, no restrictions being imposed on the exchange of sterling for other currencies.

In 1936 both the United States and France established Exchange Equalisation Accounts. In the same year a tripartite agreement was made between Great Britain, the United States and France, each country undertaking to buy its currency from either of the others in exchange for gold. Thus, when the British Exchange Equalisation Account acquired dollars or French francs they were exchanged for gold. In other words, in a modified form the gold standard was revived in the international field. These three countries also agreed not to alter the parity of their currencies without consulting one another. Rates of exchange were not rigidly fixed, as on the gold standard, but reasonable stability over a period was assured. It would have been possible for Great Britain to return to the gold bullion standard in 1933, but the new system was considered to be preferable to it.

The establishment of the British Exchange Equalisation Account brought into existence a second holder of gold in addition to the Bank of England, but whereas the Weekly Return showed how much the Bank possessed, the Exchange Equalisation Account published no return. In 1939 most of the Bank's gold was transferred to the Account, and since then the Bank has held little gold.

(ii) *After 1939.* However, on the outbreak of war in 1939, Great Britain imposed a rigid system of exchange control, and, with some modifications, this was continued for some time after 1945. During this period the aim was to maintain a fixed ("pegged") rate of exchange at a higher level than the equilibrium rate so that sterling was overvalued. In both the First and Second World Wars this course had been necessary, for it is impossible to wage a modern major war and at the same time maintain normal export trade. After the war the problem of the balance of payments was still acute. To have placed a lower value on sterling would not have reduced imports, for these were essential at first to the war effort, and afterwards to enable industry to reconvert itself to peace-time production. Nor would a lower value of sterling have encouraged exports, for the demand for British exports in the immediate post-war period was greater than could be supplied. It would therefore probably have been unwise to place a lower value on sterling.

To maintain the over-valued pound Great Britain therefore had to adopt a policy of restriction on exchange transactions. As in the pre-1939 German system, foreign currency could be obtained only through the Central Bank, although for many years after 1945 each person was allowed a small amount of foreign currency for private purposes such as holidays. Since 1959 there has been in effect little restriction on the amount of foreign currency available to British residents for foreign travel, but the Bank of England has tried to restrict private investment abroad.

V. THE INTERNATIONAL MONETARY FUND AND BANK

(14) THE SEARCH FOR A NEW SYSTEM

The policies adopted during the inter-war years had reduced international trade to meagre proportions. While the Second World War was still being fought, consideration was already being given, particularly in Great Britain and North America, to the problem of post-war international exchange. The aim was the restoration of world trade after the war and the establishment of a system of international exchange that would maximise world trade. Trade would have to be multilateral, and so bilateral agreements would have to cease; exchange rates would have to be reasonably stable, and changes in rates be agreed upon; there would have to be, too, the same rate for all purposes—that is, multiple exchange rates would have to cease, as would all other devices such as blocked accounts, invented by the exponents of exchange control. All restrictions on the acquisition of foreign currencies would have to be abolished, and all currencies made freely convertible —that is, freely exchangeable at the official rate of exchange for any other currency. The gold standard would have satisfied most of these conditions, but it was felt to be too rigid, since it required the immediate export of gold whenever a country had an adverse balance of payments, however temporary this might be. Against the gold standard there was, too, the loss of independence in internal monetary policy. Free exchange rates offered the other extreme, giving freedom over domestic policy, but fluctuating exchange rates. What was desired, if possible, was the advantages of both systems without their disadvantages—a difficult, if not impossible thing to achieve.

Simultaneously, currency plans were worked out in both Great Britain and the United States, the British plan being associated with the names of Lord Keynes. Both aimed at fostering multilateral trade through stable exchange rates and unrestricted convertibility of currencies; both favoured the establishment of an international institution to be responsible for the working of the new scheme, and the introduction of an international currency; both also favoured the retention of gold in international settlements. The main differences in the two plans were due chiefly to the different interests of Great Britain and the United States. The Keynes Plan suggested an international institution with power to grant overdrafts, to make possible an increase in the volume of international currency, and so was more expansionist than the American plan, and less dependent on gold. Keynes also desired similarity of treatment for a country having a surplus in its balance of payments as for a country with a deficit.

The two plans were discussed at an international conference held at Bretton Woods in 1944, the scheme that was finally adopted leaning rather more to the American than to the British proposals. Though included in the proposals of both countries the idea of an international currency was not adopted.

(15) THE INTERNATIONAL MONETARY FUND

The principal features of the scheme as elaborated at Bretton Woods were:

(i) *The International Monetary Fund* (I.M.F.) was set up to work the new scheme, and it began operations in March 1947.

(ii) *Rates of exchange.* By an agreed date member countries had to declare the par values of their currencies. After the great upheaval caused by the war, it was exceptionally difficult to determine with any degree of accuracy what this should be. Great Britain decided that the pound should be worth 4·03 United States dollars.

(iii) *Convertibility.* All currencies were eventually to be freely convertible, but a transition period of five years was envisaged, during which some measure of exchange control would be permissible.

(iv) *Changes of parity.* Once selected, parities were generally to be regarded as fixed, and member countries agreed to consult the Fund before making any change. The consent of the Fund, however, is not required for changes up to 10%, provided that the change is due to a fundamental disequilibrium in the member's balance of payments, that is, disequilibrium resulting from over- or under-valuation of its currency. If the balance of payments is adverse, depreciation is permitted; if the balance is favourable, appreciation of the currency is allowed. If a change of parity greater than 10% is desired, the permission of the Fund has to be obtained first, the Fund to give its decision within 72 hours, if the total change is no greater than 20%. For greater changes there is no time limit.

(v) *The pool.* The International Monetary Fund was to be provided with a pool consisting of gold and members' currencies. Member countries had to make contributions to this pool according to the quotas assigned to each. Of this quota, 75% could be contributed in the member's own currency, the remainder to be either entirely in gold or in gold and American dollars. Table LXII shows the quotas of some of the members. In 1959 most of these quotas were increased by 50%. The various contributions were placed to the Fund's credit at the central banks of the countries concerned.

TABLE LXII

International Monetary Fund Quotas[1]

Country	1945	1959
	$ million	$ million
United States	2,750	4,125
United Kingdom	1,300	1,950
France	450	787·5
West Germany	—	787·7
India	400	600
Canada	300	550
Netherlands	275	412·5
Belgium	225	337·5
Australia	200	400
Brazil	150	280
Mexico	90	180
Union of South Africa . . .	100	150
Yugo-Slavia	60	120
Norway	50	75
Chile	50	75
Colombia	50	75
Greece	40	60
etc.		

[1] In 1965 many quotas were again increased

A member country can obtain from the Fund in any one year foreign currency in exchange for its own up to 25% of its quota. Thus Great Britain could, immediately the Fund started its operations, obtain up to $325·5 million from the pool in exchange for sterling; France could obtain $112·5 million; Australia $50 million. At no time, however, must there be in the Fund currency of any member of a greater value than double its quota. When this point is reached, additional foreign currency can be obtained only in exchange for gold. To discourage members from making excessive purchases from the Fund, charges have to be paid when the Fund's stock of a member's currency exceeds 25% of its quota.

The main purpose of the pool is to allow a country to have an adverse balance of payments to a limited extent and for a limited period. Beyond these limits an adverse balance requires an outflow of gold, and steps must then be taken to restore equilibrium. To this extent the new system allows more latitude than the gold standard. It was no part of the purpose of the Fund, however, to make it possible for a country to have persistent adverse balance.

(vi) *Scarce currencies*. A widespread demand for a currency will reduce the Fund's stock of it. If this stock falls below 75% of a member's quota the Fund can declare that currency to be *scarce*, and it is then the duty of the Fund to ration the scarce currency among the countries demanding it. Two courses are then open to the Fund: (*a*) it can increase its stocks of the scarce currency by buying some of it for gold; (*b*) it can borrow from the member concerned. In the scheme as agreed less pressure was, however, to be placed on a country with a surplus in its balance of payments than on one with a deficit, whereas Lord Keynes had desired equal treatment for each. Equality of treatment seems reasonable, for if some currencies are plentiful some others must clearly be scarce.

The International Bank for Reconstruction and Development. A new International or World Bank was to be established, although the Bank for International Settlement (B.I.S.) set up after the First World War was still in existence. The International Bank (I.B.) is a separate institution from the International Monetary Fund, and obtains its funds partly from the contribution of its members and partly from the issue of dollar bonds. The purpose of the Bank is to assist countries with more serious difficulties than those for which they might seek assistance from the I.M.F. Loans can be obtained from the Bank to assist reconstruction or to further economic development. A number of countries have received financial assistance from the International Bank. Other international financial institutions include the International Finance Corporation (I.F.C.) to assist private capital investment, and the International Development Association (I.D.A.) to promote the economic development of the less-developed areas of the world and thus to supplement the activities of the World Bank.

(16) THE STERLING AREA

The division of the world into different currency areas, and particularly the strength of the dollar and the weakness of the pound for some years after 1945, gave new life to the sterling area. The members of the sterling area are those countries which have found it to their advantage to keep their currencies linked to sterling. Its membership has changed from time to time, but it has usually included most of the countries within the British Commonwealth, although Canada and Newfoundland were never members. An important feature of the sterling area has always been its flexibility and adaptability. It will be useful to trace its historical development.

(i) *Before 1914.* The origin of the sterling area is to be found in the period before 1914 when Great Britain, a mature, industrially developed country, was at the head of an empire of large, diverse, economically undeveloped territories. Great Britain's powerful economic position enabled it to devote its surplus in its balance of payments to loans to these and other countries, for Great Britain possessed the financial institutions necessary for this type of business. The trade of the British Dominions and colonies was chiefly with and largely financed by the home country. Even after the Dominions had developed their own banking systems, the Bank of England continued to act as their central bank and the place, therefore, where they kept their reserves.

(ii) *Between the two World Wars.* During the period of the restored gold standard the development of a gold-exchange standard, whereby some countries held their reserves in sterling instead of in gold, gave the sterling area a new importance. When Great Britain left the gold standard in 1931, so did all the other countries which kept their reserves in sterling. These countries formed the nucleus of a block that desired to keep their currencies relatively stable. The stability of prices in Great Britain after 1931 was in striking contrast, both to prices in the countries which remained on the gold standard, and to prices in Great Britain itself before 1931. This encouraged other countries, which preferred to keep their currencies linked to sterling rather than to gold, to join the sterling area. It was, however, an entirely voluntary association, without any central means of control, simply comprising countries desirous of linking their currencies to sterling and keeping their external reserves in London. Generally, fixed exchange rates prevailed between the members, though some of them found it necessary to change the parities of their currencies from time to time. Besides Great Britain, the members of the British Commonwealth and the Scandinavian countries, the sterling bloc at one time also included Argentina, Japan and France.

(iii) *1939-45.* On the outbreak of war in 1939 most of the neutral countries left the sterling area. For the first time it received legal recognition, and Great Britain became the official guardian of the gold and dollar reserves of the entire bloc. In 1939 strict exchange control was imposed between the area and the rest of the world, though its operation was left to individual members, thus even in war-time maintaining the voluntary character of the association. Shipping difficulties would, however, have made it difficult for any member to abuse its freedom to import goods from outside the sterling area.

(iv) *After 1945.* The post-1945 currency difficulties and the need of Great Britain and many other countries to curtail their purchases from the dollar area increased the importance of the sterling area. The drain on the area's gold and dollar reserves made necessary an agreement among members to restrict their use of dollars to the utmost, for the main preoccupation of the sterling area after 1945 became the protection of its gold and dollar reserves. As banker to the sterling area, Great Britain holds its stock of gold and dollars. When a member of the sterling area acquires U.S. dollars they are passed over to the British Treasury in exchange for sterling, with the result that when the area's gold and dollar reserves increase so do the sterling balances of the members responsible for their acquisition. Since 1945 the sterling area, though still an organisation without rules, has been given some measure of organisation by the holding of periodic meetings of members and the establishment of permanent committees in London. The sterling area owes its continued existence to the fact that its members (except the Union of South Africa) evidently consider that the advantages of membership outweigh the disadvantage of having to put all the U.S. dollars they earn into the common pool. It is no mean achievement for Great Britain to have retained its leadership of the sterling area during the changing conditions of the twentieth century.

(17) THE CONVERTIBILITY AND DEVALUATION CRISES

The Washington Loan Agreement. In December 1945 Great Britain received a loan from the United States conditional upon sterling being made freely convertible in July 1947. The purpose of the loan was to enable Great Britain to cover the anticipated deficit in its balance of payments over the next five years. There was no doubt a keen desire to get the Bretton Woods scheme working, but July 1947 was much too soon. Even the transitional period of five years originally suggested eventually proved to be too short a period for most countries. Parities selected before peace-time conditions were restored were bound thereby to be arbitrary.

The facilities provided by the International Monetary Fund were sufficient to cover only a very small adverse balance of payments. Great Britain, for example, with its original quota, could for a period of four years obtain currency from the Fund to cover an annual adverse balance of about £80 million. A glance back at p. 463 will show that even in 1938 Great Britain had an adverse balance of £70 million. Allowing for the rise in prices, the adverse balance permitted by the Fund was very small indeed. The delegates who met together at Bretton Woods grossly underestimated the extent to which economies of Western Europe had been dislocated by the war.

The 'Convertibility' Crisis (1947). The I.M.F. began operations in March 1947. Great Britain carried out the Washington Loan Agreement by making freely convertible all sterling acquired as a result of current transactions, the sterling balances accumulated during the war remaining blocked. Many countries at this time found it necessary to build up their stocks of all kinds of goods, but few countries other than the United States were as yet able to produce goods for export. Most countries, therefore, were short of dollars. Consequently, when sterling became convertible there was a general demand from those holding it to exchange it for U.S. dollars, with the result that after only five weeks Great Britain had to suspend convertibility. For five weeks it had been tantamount to Britain having to pay for all its imports in dollars, and this almost exhausted what little was left of the American credit.

The failure of Great Britain to maintain convertibility of sterling made the United States realise the seriousness of the blow dealt to the British economy by the war. Marshall Aid to Great Britain and other countries of Western Europe was the result, American assistance speeded up European recovery. Meanwhile purchases of dollars from the International Monetary Fund were suspended.

Effects of the failure of convertibility. In its effort to bring its balance of payments into equilibrium, Great Britain—like many other countries—reduced its imports from the United States to a minimum consistent with its industrial recovery. In Great Britain severe restrictions were placed on the acquisition of American dollars, and imports from the United States were strictly controlled. Purchases were therefore not always made in the cheapest markets, since the currency in which payment was made became of greater importance than the price of the commodity. Thus there was further interference with the working of the Principle of Comparative Cost. Instead of one world price for goods entering into international trade, there were two sets of world prices. Many bilateral agreements were made, and multilateral trade as an objective appeared to be even more remote than in 1938. By 1951 there were few countries that did not impose some degree of exchange control and there were also several cases— Argentina and Spain, for example—of multiple exchange rates. France twice devalued its currency without consulting the Fund. Thus, within five years of the signing of the Bretton Woods agreement,

R

most of the practices condemned as detrimental to multilateral trade were again in operation. The International Monetary Fund was not suited to the unsettled conditions of a post-war world; it had commenced its operations too soon.

The devaluation of the pound (September 1949). It came to be felt in many quarters that the disequilibrium in Great Britain's balance of payments was of a "fundamental" kind, and therefore to be overcome only by a devaluation of the pound. The choice of a rate of £1 = $4·03 had been more or less arbitrary, but it soon became clear that this rate greatly over-valued the pound. The advantages of an over-valued currency immediately after a war have already been noticed. Even if, by chance, the pound had originally been fairly valued at $4·03, its value might still have been reduced by inflation at home. It is not possible to construct an international monetary system that will confer the advantages of both stable exchange rates and complete freedom over internal monetary policy, for the internal situation affects the external. Inflation at home raises prices and wages, stimulates imports and checks exports, and in the end the strain on physical controls becomes too great. Inflation in Great Britain after 1945 has already been discussed. During 1945–47 the internal value of the pound in terms of goods and services continued to fall. In spite of official denials that devaluation was contemplated, fear of it made merchants in dollar areas postpone purchases from Great Britain, especially since at that time a trade recession in the United States was feared. In September 1949, therefore, the value of the pound was reduced from $4·03 to $2·80—that is, by about 30%. At the same time a number of other countries devalued their currencies. Devaluation can succeed in correcting an adverse balance of payments only if imports, by becoming dearer, are checked, but this will not occur if the demand for imports is inelastic. Nor will exports be stimulated by the fall in their price unless foreign demand for them is elastic. Again, if rising prices, resulting from devaluation, lead to wage increases the inflationary spiral will be set in motion and the problem will recur. Devaluation is a remedy to be tried only in an extreme case, and should not be repeated, otherwise confidence in a currency will be destroyed.

The European Payments Union. Part of the dollar allocations to European countries under Marshall Aid was dependent on the recipients making available some of their own currencies for the use of others, the aim being to assist Europe to help itself. As there appeared to be little hope of achieving free convertibility between European currencies and the U.S. dollar for some considerable time, the aim instead became convertibility between European currencies themselves in order to encourage multilateral trade between the nations of Western Europe. In 1950, therefore, The Organisation for European Economic Co-operation (O.E.E.C.) set up the European Payments Union (E.P.U.). This was somewhat similar to the International Monetary Fund, but on a regional basis. The scheme was operated through the Bank for International Settlements, the members settling their accounts monthly, not with one another but through the E.P.U.

(18) THE CONVERTIBILITY OF STERLING

The failure of the premature attempt of 1947 to make sterling convertible made the British monetary authorities reluctant to risk a second failure, which might have a disastrous effect on the commercial and financial prestige of this country. The development of multilateral trade is, however, impossible unless currencies are convertible, and so the achievement of convertibility remained the aim, though not to be attempted until the Government was assured of the economic strength of the country. Thus, every time a favourable balance of payments occurred it encouraged hopes of an early restoration of convertibility, but such hopes were immediately dashed whenever the balance became adverse. The crux of the problem was that after 1945 Great Britain's gold and dollar reserves, even in the best years, were never felt to be adequate.

Steps towards convertibility. It therefore became British policy to relax the restrictions on the convertibility of sterling by easy stages in order to test the ability of the currency to stand up to each additional strain. For a time, therefore, sterling became convertible only among the members of the Sterling Area. Gradually, however, two other areas of convertibility were built up, these being known as the American Account area and the Transferable Account area. The area of the American Account included the United States, Canada and some other countries of Central America; the Transferable Account area had been expanded by 1955 to include the rest of the world outside the Sterling Area. Within each of these areas sterling was convertible. Thus Canada could exchange sterling for U.S. dollars, France could convert sterling into German marks or Italian lire, and of course within the Sterling Area the currencies of the members were freely convertible. There was also one-way convertibility between the three areas. For example, the countries of the American Account could exchange sterling for any other currency, and those of the Transferable Account with members of the Sterling Area, but convertibility in the opposite direction was not permitted, the countries of the Sterling Area being restricted to convertibility with one another, and those in the Transferable Account not being allowed to exchange sterling for currencies in the American Account area. The administration of this system left many loopholes for unauthorised dealings in sterling, but these came to be regarded as the testing ground for the full convertibility of sterling. Meanwhile, many other restrictions on sterling were relaxed. Most important has been the re-opening of the foreign-exchange market, and although the British monetary authorities through the Exchange Equalisation Account intervene to keep sterling fluctuations with the U.S. dollar within the range of 2·82 and 2·78, this provides an indicator of the strength of sterling. If sterling is in great demand the market rate will be near the upper limit and there will be a tendency for the reserves to increase, but if the rate is near the lower limit this indicates a demand to sell sterling with a consequent fall in reserves.

Non-resident convertibility. Finally, in January 1959 sterling was given "non-resident" convertibility, that is it was made freely convertible to all foreigners by the amalgamation of the American and Transferable Accounts. At the same time the E.P.U. came to an end. From 1959 to 1966 British people could obtain as much foreign currency, including U.S. dollars, as they wished for ordinary commercial or private purposes. Restrictions on foreign travel were re-imposed in 1966. Then in 1967 sterling was again devalued from $2.80 to $2.40 to the £, and bank rate was raised to 8%.

(19) RECENT INTERNATIONAL MONETARY PROBLEMS

The period since 1951 has been punctuated by a series of sterling crises during which lack of confidence in sterling as an international currency has led to heavy withdrawals from London. Crises of this nature occurred in 1951, 1955, 1961 and 1964. On each of these occasions Great Britain was in difficulties with its balance of payments on current account, generally the result of an internal upsurge of inflation. At such times the inadequacy of the country's reserves brings fear of a devaluation of sterling. In 1961 Great Britain's difficulties were brought on by the revaluation of the West German deutschemark. In both 1961 and 1964–65 Great Britain was assisted, not only by the International Monetary Fund, but also by joint action on the part of the leading central banks. Bank rate on these occasions was raised to 7%.

In recent years it appears to have been realised that the facilities offered by the I.M.F.—although over the years operating with increasing success—are insufficient to meet present-day temporary difficulties that have beset many countries in connection with their balances of payments. Even the increases in the quotas of members made in 1959 and 1965 have done little more than merely offset the rise in world prices. The result has been demands for an increase in "international liquidity." To this end the leading central banks of the world have co-operated as the Group of Ten—those of Great Britain, the United States, France, West Germany and six others—and have agreed to lend to the I.M.F. if that institution finds itself short of funds.

At the present day, both sterling and the U.S. dollar function as international currencies, and in consequence both at times have been subjected to severe strain. Both Great Britain and the United States have had difficulties with their balances of payments in recent years. In the case of the United States this has been almost entirely due to the enormous assistance given by that country to developing nations, its balance on current account invariably being favourable. In the case of Great Britain, expenditure on economic aid abroad has exaggerated the country's difficulties with its balance of payments. Thus, while Great Britain has found its reserves of gold and convertible currencies inadequate to its present-day needs, the United States has experienced a severe drain on its gold reserves, formerly so huge.

RECOMMENDATIONS FOR FURTHER READING

G. Crowther: *An Outline of Money*, Chapters 7–10.
J. L. Hanson: *Monetary Theory and Practice*, Chapters 7–9, 18, 19.
R. S. Sayers: *Modern Banking*, Chapter 6.
White Papers on *Balance of Payments*.

QUESTIONS

The Gold Standard

1. What is meant by the gold standard? Give *two* variations of it and indicate under what conditions each might be used. (I.H.A.)

2. What do you mean by the gold standard? What was the difference between the gold standard of 1913 and that of 1925–31? (I.B.)

3. What case was or could be made for the return to the gold standard in 1925? How far did subsequent events expose weaknesses in the case? (Final Degree.)

4. Give a brief account of the underlying and immediate causes of this country's abandonment of the gold standard in 1931. (Final Degree.)

Free Exchange Rates

5. Consider the advantages and disadvantages of flexible exchange rates. What might be done to reduce the disadvantages? (C.I.S. Inter.)

6. What determines the external value of a country's currency in a freely operating foreign-exchange market? (G.C.E. Adv.)

7. Discuss the relationship between the internal level of prices in a country and the foreign-exchange value of its currency, assuming a free foreign-exchange market. (G.C.E. Adv.)

8. Compare the advantages and disadvantages of fixed exchange rates and of flexible exchange rates. (C.C.S. Final.)

9. Do you consider the purchasing-power parity theory to be an adequate explanation of the equilibrium rate of exchange between national currencies? (Final Degree.)

Exchange Control

10. Describe the events leading to the formation of the Exchange Equalisation Account and how it has been operated. Is the Account still operating? (L.C. Com. B. & C.)

11. Write a short essay on the transition from the international gold standard system as it worked before 1914 to the managed currency systems of the present time. (S.I.A.A.)

12. In what circumstances would you recommend a country to raise the foreign-exchange value of its currency? (Final Degree.)

13. What is the system known as the Sterling Area? Consider in relation to it the position of (a) Canada, and (b) South Africa. (Final Degree.)

The Post–1945 System

14. In your estimate would it be possible to create an international currency, and if such a currency system were introduced would it have any practical advantages? (L.C. Com. B. & C.)

15. Describe briefly the functions of the International Bank established under the Bretton Woods Agreement. Having regard to these functions, do you consider it correct to describe the institution as a bank? (I.B.)

16. It has been contended that the Bretton Woods Agreement is tantamount to a return to the gold standard. Give your reasons for agreeing or disagreeing with this contention. (D.P.A.)

17. In what circumstances will a country benefit from currency devaluation? (G.C.E. Adv.)

18. Compare the rôle of gold under (a) the gold standard, and (b) the International Monetary Fund. (Final Degree.)

19. The International Monetary Fund Agreement used the concept of "a fundamental disequilibrium" in the foreign-exchange value of a currency. Discuss the economic conditions lying behind such a situation and the difficulties of identifying it. (Final Degree.)

PART EIGHT

ECONOMICS AND THE STATE

CHAPTER XXVIII

THE EXPANSION OF THE ECONOMIC ACTIVITY OF THE STATE

I. FROM LAISSEZ-FAIRE TO NATIONALISATION

(1) *LAISSEZ-FAIRE* AND ITS DECLINE

The adoption by Great Britain of a policy of *laissez-faire* in the nineteenth century was largely due to the influence of Adam Smith. By *laissez-faire* is meant a policy of non-intervention by the State in the economic life of the country. Economic intervention by the State was condemned by Adam Smith as "folly and presumption." It was a comparatively new idea at the time when he wrote, for he was criticising the views of the Mercantilists, up to then widely prevalent. The emergence of the nation-state in the fifteenth and sixteenth centuries had led Governments to seek to regulate trade, and particularly to restrict imports.

Gradually, however, during the nineteenth century State interference increased, and the way was prepared for the complete abandonment of *laissez-faire* in the twentieth. It was only with great reluctance that the State at first intervened to regulate the employment of women and children in the mines and factories. It was only slowly, too, that it took upon itself the task of providing free education for all. By 1914, however, a comprehensive body of factory legislation had been built up, elementary education was free, secondary education inexpensive, many regulations existed for safeguarding the health of the people, and a limited scheme of national insurance covering old age pensions, sickness and unemployment had been introduced. Throughout the nineteenth century Parliament kept a watchful eye on the activities of the railways, to prevent the development of monopoly, and railway rates were controlled. Amalgamations of railways were frowned upon, just as were bank amalgamations later. The issue of bank-notes was restricted by the *Bank Charter Act*, 1844. The development of the limited company eventually led to the growth of a body of company law for the protection of the public. In the sphere of foreign trade, however, the doctrine of free trade, at least in Great Britain, remained triumphant for a few years longer. In these various ways the State began to take an active interest in the social and economic life of the nation.

(2) NEW FORMS OF STATE ACTIVITY, 1919-39

Between the two World Wars the intervention of the State in economic affairs still further increased. In 1932 Great Britain at last abandoned free trade. During the twenty years, 1919-39, the link between the Treasury and the Bank of England became closer, the policy pursued by the Bank being influenced by the Treasury to a greater extent than ever before. During the First World War the Treasury had undertaken the issue of £1 and 10s. notes, but the Bank of England took over the issue in 1928. Shortly after Great Britain had left the gold standard the Government established the Exchange Equalisation Account for the purpose of buying or selling foreign currencies or sterling in order to influence the exchange rate of sterling. The world trade depression was responsible for the Government's promoting the setting up of Marketing Boards for milk, potatoes, etc., regulating the import of bacon and some other commodities by import quotas.

Social Insurance was extended in 1929 to cover widows' pensions, and in 1937 the scope of the scheme was widened to include salaried workers. A number of monopolies, such as broadcasting, came to be managed by a new type of organisation, the public corporation.

(3) THE DEVELOPMENT OF THE STATE PLANNED ECONOMY

During both World Wars the economic life of this country was brought to a great extent under State control. By means of exchange control and control of imports, foreign trade was regulated by the Government. Industries not essential to the war effort were curtailed, and by direction the distribution of labour among different industries was controlled. Many prices were controlled and the commodities concerned rationed. Investment, too, was controlled, so that the diversion of real resources to less essential forms of production could be prevented. The greatest advance in the acceptance by the State of responsibility for economic affairs, however, occurred in 1944 when the Government for the first time assumed responsibility for the maintenance of full employment, a policy on which all three political parties in Great Britain were agreed.

All parties, too, were agreed that a more comprehensive scheme of social insurance should be provided. Family allowances were introduced in 1946, and the full scheme came into operation two years later. All classes of people, irrespective of income, and whether employed or self-employed, were brought within its scope. Benefits include payments during sickness and unemployment, retirement pensions, widows' pensions, maternity and funeral grants. It is more correctly a scheme of social security rather than of social insurance, for its financing—especially the National Health Service—has required an increasing contribution from the national exchequer, in addition to large weekly contributions by employers and employees.

An important step towards greater State planning in Great Britain took place in 1962, when the National Economic Development Council (usually known as "Neddy") was established. The main functions of this body are (i) to advise the Treasury; and (ii) to consider obstacles to Great Britain's economic growth. During 1964–65 the N.E.D.C. delegated work appertaining to particular industries to a number of Economic Development Committees ("Little Neddies"), as, for example, for the machine-tool industry, building, wool textiles, chemicals, mechanical engineering, etc. Then, in 1965 the Ministry of Economic Affairs published its National Plan. This showed the Government's aim to be to increase total output by 25% by 1970, and outlined the measures it considered necessary to achieve this objective.

The extent of the State's intervention in economic and social affairs in Great Britain is indicated by the fact that in 1964–65 there were no fewer than fifteen Government departments, headed by ministers of the Crown, concerned with these matters—the Exchequer, Economic Affairs (DEA), Labour, Trade, Agriculture Fisheries and Food, Transport, Power, Aviation, the Post Office, Technology, Land and Natural Resources, Education and Science, Health, Housing, and Pensions and National Insurance.

Nowadays, too, all parties agree that some State planning is necessary, though they differ as to the amount of control the State should undertake. At one extreme is the Communist State, where there is a maximum amount of planning; at the other extreme there is the State that allows the maximum amount of freedom to private enterprise, the price mechanism being subject only to those restrictions necessary for the protection of the community. Between these two systems is the "middle way," taken by Great Britain and most non-Communist countries since 1945, an economic system with both a public and private sector, a "mixed" system, as it is sometimes called. By 1965 the public sector employed 25% of the total labour force, and owned 40% of the total capital assets of the country.

In earlier chapters of this book we have seen how the British Government has widened its interest in economic affairs in recent years. In Chapter VIII we saw how it has attempted to influence the location of industry, at first by the creation of Development Areas and more recently through its proposals for regional planning. Its interest in the National Income (Chapter XVI), too, has increased, as it is greatly concerned to stimulate economic growth—hence the Government's National Plan, published in 1965. Throughout the period since 1945 it has attempted to keep inflation in check (Chapter XXI), and to that end it has taken a more active part in promoting monetary policy (Chapter XXIV) than ever before. Anxiety to control inflation led to efforts in 1964–65 to obtain the agreement of the trade unions to an "incomes policy" in an effort to relate increases in wages to increased production. Matters affecting the balance of payments (Chapter XXVI) are also now a prime Government concern.

II. STATE OWNERSHIP OF INDUSTRY

(4) NATIONALISATION IN GREAT BRITAIN

The sole commercial enterprise operated in Great Britain by the State for a long time was the Post Office, established as long ago as 1660. Towards the end of the nineteenth century nationalisation of "the means of production" became one of the chief items of socialist policy.

Public ownership and control of an industry can be supported on a number of grounds:

(i) as a means of protecting the consumer against monopoly;

(ii) where competition is wasteful it may be better to create a state-owned monopoly, as when road haulage was nationalised;

(iii) it is in the national interest that basic industries such as coal, iron and steel, and transport should be brought under public control;

(iv) where it is clear, as with airlines, that the industry for many years would have to be subsidised by the State;

(v) where an industry is clearly technologically inefficient, as was the case of coal-mining, and where the private owners appeared to be unwilling or incapable of improving it;

(vi) where labour relations are particularly bad, as also in the case of the coal-mining industry;

(vii) where, because of economies of scale, a service can be provided more efficiently nationally than locally, as with electricity;

(viii) where it is felt that control is necessary to the carrying out of Government policy, as in the case of the Bank of England;

(ix) where it might be to the public danger to allow an industry to be privately controlled, as with atomic energy.

After 1945 an extensive programme of nationalisation was embarked upon in Great Britain, partly for political reasons and partly because, for one or other of the reasons listed above, it was considered that certain basic industries could be better operated by the State. An economist's attitude to nationalisation will depend, however, on the answer to the question: will the industry be more efficiently run by the State than by private enterprise? First came the nationalisation of the Bank of England (1946), closely followed by the coal industry and public transport (1947), electricity (1948), gas (1949) and iron and steel (1951). Road transport (partially) and the iron and steel industry, however, were both denationalised in 1953. The iron and steel industry was renationalised in 1967. A public corporation was set up to manage each nationalised industry. The two principal British airlines—British European Airways and British Overseas Airways—were already operated by public corporations. In 1954 two more public corporations were established—the Independent Television Authority, to break the monopoly of the B.B.C., and the Atomic Energy Authority, to promote the development of atomic power. In the case of atomic energy all three of the British political parties favoured State control. By 1965 the public sector in Great Britain had a combined income equal to 26% of the country's national income.

Financial aspects of nationalisation. The previous owners of the firms comprising the nationalised industries were paid compensation except where they happened to be local authorities. The stock-holders of the Bank of England, for example, received 3% Government Stock, giving them an income equal to that which they had been previously receiving. In the case of the coal industry, compensation was fixed at £114,160,000 in Treasury Stock, this sum being divided first among the nine regions of the Coal Board, and then distributed among the firms in each region. Transport Stock to the value of £1,024 million was allotted to the shareholders in the railways and canals. Individual agreements were made with road-haulage firms. Some gas and electricity undertakings were owned by municipal authorities and some by joint-stock companies, but compensation was given only to the shareholders in the company-owned concerns in the form of Gas and Electricity Stock.

Compensation in the form of Government Stock has vastly increased the volume of the country's reproductive debt. From the point of view of the nationalised industries, they are all burdened with heavy fixed charges, which have to be covered in bad times as well as good, whereas previously dividends paid to shareholders varied directly with profits. Upon the railways was at first placed the additional burden of having to make payments to a stock redemption fund.

From the beginning the National Coal Board was financed directly by the Exchequer, but the other nationalised industries, particularly the Central Electricity Generating Board, the Gas Council and the Transport Commission, at first obtained additional capital by the issue of long-term guaranteed stocks. Since 1956, however, all nationalised industries have been financed by the Exchequer.

(5) PRICE AND PROFIT POLICY OF NATIONALISED INDUSTRIES

All the British nationalised industries (except road haulage) are monopolies or near-monopolies, though some of them, such as coal, gas and electricity, compete against one another and against oil, while the railways also compete against road passenger services, airlines and the private motor car.

The price and profit policies of the nationalised industries are matters of great economic importance. The constitutions of the public corporations operating the nationalised industries do not state that they should be run for profit, although they are expected to pay their way over a number of years. Public ownership of an industry implies that it should provide a service and so be operated in the national interest rather than that the aim should be to make a profit. The phrase "in the public interest," however, has no precise meaning, and if the question of profit or loss is completely ignored no satisfactory economic test of the efficiency of an industry can be applied. It has been suggested, therefore, that since to earn a profit is not the primary aim of a nationalised industry, some kind of audit of efficiency by an audit commission should replace profit as a test of its efficiency.

If problems of output, price and profit are to be decided solely on economic grounds, it is important that a nationalised industry should attract to itself that quantity of factors of production—neither more nor less—that is economically desirable. Thus, prices should be related to costs, particularly where nationalised industries are in competition with one another. Many economists, therefore, think that the aim should be to break even, thus avoiding either a large profit or a heavy loss. If prices are too high, this will check the development of the industry; if too low, there will be over-expansion at the expense of other forms of production. Under perfect competition it has been seen that price is equal to marginal cost, and if economic considerations are to prevail this might appear on theoretical grounds to be the price a nationalised industry should charge to its consumers. Most of the nationalised industries, however, have heavy fixed costs in proportion to their variable costs, and in such cases average costs fall as output increases, so that marginal cost tends to be below average cost. In these circumstances, therefore, a loss will be incurred if a price equal to marginal cost is charged.

If the price to be charged is based on average cost it means that the more profitable activities of a nationalised industry have to subsidise the less profitable. This principle is observed by the Post Office. Thus it costs the same to send a letter from London to an isolated farm in the Western Highlands of Scotland as from Westminster to Chelsea. Average cost, and therefore price, can be reduced by ceasing to operate unremunerative activities—the policy for the railways outlined in the Beeching Report—though some may be retained on the ground that all sections of the community are entitled to the service.

A further difficulty arises because most nationalised industries produce goods or services in fairly inelastic demand. In such cases it is easy to pass on increased cost to the consumer, and this can have serious effects, for most of these industries help to produce capital goods on which other industries depend. Increased charges for power, transport, and iron and steel, therefore, will increase the costs of all other producers.

It is sometimes argued that, for reasons other than economic, some nationalised industries should be run deliberately at a loss because it is socially desirable that they should do so or because they are of strategic importance or essential to a country's defence. The railways might be considered to fall within this category. Any decision to run at a loss, however, must be the responsibility of Parliament, but if such a course is decided upon it then becomes almost impossible to test the efficiency of the industry. In practice, the State may impose its own price policy. A Standing Committee reporting on the pricing policy of nationalised industries recommended that the two British Airways Corporations should continue to operate certain routes at a loss,[1] and yet these corporations are expected to make a profit. The argument has also been employed in connection with the railways. On a number of occasions the National Coal Board has complained that it has had to charge too low prices for some grades of coal.

(6) SOME NATIONALISED INDUSTRIES

Let us now take a brief glance at some of the nationalised industries:

(i) *Coal*. The nationalisation of the coal-mining industry was recommended by the Sankey Commission as long ago as 1919. The Act to nationalise the coal industry brought 1,500 mines under the control of the National Coal Board on 1st January 1947. Some 400 mines, each

---

[1] For example, B.E.A. to the Western Isles and B.O.A.C. to Kuwait.

employing fewer than 30 underground workers, retain their independence, although they had to be licensed by the Coal Board. The industry is administered by nine regional Coal Boards, and under them are 48 area managements. The *Coal Mines Nationalisation Act* (1946) declared the policy of the National Coal Board to be the efficient development of the industry and the provision of coal in such quantities and at such prices as to "further the public interest."

Throughout the nineteenth century and down to 1913 the output of coal from British mines continued to increase. From a mere 10 million tons in 1800, production expanded to 80 million tons in 1860, and reached its maximum of 287 million tons in 1913. During the last two decades of this period the export trade in coal was developed. Since 1913 the industry has felt the impact of two world wars and a prolonged trade depression. The Great Depression severely affected the industry, for when the home demand for coal fell off it was found difficult to revive the export trade, particularly since the depression was world-wide. Germany and Poland, too, had become serious rivals to Great Britain in foreign markets, and the development of the production of hydro-electric power in the Alps and Scandinavia, and more economical methods of using coal in industry, reduced the demand for it. Consequently, between the wars, coal-mining in Great Britain was a declining industry, and there was a contraction of its labour force. Therefore, after the outbreak of war in 1939 compulsion had to be adopted in order to increase the labour employed in the mines. The *Coal Mines Act* of 1930 had recommended the amalgamation of mines, but this policy met with little success, the owners of the more efficient mines being unwilling to combine with the less efficient—hence the large number of separate firms at the date of nationalisation. During both wars and both immediate post-war periods, however, there was little coal to spare for export, and on several occasions after 1947, coal actually had to be imported.

For many years the great problem of the industry was to keep up output of coal to meet the demand for it in a period of full employment. Table LXIII shows the output of coal in recent years.

There has been some extension of mechanisation in the mines, and this has raised the average output per man shift from 1·14 tons in 1938 to 1·33 in 1958 and 1·7 in 1964. However, the problem for many years has been labour difficulty, the labour force in the industry falling steadily since 1945 to 602,000 in 1960 and to 498,000 in 1964. Successive increases in miners' wages have not attracted labour. In fact, the supply curve for labour in this industry is probably regressive, so that high wages, coupled with a high level of employment, have tended

TABLE LXIII

Coal Production in Great Britain

Year	Million tons
1913	287
1938	217
1948	200
1950	216
1952	223
1954	222
1956	222
1958	216
1960	194
1962	189
1964	186

to increase absenteeism. Uniform prices for coal throughout Great Britain would be economically unsound, and so the National Coal Board favours uniform prices only within particular areas. The National Plan, published in 1965, allowed for a fall in both output and in the labour force in the coal industry by 1970.

Coal is no longer the sole source of power, though it still ranks first in importance both for industrial and domestic purposes. It can be used directly or for the production of gas or electricity. In the future, atomic energy is likely to become more important in the production of electricity. In recent years oil has become a greater rival to coal than formerly. In consequence, the price policy of the National Coal Board acquires increased significance, and to reduce the average cost of producing coal a number of uneconomic mines have been closed.

(ii) *Iron and steel.* The iron and steel industry is, like coal, one of the basic industries, and it was for this reason that its nationalisation was suggested. It is, too, one of the first industries to be affected by the onset of either a boom or a slump. The older centres of the industry are located on the coalfields, because in earlier days a large amount of coal was used in the smelting of iron ore. The newer centres of the industry, at Scunthorpe in North Lincolnshire and at Corby in Northamptonshire, are near supplies of iron ore.

Down to 1913 the iron and steel industry enjoyed almost continuous expansion, and to meet the needs of the first World War the industry was enlarged to such an extent that there was excess capacity when the war was over. By 1924 the output of the industry was only half of what it was capable of producing, and there followed a period of "rationalisation" when the industry was deliberately reduced by the closing down of many plants. The rise in the demand for basic steel and the fall in the demand for wrought iron reduced considerably Great Britain's advantages over its rivals, and the output of both the United States and Germany went ahead of that of Great Britain. The iron and steel industry is one in which economies of scale are to be enjoyed, and in all three countries it has been a large-scale industry for a long time. In the United States there is a huge concern known as the United States Steel Corporation, in Germany there are large cartels and in Great Britain, too, there are huge combines of the cartel type.

The British iron and steel industry was nationalised in 1951. The firms involved numbered 96, and comprised companies producing 50,000 tons of iron ore or 20,000 tons of pig-iron or steel in one year. All the completely owned subsidiaries of the 96 companies named in the Act, of which there were about 150, were also taken over. In order to preserve the goodwill of the old firms, they were allowed to retain their original names, and their entire capital was vested in the Iron and Steel Corporation of Great Britain, a holding company under the Ministry of Supply. Thus the companies became publicly owned, each with a single shareholder—the State. Medium-sized firms outside the scheme were not permitted to expand beyond double their size at the time of the passing of the Act, except under licence. The iron and steel industry, therefore, remained what it had been before nationalisation—a cartel—and with the same drawback that the more efficient firms would have to subsidise the less efficient.

The iron and steel industry was denationalised in 1953, though it took seven years to return the constituent companies to private ownership. Denationalisation was easy to accomplish, since the general structure of the industry had not been seriously disturbed under nationalisation. After its denationalisation a measure of supervision over the industry was, however, retained, the Iron and Steel Board being established for this purpose. In 1964, and again in 1966, it was announced that the industry would be renationalised.

(iii) *Electricity*. At the time of nationalisation two-thirds of all the electricity undertakings in Great Britain were operated by local authorities (mostly county boroughs), the remainder being in the hands of public companies (mostly in county areas). Before nationalisation some measure of co-ordination by the linking up of one area with another had been achieved under the Central Electricity Board. The Act of Nationalisation established the Central Electricity Authority (later known as the Central Electricity Generating Board), but the setting up of fourteen area boards—for example, the Yorkshire Electricity Board, whose members were appointed by the Minister of Fuel and Power, and not by the Central Electricity Generating Board—provides considerable decentralisation. Each area board keeps its own separate accounts, and has at its disposal—subject to the approval of the parent authority—any surplus it may earn. Before nationalisation there were almost as many different scales of charges as there were undertakings. Greater uniformity has meant increased charges in the towns and lower charges in the country. A serious drawback to uniformity of charges is that it is liable to lead to uneconomic location of industry. Shareholders in the former electricity companies received compensation in the form of Electricity Stock, but undertakings owned by municipal authorities were taken over without compensation.

(iv) *Gas.* Before nationalisation many local authorities owned gasworks, but a great many were operated by joint-stock companies, a large number being controlled by a single combine, the Gas, Light & Coke Co. Ltd. The nationalisation of the industry instituted a form of organisation similar to that for electricity, but the twelve gas boards are even more independent of the Gas Council, which comprises the twelve chairmen of the area boards, than are the area electricity boards of the Central Electricity Generating Board.

Most local authorities made a profit from supplying gas and electricity, and this was partly used for the relief of rates. One effect, therefore, of the nationalisation of gas and electricity was to increase the rates of many local authorities.

III. INLAND TRANSPORT

(7) DEVELOPMENT OF COMPETITION BETWEEN THE RAILWAYS AND ROAD TRANSPORT

Consideration of the nationalisation of transport provides a convenient opportunity for a more detailed discussion of some of the economic problems associated with inland transport. Industrial development has gone hand in hand with the development of means of communication, for exchange is the corollary of territorial division of labour. The Industrial Revolution was both a cause and a result of improvements in transport. In many countries, in contrast to Great Britain, where even the building of roads had been left to private enterprise, the State assisted this development, mainly because means of transport are of strategic as well as economic importance. In most countries railways are now State-owned, the main exceptions being the United States and the Netherlands.

The British railways were mostly built in the first place to satisfy local needs, but the amalgamations of local lines resulted in the development of the first railway systems in this country. Parliament, through fear of monopoly, encouraged competition by sanctioning the building of competitive lines, with the result that a measure of excess capacity was created. In spite of amalgamations, Great Britain, as late as 1914 was still served by 25 railway companies of medium size, in addition to over 75 small concerns. An Act of 1921 made compulsory their amalgamation into four groups,[1] the grouping being so arranged that some measure of competition remained.[2] During both World Wars the State took over the operation of the railways.

The return to the roads. The development of the railways during 1844-70 had driven nearly all inter-town traffic off the roads. The first competitors of the railways were street tramways, which became their rivals for suburban traffic. It was not, however, until the perfection of the petrol engine that road transport became a serious competitor of the railways. A few motor omnibuses were in service before 1914, but after 1922 a rapid expansion of this form of transport began. Many of these road-passenger transport firms were run by small operators, each with only two or three vehicles. It is important to emphasise that many of these operators, like most of the tramways before them, were at first developing new traffic, and not taking traffic from the railways. By expansion and amalgamation many large companies developed, such as the West Yorkshire and Ribble and United companies in the north, and the Southern and Western National companies in the south. All over the country small operators of goods services also sprang into existence about the same time, the small amount of capital initially required making it easy for them to establish themselves. Just as large omnibus companies came to be established, so large haulage firms soon appeared. Both long-distance passenger and goods services were developed, many of the goods vehicles travelling through the night. Alarmed by this development, the railways in 1928 obtained powers to operate road-transport services, but instead of putting competing services on the road, they preferred to acquire substantial holdings in the larger of the existing road-transport concerns. The railways then began to close some small country stations and short branch lines.

The increasing amount of traffic on the roads made it necessary to restrict competition between road operators, both passenger and goods services. The *Traffic Acts* of 1930 and 1933 regulated road transport by

---

[1] The Great Western Railway, the London Midland and Scottish Railway, the London and North Eastern Railway and the Southern Railway.

[2] For example, the L.M.S.R. and L.N.E.R. were competitors for traffic between London and Scotland, the G.W.R. and L.M.S.R. between London and Birmingham, the G.W.R. and S.R. between London and Plymouth.

introducing a system of licensing for road services. The Act of 1930 divided the country into areas, each with a body of Traffic Commissioners, whose first business was to restrict the number of bus operators over each route, and to consider applications from operators wishing to establish new routes. Thus existing operators were given a monopoly, but their time-tables and charges were subject to sanction by the Traffic Commissioners. For goods vehicles there were three categories: A—general hauliers; B—firms carrying their own goods, but also having some general haulage business; C—firms delivering only their own goods. The Act of 1933 restricted the number of hauliers in groups A and B, but C licences were granted to all applicants entitled to apply for them. As a result, freedom of entry to the main branches of road transport was removed.

(8) ROAD v. RAIL

During the past thirty years keen competition between road and rail operators has developed.

Advantages of road transport. (i) For distances up to at least 200 miles, road haulage of goods is speedier than the railway. (ii) The road transport unit is small, and so small loads can be expeditiously dealt with, whereas the railway has to build up whole train-loads, and this involves a complicated system of marshalling. (iii) Road transport can offer a door-to-door service, whereas transport by rail involves collection and delivery. For many goods road hauliers charge lower rates than the railway. Many manufacturers—especially those making branded goods—prefer to deliver their products in their own vans. For passengers, the bus often has the advantage over the railway of a more frequent service at regular time intervals. The railways often suffer from the disadvantage of having inconveniently situated stations, frequently situated miles from the village they are intended to serve.

The operation of railway and road transport. The construction of railways involved heavy capital investment, whereas the initial outlay of the small road operator was often little more than the cost of a single vehicle, and even that might be acquired on the hire-purchase system. Operational costs of a railway are heavy, for it is solely responsible for the upkeep of its "road" and the maintenance of signalling, stations, etc. Motorways for the use of road vehicles are constructed at the cost of taxpayers. The road operator had merely to pay for a road fund licence and insure his vehicle, and then (until 1930 or 1933) he could run wherever he pleased.[1] The marginal cost of railway transport,

[1] In the case of passenger services licences to operate had to be obtained from the Local Authorities through whose areas the route lay.

however, is low, for the cost of running an additional train is small; on the other hand, marginal costs of the road operator are relatively heavy, and nearly proportional to any increase in his traffic. As has already been noticed, railway rates until 1963 were based on the principle of charging what the traffic will bear, goods being arranged in 21 classes. Another important feature of railway charges is their publicity and their subjection to public control, these features being the result of efforts to curb their possible misuse of monopoly power. In road haulage keen competition prevailed, and so for a long time it was free from control. Railway charges were based on average costs for the whole railway; road charges were based on the costs of particular journeys, exceptionally low rates sometimes being charged for return loads, a load at almost any price being preferable to the running of an empty vehicle. The railways complained that road operators confined themselves almost entirely to the carriage of goods in the more expensive categories of railway classification, and to routes where density of traffic was high.

(9) NATIONALISATION OF INLAND TRANSPORT

In 1947 an Act was passed to nationalise inland transport. This act set up the British Transport Commission, whose work was distributed among five executives covering: (i) railways, (ii) docks and inland waterways, (iii) road transport, (iv) London Transport and (v) hotels. On 1st January 1948 British Railways acquired the four main-line railways, British Waterways took over the inland waterways and docks, some of which had previously been owned by the railways and London Transport Executive[1] took over London Transport. An Act of 1963 transferred the functions and property of the Transport Commission to the following four boards—Railways (British Rail), London Transport, British Waterways and the British Transport Docks and the newly created Transport Holding Company, in which are vested shares in road haulage (British Road Services), many bus companies in England, Scotland and Wales, some shipping companies and travel agencies. Except for the haulage firms acquired by British Road Services, these companies continued to operate under their own names as, for example, Pickford's, Thos. Cook & Son Ltd. Some decentralisation of the railway system was achieved by dividing the railways into six regions,[2] the work of the six regional boards being co-ordinated by a central committee.

---

[1] With the abolition of the British Transport Commission by the Act of 1963 the various transport executives were replaced by boards, e.g. British Railways Board, etc.
[2] Southern, Western, London Midland, Scottish, North-Eastern and Eastern.

Road transport presented a more complicated problem, owing to the huge number of firms involved.[1] British Road Services were given power to acquire road-transport undertakings by individual bargaining with the firms concerned. Holders of "C" licences were exempt from nationalisation. The Road Haulage Executive had its headquarters in London, with eight regional divisions, further subdivided into 31 districts. Each operational group of about 150 vehicles is under a Group Manager. Road transport was denationalised in 1953, but fear of renationalisation made business men unwilling to return to road transport. In consequence, only 54% of the vehicles were returned to private enterprise, the remainder having to be retained by British Road Services. Road passenger operation was not much affected by nationalisation on account of the delay caused by local interests having to be given an opportunity of putting forward objections.

The problem of co-ordination. Competition from road transport in the 1930s brought about increasing co-operation between the four railways —for example, inter-availability of tickets between towns served by more than one railway. After the railways had acquired interests in some road services inter-availability was extended to include some bus services. Considerable co-ordination of both routes and time-tables by bus operators resulted from the Act of 1930. It was said that one advantage of nationalisation of all forms of inland transport was that it prepared the way for a degree of co-ordination not previously possible. One difficulty is the absence of a uniform system of calculating operational costs, without which comparison of the efficiency of different forms of transport is impossible. It may be that short-distance traffic, both passenger and goods, can best be left to road transport, and that long-distance traffic is more suited to the railway. It may be that fast traffic can best be dealt with by the railway, and road transport used for distribution from focal points on the railway system, as suggested in the Beeching Report of 1963. Such decisions should depend primarily on economic factors, though social considerations, such as the congestion of town streets by through heavy traffic, ought to be taken into account.

The exemption from nationalisation of the "C" licence-holders, who together operate five times as many vehicles as the Road Haulage Executive, and the increasing number of private motor cars means that the nationalised industry is not free from outside competition. The problem of co-ordination of the various forms of inland transport was further complicated by the denationalisation of road transport.

---

[1] Some 20,000 firms with an average of between two and three vehicles each.

(10) THE PRESENT PROBLEM

In their efforts to compete successfully against road operators British Railways have tried to reduce their average costs by closing unremunerative branch lines, a policy accelerated under the Beeching Plan, 1963–65. Where diesel services at regular intervals have been introduced, there has been some return of passenger traffic to the railways. Express goods services, too, have had some success. Though their local traffic has declined, the railways are still the main carriers of coal, and their long-distance express passenger trains are usually well-filled.

The decline in passenger travel by railway is not confined to Great Britain. Two new competitors of both the railway and the motor bus have come into the field—the private motor car and the aeroplane. The huge increase in the number of privately owned motor cars in Great Britain has reduced the number of people using both the railways and suburban bus services. The shortness of the distances has retarded the development of internal airlines in Great Britain, but in the United States 25% of all travellers go by air, 50% in their own cars, and only 25% by bus or railway.

The Beeching Report (1963). This Report was the work of Dr. (now Lord) Beeching, who was appointed by the Minister of Transport to study the problem of the railways. Its main recommendations, known as the Beeching Plan, were: (i) non-remunerative branch lines should be closed; (ii) on many routes stopping trains should be withdrawn; (iii) speedy, regular (liner) freight services should be introduced; (iv) main-line traffic should be concentrated on the most direct routes and some alternative routes closed. The aim was to use the railways for the traffic for which they were most suited, so that by 1970 the railway deficit would be wiped out.

The increasing difficulty of covering their costs of operation has led to suggestions that both railways and local buses should be operated as services and not with the aim of making a profit. In such a case one of the first problems is to decide how much service to provide—for example, should there be as frequent a service of trains from London to Leeds as from London to Brighton? The greatest problem, however, is that once the aim of making a profit is removed, it becomes very difficult to test the economic efficiency of an industry.[1]

RECOMMENDATIONS FOR FURTHER READING

G. C. Allen: *British Industries and their Organisation*, Chapters 3, 4, 8–11.
W. A. Robson: *Nationalised Industry and Public Ownership*, Chapters 1–5, 8.
G. Walker: *Road and Rail*.

[1] See p. 498.

M. R. Bonavia: *Economics of Transport.*
W. Hagenbuch: *Social Economics,* Chapters 9, 10.

QUESTIONS

1. Argue the case for and against a nationalised industry making a profit. (L.C. Com. C. & F.)

2. What are the economic arguments for and against State ownership of industries? (C.I.S. Inter.)

3. In what types of industry does the case for public ownership seem to you to be strongest? Give examples. (C.C.S. Final.)

4. What are the principal reasons for the increased expenditure by the State in recent times? (C.C.S. Final.)

5. What rules should a State adopt in fixing the prices of nationalised goods and services? (C.I.S. Final.)

6. Examine, from the economic point of view, the expenditure by the State of large sums on "social services." (Exp.)

7. "Social security is a much larger issue than national insurance against particular risks." Discuss this statement. (I.T.)

8. "Economic planning is suited to backward countries but not to advanced ones." Discuss. (G.C.E. Adv.)

9. Does economic theory indicate any rules which should govern the policies pursued by the nationalised industries? (C.I.S. Final.)

10. If the railways make a loss, what remedies do you suggest? (C.C.S. Final.)

11. "Publicly owned undertakings should always be guided by the rule that price must be equated to marginal costs." Discuss. (Final Degree.)

CHAPTER XXIX

THE TRADE CYCLE AND FULL EMPLOYMENT

I. INDUSTRIAL FLUCTUATIONS

(1) THE TRADE CYCLE IN THE NINETEENTH AND TWENTIETH CENTURIES

The trade or business cycle is the name given to the tendency of business activity to fluctuate from boom to depression and back to boom and depression again. These alternating periods of prosperity and slump were a characteristic feature of the industrial history of Great Britain in the nineteenth century and down to 1913. During the nineteenth century periods of boom and depression followed one another with great regularity. Lord Beveridge has compiled a table to show the crests and troughs of business activity from 1792 to 1913.[1] During this period of 121 years the intervals between booms were as follows:

11, 7, 8, 7, 11, 9, 8, 7, 5, 9, 8, 7, 10, 7, 7 years.

This gives an average of eight years between one boom and the next. A study of the time intervals between crests and troughs is instructive. Taking first the down-swing, that is, the interval between boom and slump—the intervals are as follows:

5, 5, 6, 3, 7, 6, 4, 5, 2, 2, 5, 4, 4, 4, 2 years.

This gives an average of 4·26 years. The up-swing of the cycle shows the following intervals:

6, 2, 2, 4, 4, 3, 4, 2, 3, 7, 3, 3, 6, 3, 5 years.

This yields an average of only 3·66 years. These figures show clearly the business cycle during the period 1792–1913 (see Fig. 74, p. 360). A feature, therefore, of the period down to 1914 was a fairly regular cycle of alternating trade booms and depressions, neither lasting longer than a few years at a time. The First World War, however, completely upset the rhythm of the cycle, and during the war itself business activity soared to a higher level than ever before.

Although there were indications of cyclical conditions at each end of the inter-war period (in 1919–25 and again in 1935–39), these years

[1] W. H. Beveridge: *Full Employment in a Free Society*, p. 281.

were characterised by a world-wide trade depression of a severity, length and extent never previously experienced.

The periods of depression before 1914 were very short compared with the long inter-war depression. Before 1914 the population of Great Britain was expanding rapidly, and the consequent expansion of the economy soon brought a depression to an end. The world economy, too, during the nineteenth century was being rapidly enlarged by the opening up of new countries. In such conditions declining industries often do not decline absolutely, but only relatively to

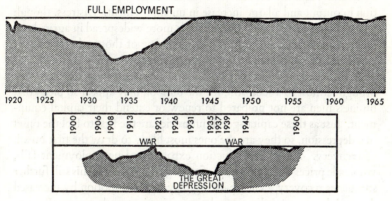

FIG. 80.—EMPLOYMENT.

the expanding industries. Even when recovery from the Great Depression at last occurred and the trade cycle appeared to be reasserting itself, the so-called boom of 1937 was accompanied by unemployment at a higher level than in any pre-1914 depression. During the Second World War it took several years of expanding production for war purposes to reach full employment, but eventually a level of output and employment was achieved greater than at any time before.

The years since 1945 have been characterised in Great Britain, the United States and most European countries by a period of almost continuous boom conditions. In Great Britain average unemployment for the country as a whole has never approached 5%, and in many areas it has been below 2%. For most countries, too, it has been a period of record economic growth. A number of mild recessions, however, have occurred, as in 1948–49, 1953–54, 1957–58 and 1961–62 in the United States, and 1951, 1955 and 1960–61 in Great Britain. The British recessions were all associated with curbs on credit following periods of severe inflationary pressure and difficulty with the balance of payments.

(2) SOME GENERAL FEATURES OF THE CYCLE

In addition to its regularity, there are certain other features common to each phase of the trade cycle. Periods of depression are characterised by low industrial production and unemployment of resources, both human and material. The national income is low, partly because of unemployment, and partly because the average income of those who succeed in avoiding unemployment is low. In agriculture output may fall little, but prices and farmers' incomes fall considerably. In manufacturing industry prices also fall, but not to the same extent as in agriculture, and the depression there manifests itself in a severe reduction in output and a large increase in unemployment. Distress, though generally less severe and less obvious, is more widespread in agriculture than in manufacturing industry, where some of those who remain at work actually find that their *real* wages increase.

In the capital-goods industries, for example, production may be brought almost to a standstill, for the outlook may appear so bleak that business men are not prepared to renew or extend their capital equipment. Just as these capital-goods industries are the first to feel the onset of a depression, so they are the ones most likely to draw the first breath of recovery. Then, as production expands and unemployment falls, wholesale prices begin to rise, profit margins widen, and this still further stimulates recovery. The up-swing may be set in motion by increased demand due to expanding population, as in nineteenth-century Britain, or by the development of some new line of investment, such as the housing boom in Great Britain in the 1930s. Encouragement to recovery may be given by a low rate of interest—though this may have little effect at the bottom of a depression—for an expansion of bank credit is characteristic of the up-swing of the cycle, just as a contraction of credit is a feature of the down-swing. Stock-exchange prices reflect the attitude of investors towards future trade prospects, and the optimistic or pessimistic feeling engendered by their movement may be infectious. Retail prices generally rise slowly until the later stages of a boom, but if full employment is reached and the boom is unchecked inflation will result. In such a case, once the unsoundness of the position has been realised, the boom may end in a crash, and the return to depression may be precipitous. Prices fall, profit margins are reduced or wiped out, entrepreneurs cautiously curtail their output and unemployment becomes widespread throughout industry.

(3) THE ORIGIN OF THE TRADE CYCLE

The late-nineteenth-century economists—Jevons and Marshall, for example—were aware of the swing of the pendulum of business activity, but it was the length and the severity of the Great Depression of 1929–35 that really focused the attention of economists upon this economic problem. Much was written on the question both by professional economists and by amateurs, the former group seeking to find some satisfactory explanation of the cycle, the latter more often looking round for some institution or section of the community on whom to lay the blame for the troubles of the time. The commonest scapegoat was the banks, but others blamed the Government or the timidity of business men, or pointed an accusing finger at the thrifty for saving too much. Some said the cause was to be found in over-production, others in under-consumption. Some wanted to deflate prices and wages; others wished to inflate. The multiplicity of explanations put forward shows that there was not a single cause, but many causes.

So although many different theories of the trade cycle have been advanced, the acceptance of one theory does not necessarily imply a complete rejection of all the others, for the true explanation of the cycle is probably made up of elements from many theories.

The features of some of the more important theories of the trade cycle must now be considered.

II. REAL CAUSES OF BUSINESS FLUCTUATIONS

(4) AGE DISTRIBUTION OF DURABLE CAPITAL

There appear to be inherent causes of fluctuations in industries producing capital goods because of the durability of such goods. If an industry making commodity A requires seventy units of capital B to produce it, and if each unit of B has a "life" of seven years a fixed stock of this type of capital can be maintained if ten units of it are replaced each year. Provided that no change in demand takes place, production of capital B can be kept at a steady output of ten units per year, and in any given year, at the moment of replacement there will be ten units aged one year, ten aged two years, ten aged three years and so on, the oldest ten units being seven years old and due for renewal. To cover this replacement will require the production of ten units of capital B each year.

Provided that no other disturbing factors arise, the provision of capital for the manufacture of commodity A can proceed smoothly, but if, for any reason, this rhythm of production is upset a permanent wave of fluctuation may be set in motion. Such a disturbance could be caused by a temporary change of demand. Suppose that an expansion of demand occurs for commodity A, to produce which twenty additional units of capital B are required, and then suppose that the following year demand drops back to its former level. No new capital will be needed for two years, so that in future, instead of an equal amount of capital (viz. ten units) having to be renewed each year, there will be one year when thirty units have to be renewed and two years when no renewals take place. The following table will make this clear:

TABLE LXIV

Age Distribution of Capital

Year	Ages of units of capital							Total	Annual production
	1 year	2 years	3 years	4 years	5 years	6 years	7 years		
1	10	10	10	10	10	10	10	70	10
2	30	10	10	10	10	10	10	90	30
3	0	30	10	10	10	10	10	80	0
4	0	0	30	10	10	10	10	70	0
5	10	0	0	30	10	10	10	70	10
6	10	10	0	0	30	10	10	70	10
7	10	10	10	0	0	30	10	70	10
8	10	10	10	10	0	0	30	70	10
9	30	10	10	10	10	0	0	70	30

This table shows that in Year 1 the industry has a total stock of seventy units of capital, equally distributed among the seven age-groups, and that ten units are produced that year. In Year 2 the increase in demand results in thirty units being produced, but in Years 3 and 4 production falls to nil. Before this disturbance took place ten units of capital were produced each year; afterwards production varies from none to thirty units per year, and assuming no futher disturbance occurs, production will then rise and fall in a regular cycle (Fig. 81). These fluctuations will be further exaggerated when transmitted to the industry making the machine tools to produce capital B—hence the term "acceleration principle." From such fluctuations in the production of durable capital goods some people believe that the trade cycle is born.

The greatest recent disturbances to the economic system have been the two world wars. In time of war there is a tendency to live on capital, in order to concentrate production on the essentials of war, a combatant country hoping the war will end before failure to make good depreciation dislocates production. Capital goods are made to last longer, and no regular yearly renewals take place, so that immediately the war ends it is necessary to embark upon a big programme

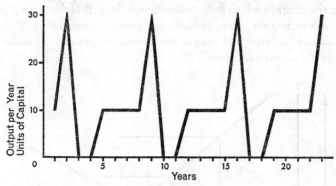

FIG. 81.—OUTPUT OF CAPITAL GOODS.

of capital replacement. The age distribution of many capital goods may then be as follows:

	Ages of units of capital							Total	Annual production
	1 year	2 years	3 years	4 years	5 years	6 years	7 years		
Pre–war	50	50	50	50	50	50	50	350	50
Post–war	200	0	0	0	50	50	50	350	200

For the next three years production will be at the pre-war level of 50 per year, but after that there will be three years when none of this type of capital requires replacement. This distortion of the age distribution of capital is particularly noticeable in capital-producing industries, where the demand for a commodity is derived from the demand for another commodity.

(5) FLUCTUATIONS IN AGRICULTURAL OUTPUT

Violent fluctuations in output are liable to occur in any industry where supply adjusts itself slowly to changes in demand, because a long period must elapse between the taking of the decision to produce, and the beginning of the flow of the product on to the market. The immediate effect of an increase in demand is a steep rise in price, because in the short period supply is fixed. This high price makes producers over-optimistic, so that they plan for a larger output than is justified by the change in demand. When this extra supply comes on to the market a steep fall in price occurs, and this then makes producers over-pessimistic, with the result that production is seriously curtailed.

The rise in prices which follows sets the whole cycle of fluctuating production in motion again. The diagrammatic representation of these fluctuations in price and output has a cobweb appearance—hence its name of "cobweb theorem":

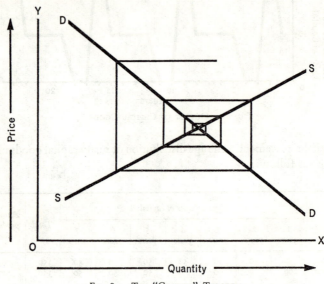

FIG. 82.—THE "COBWEB" THEOREM.

The fluctuations in output may have their origin in a temporary reduction of supply due perhaps to an exceptionally bad harvest. Price rises, and this encourages over-production, and price then falls, leading to a reduction of output and so on. The cobweb theorem is doubtless a gross exaggeration, possibly because it can be effectively represented by a diagram only if the fluctuations are excessively violent. A more correct representation would merely show a ring of small oscillations round the point of intersection of the supply and demand curves. If these fluctuations in production have their origin in a change in demand it is probable that they will gradually diminish in intensity, as shown in Fig. 83, and finally disappear as a new position of equilibrium is established.

(6) IRREGULARITY OF ECONOMIC PROGRESS

In a progressive economy there will always be some forms of production that are declining while new forms are being developed. Such changes require resources—land, labour, capital and the entrepreneur—to be transferred from old to new occupations, and the more specific the factors of production, the more difficult the transfer becomes.[1] It cannot be denied that this is a real cause of fluctuation in production, for economic development is irregular, periods of rapid and slow progress alternating with one another, although there has been a general tendency for technical progress to become increasingly rapid. There is, however, little to show that these fluctuations are cyclical.

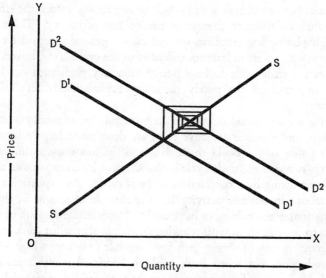

FIG. 83.—DECLINING FLUCTUATIONS.

It is clear, nevertheless, that there are a number of real causes why production and employment vary from year to year, some of which show a short-period cyclical trend. Jevons attempted to explain the trade cycle in terms of real causes. His was a theory based on harvest fluctuations—sometimes called the "Sun-spot theory" because it was thought that harvests were influenced by sun-spots. He noticed that periodically there was a poor harvest, and he thought that when this occurred its influence was transmitted to other industries. There is no doubt that agricultural output due to vagaries of the weather is subject to wide unforeseen fluctuations from one year to another, but it has already been seen that farmers and, indeed, all producers of commodities for which there is a fairly inelastic demand often enjoy larger incomes in a poor season, when supplies are small, than in a season of bumper harvest.[2] That there are real causes of the trade cycle few people will deny, but no one today would try to explain the cycle solely

[1] See pp. 45–47. [2] See pp. 188–190.

s

in real terms. On the other hand, there are others who, attaching little importance to real causes, regard the trade cycle as a purely monetary phenomenon.

III. OTHER THEORIES OF THE TRADE CYCLE

(7) PURELY MONETARY THEORIES

A number of writers on trade-cycle theory strongly stress the effect on business activity of changes in the volume of money. The rest, though placing less emphasis on this factor, generally consider that monetary causes are at least contributory to the cycle. Few, however, believe the trade cycle to be a purely monetary phenomenon. The chief exponent of the purely monetary explanation is Sir Ralph Hawtrey.

In the modern economic system the principal kind of money is bank deposits, and these, as we have seen, are determined largely by the credit policy of the banks themselves and the monetary authorities. The up-swing of the trade cycle is characterised by an expansion, and the down-swing by a contraction, of bank credit. An explanation of fluctuations in business activity has therefore been sought in these fluctuations in the volume of bank credit. Many businesses look to the banks to provide them with working capital, so that when bank loans are relatively easy to obtain, such firms are able to finance a high level of production, but when bank credit is restricted many firms are unable to obtain the funds necessary for the purchase of raw materials or the payment of wages, and so are compelled to curtail production. It is said that banks periodically tend to expand credit to excess, the fact that advances to customers are their most profitable activity often inducing them to do so. This tendency is encouraged by competition between different banks, a bank often being unwilling to refuse to lend to a customer, for fear he should be driven to one of his rivals. We have seen that a single bank cannot by itself expand credit, though, subject to the restraining influence of the monetary authorities, all banks together can do so. The action of one bank in expanding credit may, however, encourage others to do so, since the increase in their reserves at the central bank resulting from one bank's expansion of credit will enable the others also to expand credit.

The principal instrument employed to influence credit expansion or contraction was the rate of interest. In a boom, however, optimism regarding the future trend of business may run so high that the rate of interest would have to be exceptionally high in order to discourage borrowers; in a depression the outlook may appear so dark that business men will not borrow at any price. In the case of credit contraction, this can be supported by more direct action: the bank can become more eclectic in its choice of borrowers. Thus the monetary authorities could more easily terminate a boom than initiate recovery from a depression. Sir Ralph Hawtrey thinks, however, that the rate of interest makes its influence felt through its effect on merchants rather than on manufacturers. To them even a slight change in the rate of interest affects the cost of financing the holding of stocks, and consequently their desire to borrow from banks. A rise in the rate of interest will cause the merchant to allow his stocks to run down, with the result that manufacturers suffer a reduction in orders; a fall in the rate of interest has the opposite effect, merchants building up their stocks, and their orders to manufacturers stimulating production. The effect is cumulative, and from small beginnings boom or depression results. It is only because there are limits to the creation of credit (again according to Hawtrey) that the boom changes to depression, and, since the supply of cash is more rigidly fixed on the gold standard, the ending of the even rhythm of the cycle, and the departure from the full gold standard in 1914, are not unrelated events.

It is quite true that bank deposits are a fairly accurate barometer of business activity, rising as business improves and falling as it slackens, but this does not necessarily mean that there is a causal connection between them. According to Prof. Sayers,[1] the bank plays a passive rôle in the trade cycle, for usually, he says, bank advances begin to increase only after the up-swing of the cycle has developed, and to decrease only after business activity has passed its peak. The banks may, of course, intervene to check a boom which is in danger of passing into an excessive inflationary phase, but if so they do not cause the down-swing, but merely prevent the occurrence of a more serious crisis.

Saving, it has been seen, makes possible the production of capital goods, because it enables factors of production to be transferred from making consumers' goods, the demand for which falls as saving increases. Inflation caused by an expansion of bank credit brings about a rise in prices, and similarly curtails the demand for consumers' goods, thereby releasing factors for the production of capital goods. Since this has the same economic effect as saving, it has been called "forced saving." Sir Dennis Robertson took the view that periodic inflation by the banks might be advantageous at times when it was desirable to supplement voluntary by forced saving.

Excessive creation of credit by banks, said Wicksell, may be due to the fact that the *natural* rate of interest often diverges from the actual or

[1] R. S. Sayers: *Modern Banking*, Chapter IX.

market rate. By natural rate he meant the equilibrium rate which would equate the demand for loans with the supply of loanable funds. The market rate is the actual rate charged by banks to borrowers, and this may be above or below the natural rate. If the two rates are not identical it must be due, he thought, to an error of judgment on the part of the banks. If the market rate is below the natural rate there will be an excessive demand to borrow from the banks and a tendency for an over-issue of credit to take place.

(8) OVER-INVESTMENT THEORIES

The first industries to feel the effect of the onset of a boom or depression are industries making capital goods, and therefore the explanation of the trade cycle may perhaps be found in these fluctuations of real investment. Members of the Austrian School of economists consider that monetary causes are only partly responsible for the cycle. Prof. Hayek starts from the influence of the rate of interest, but to him its principal effect is on the structure of production. If the rate is low this encourages a lengthening of the structure of production—that is, production becomes more specialised, more capitalistic or more "roundabout," because greater division of labour is introduced. The reduction in the rate of interest may be brought about by an increase in saving, voluntary or forced, the increased saving expanding the demand for producers' goods relatively to the demand for consumers' goods, for saving decreases the demand for consumers' goods, thereby releasing factors of production for making producers' goods. At the lower rate of interest many lines of investment become profitable that were previously unprofitable. Over-investment, however, results, for there is a tendency for too many forms of investment to be undertaken and for the structure of production to be unduly lengthened, with the result that the stock of capital is greater than is required to produce the consumers' goods demanded. When the rate of interest rises it becomes necessary to shorten the structure of production, some intermediate stages being no longer profitable.

One of the difficulties of this approach is that it associates an increased demand for consumers' goods with a falling off in the production of producers' goods. Obviously, factors of production cannot at the same time be used for the production of both consumers' goods and producers' goods, and if more factors are used in one branch of production, there are clearly fewer factors available for the other. The demand for producers' goods, however, is derived from the demand for consumers' goods, and where the producers' goods are raw materials the two demands are even more closely related, since the demand for raw materials is directly related to the demand for the finished goods made from them. It is difficult to see, therefore, how an increased demand for consumers' goods can cause a fall in the demand for producers' goods.

(9) UNDER-CONSUMPTION THEORIES

The notion that there is a tendency for purchasing power permanently to fall short of the amount required to purchase what has been produced is the main feature of under-compensation theories. As a result of technological improvements and capital accumulation there is a secular—as distinct from a cyclical—expansion of production, and the volume of purchasing power fails to keep pace with it. The reason for this, it is said, is that some purchasing power is lost to the economic system because all costs of production do not return to consumers as purchasing power. The supporters of the cruder versions of the theory declare therefore that the quantity of purchasing power needs to be continuously increased, and they suggest that this should be accomplished by periodic gifts of money to the community at large, the amount in some way, perhaps, being dependent on the volume of production.

Purchasing power is lost, it is said, when producers purchase raw materials or new capital, when sums are put aside to cover depreciation, or when interest payments or repayments of loans are made to the banks. The fallacy of lost purchasing power can easily be demonstrated by the following diagram, showing the distribution of costs of production at various stages between payments for wages, rent and profits, and payments for raw materials:

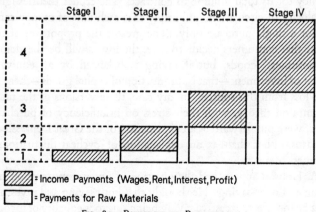

Fig. 84.—Payments to Production.

Stage IV is the final stage in the process of production of some commodity—for example, worsted cloth. Stage I will, then, consist of the production of the raw material by sheep-farmers. In order to simplify the diagram, the many intermediate processes have been combined, and reduced to two—Stages II and III. At the final stage, as the under-consumptionists say, only part of the costs of production—wage payments, rents, interest and profits—become income to consumers. Costs incurred in the purchase of partly processed materials at Stage IV become revenue to the producers at Stage III, whose costs can again be divided between income payments to owners of factors of production and payments to partly processed goods. The payments made at every intermediate stage can be similarly analysed. At the primary stage (Stage I) in the production of any commodity in an extractive industry —mining, some branch of farming, lumbering, fishing, etc.—where the costs of production may consist entirely of wage and other income payments.

It is clear, therefore, that the whole of the costs incurred in producing this piece of cloth have already become income to those who assisted in its manufacture. It will be remembered that it is just because this is so that the national income can be calculated either as the total volume of production or as the sum of all individual incomes.[1] Every commodity is nothing more than a "bundle of services," the cost of each process in its manufacture being merely the price of a particular service. There is thus no loss of purchasing power because costs of production include payments for raw materials or partly processed goods. Nor is there any such loss from the repayment of bank loans, for though the volume of bank credit fluctuates from time to time, there is no general tendency for its total volume to contract. The cruder theories ignore the velocity of circulation, and imply that each unit of money can be used for a single purchase only. The greater the proportion of their income that consumers decide to save, the lower will be the demand for consumers' goods, but if saving is balanced by an equivalent amount of investment—that is, production of capital goods—there will be no loss from this source. In any case, these versions of the under-consumption theory, with their stress on insufficiency of purchasing power, were put forward as an explanation of the Great Depression of the 1930s rather than as an explanation of cyclical fluctuations in consumers' demand.

J. A. Hobson approached the question of under-consumption from the angle of over-saving. He thought that both saving and investment might be too great, excessive saving being due to inequality of incomes, for generally the higher the income, the greater the proportion of it that is saved. This would mean that a high level of investment would

[1] See Chapter XVI.

lead to underconsumption and depression. Against Hobson's theory is the fact that high investment is a feature of boom years, just as a low level of investment is characteristic of a depression. Further, it is the insufficiency of demand, and not a glut of consumers' goods, that turns a trade boom into a depression.

IV. SAVING, INVESTMENT AND CONSUMPTION

(10) DEFINITIONS OF SAVING AND INVESTMENT

Saving. As we have seen, saving reduces the demand for consumers' goods and sets free resources for the production of producers' goods. That part of income not spent on consumers' goods can be said to be saved. Thus saving means refraining from consumption. The amount saved depends on several factors: the keenness of people to save (the propensity to save), the total income of the community and the way in which it is distributed. The marginal propensity to consume is the extra amount of consumption that takes place as a result of the smallest possible increase in income. The motives for saving have already been discussed.[1] It was seen then that the rate of interest has much less influence on the rate of saving than was once thought. Of much greater importance than the rate of interest is the size of a person's income. The larger one's income, the larger the proportion of it one is likely to save. For this reason the less the inequality of income between different groups of people, the less that community is likely to save. Total income depends on the level of business activity.

Investment. By investment is meant the actual production of capital goods—the building of a railway, a motorway, a road bridge or a road tunnel, the erection of a new electric generating station, building up stocks of raw materials, the manufacture of machinery, etc. Investment is thus the amount of real capital produced during a period, some of this, of course, being required to make good depreciation. The volume of investment depends partly on the rate of interest and partly on the expectations of entrepreneurs regarding the trend of business in the immediate future. If it is thought that the rate of profit is likely to be less than the rate of interest, investment will not take place. If prices are rising, profit margins will also tend to rise, and business men, taking an optimistic view of the future, will wish to increase their investment. But if prices are falling the reverse will happen, and however low the rate of interest, pessimism regarding the future will make business men generally unwilling to undertake investment.

Saving is carried out by the community at large—by individuals

[1] See pp. 330-2.

and corporate institutions; investment is partly undertaken by entre-preneurs in the private sector and partly by the State for the public sector. According to the supporters of the earlier theories of saving and investment, it was because saving was left to one group of people and investment to another that the equilibrium of the economic system was disturbed. Saving was a pre-requisite of investment, but a given amount of saving did not guarantee an equal amount of investment. In other words, fluctuations in production occurred, it was thought, because sometimes saving exceeded investment, when there would be a tendency towards a curtailment of production, and sometimes invest-ment exceeded saving, with the probable development of a boom. The problem was complicated because saving was a *monetary action* (though it has *real* consequences), whereas investment was a *real* thing.

(11) THE DETERMINATION OF INCOME AND EMPLOYMENT

Lord Keynes showed that the level of business activity and employ-ment depends on the level of income, which also determines the extent of both saving and investment. Thus Saving, Investment and Income are mutually dependent on one another. The level of consumption too depends on Income. The main influence, however, is Investment, the extent of which is mainly responsible for the level of Income. Invest-ment generates Income, and Income then determines the maximum extent of Saving and Consumption. The level of employment, there-fore, is dependent partly on the production of capital goods (Invest-ment) and partly on the production of consumers' goods (Consump-tion). A high level of Consumption, too, stimulates further Investment:

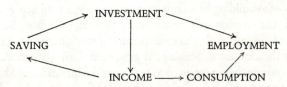

Equilibrium can occur at any level of employment, and so the objective becomes the achievement of equilibrium at full employment.

Keynes's psychological influences. Keynes stressed the importance of a number of psychological influences on saving, investment and con-sumption. Three sets of causes of the trade cycle can therefore be dis-tinguished—real causes, monetary factors and psychological influences. It has already been pointed out that the trade cycle cannot be satis-factorily explained in terms of any one of these sets of causes, but only in a combination of them. The following are the psychological influences of Lord Keynes:

(i) *The propensity to consume,* that is, the keenness or otherwise of people to buy consumers' goods.

(ii) *The propensity to save,* that is, the keenness or otherwise of people to refrain from the purchase of consumers' goods.

(iii) *Liquidity-preference,* which indicates people's demand for money as distinct from investing it. Three reasons for holding money were distinguished by Keynes, the third—the speculative motive—being psychological in character and dependent on estimates of the future trend in the rate of interest.

(iv) *Expectations.* An important influence on the level of investment is the expectation of business men regarding the future level of business activity. This was no new idea, as A. C. Pigou had previously referred to business men being influenced by alternating waves of optimism and pessimism. Keynes, however, related expectations to the prospective yield of capital. The amount of investment undertaken in a period depends on whether entrepreneurs expect the yield from capital investment to exceed the rate of interest. This Keynes termed *the marginal efficiency of capital,* which he defined as the relation between the prospective yield of one more unit of capital and the cost of producing it.

The following diagram summarises the situation:

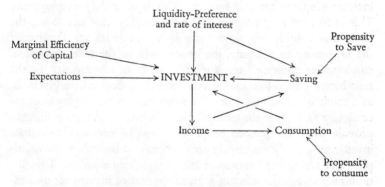

The diagram shows that there are five influences on investment—expectations, the marginal efficiency of capital, the rate of interest, saving and consumption. Three influences on saving are distinguished—income, the rate of interest and the propensity to save. Two factors are shown as influencing consumption—income and the propensity to consume.

Keynes developed his theories during the most severe trade depression ever experienced, his aim being to show how a high level of employment could be maintained. He refuted the argument of Say (the

Law of Markets) that supply created its own demand, that production itself instigates a demand for what has been produced. Thus Keynes can be described as an under-consumptionist, but unlike the exponents of the crude under-consumption theories, he did not propose to increase directly the amount of purchasing power in the hands of consumers. Instead, this would occur indirectly as a result of increased investment.

The concept of the multiplier. A given amount of investment, whether private or public, will create a greater amount of employment than that directly concerned with the actual production of the additional capital goods. For example, suppose that 1,000 men are employed upon a new Government project. Part of the expenditure is directly incurred in paying wages to these men, part is profit to the entrepreneur and part is devoted to the purchase of raw materials. It was seen above that all the expenses of production eventually become income to some people.[1] The amount of employment directly created in this way is termed primary employment. Because of their increased incomes, these people increase their expenditure on consumers' goods. A proportion of these incomes, however, may be saved, and so the expansion of demand will depend on the propensity to consume. The increased demand for consumers' goods will stimulate demand and increase employment still further. This is secondary employment. This in its turn may produce still more employment and so on, the amount of additional employment at each stage declining. The greater the propensity to consume, the greater will be the total amount of employment resulting from a given amount of investment. To the ratio between these two amounts the term *multiplier* has been given. If, as a result of providing work for 1,000 men, total employment increases by 3,000, then the multiplier is 3. In such conditions in order to provide work for 300,000 people it would be necessary to initiate investment directly employing only 100,000. It is through the multiplier that saving and investment are brought into equality. Thus the multiplier shows the effect of a given amount of investment on consumption in contrast to the acceleration principle, which shows the effect of consumption on investment.

(12) THE EQUALITY OF SAVING AND INVESTMENT

Lord Keynes, in his most famous work, *The General Theory of Employment, Interest and Money*, declared that saving and investment are always equal. Consider his proof of this assertion. Personal income can either be spent or saved. Since, therefore, part of the total of

---

[1] See p. 521.

personal incomes—the national income—will be spent on consumers' goods and part will be saved, it follows that:

$$\text{National income} = \text{Amount spent on} + \text{Amount} \atop \text{consumers' goods} \quad \text{saved}$$

that is:

$$\text{Income} = \text{Consumption} + \text{Saving.}$$

Therefore:

$$\text{Saving} = \text{Income} - \text{Consumption.}$$

Regarding national income now in real terms as the volume of production, which consists partly of consumers' goods and partly of producers' goods, we have the following equation:

$$\text{National income} = \text{Amount of con-} + \text{Amount of pro-} \atop \text{sumers' goods} \quad \text{ducers' goods} \atop \text{produced} \quad \text{produced}$$

The production of producers' goods is known as investment, and so:

$$\text{Income} = \text{Consumption} + \text{Investment.}$$

Therefore:

$$\text{Investment} = \text{Income} - \text{Consumption.}$$

By the first line of reasoning Income − Consumption is equal to Saving, and by the second Income − Consumption is equal to Investment. Therefore:

$$\text{Saving} = \text{Investment}$$

In the case of someone like Robinson Crusoe, saving and investment would always be equal, because the two actions of saving and investing could be performed only at one and the same time. He would simply transfer his efforts from one form of production to the other. But in a modern society saving and investment are undertaken by different groups of people, and the factors that influence the propensity to save are not the same as those which influence the propensity of entrepreneurs to undertake investment.

Keynes, however, contended that if any new investment occurs there must be an equivalent amount of saving, for if people save, instead of spending, stocks of goods (investment) will increase by exactly the same amount. If saving declines, investment will be similarly reduced, for stocks will not require to be replenished, and so production will be curtailed by the same amount as that by which saving has declined. If the money value of investment is reduced by a fall in prices the incomes of sellers will be reduced, and consequently saving also, since saving depends on income. Therefore it is through changes in income that equality of saving and investment is brought about.

It is only recently that the great controversy arising from Keynes's assertion that saving and investment are always equal has died down. The two opposing views, (i) that booms or slumps are the result of saving and investment not being equal, and (ii) that saving and investment are always equal, have been reconciled by the British economists, Sir Dennis Robertson and Sir Ralph Hawtrey, and Professor Ohlin of Sweden, by the so-called period analysis. Income received in one period becomes available for spending only in the next period. Therefore the amount of saving and consumption undertaken in one period both depend on the income generated by the investment of the previous period. Thus, though the saving of one period is equal to the investment of the previous period, saving and investment will rarely be equal to one another in the same period.

V. FULL EMPLOYMENT

(13) CAUSES OF UNEMPLOYMENT

There are various causes of unemployment. Therefore, before plans can be formulated for maintaining full employment, it is necessary to distinguish between these different causes, for only after this diagnosis has been made can the appropriate remedy be applied. The following types of unemployment can be distinguished:

(i) *Mass unemployment.* Sometimes known as cyclical unemployment, on account of its association with the trade cycle, it is the most serious type, for it is characterised by a general deficiency of demand. The result is that it affects nearly all industries at one and the same time —though not all to the same extent—and it produces widespread unemployment. During the nineteenth century neither boom nor slump lasted very long, the level of unemployment in a slump rarely exceeding 10%. During that period 1879 was the year of severest slump, with over 10%.

The most serious example of mass unemployment occurred between the two world wars, when there was a period of prolonged depression, during which unemployment among insured workers fell below 10% only in 1927, when it was 9·7%. In 1937, which marked the peak of recovery, 10·8% of insured workers were still unemployed. In the inter-war period therefore unemployment was at a higher level in the best years, than it generally was in the worst years before 1914. In the worst of the depression years unemployment rose to 17% in 1921, and to 22·1% in 1932. It was not only the gravity of unemployment which characterised the inter-war slump but the length of time it lasted, for Great Britain suffered some years of depression before the onset of the world slump in 1929.

(ii) *Frictional unemployment.* The economic development of a country frequently requires factors of production to be switched from one form of employment to another. If all factors, including labour, were non-specific transfer would be easier: it is mainly because this is not so that economic frictions occur, and factors become unemployed because the demand for their services in their present occupations has fallen off, although at the same time there may be a demand for labour in other occupations. This is the essential feature of frictional unemployment. Since so much labour is immobile, in both the geographical and the occupational senses, labour is particularly prone to this kind of unemployment. Economic friction arises from a variety of causes:

(a) *Change of demand.* This may occur for no other reason than a mere change of taste, as for example a preference for prepared breakfast cereals instead of oatmeal porridge. Or a change in demand may be the result of economic progress, some new commodity superseding an older one because it is superior to it in some way. The building of railways, for example, stimulated the demand for all kinds of railway equipment, but caused a fall in the demand for horse-drawn vehicles. As a result, most of the old coachmen, who formerly had carried the mail so proudly to its destination on time, soon found themselves out of work, for the "mechanics" who built or drove the new steam locomotives were men of a different stamp from the coachmen.

We have already seen that there are many causes of change in demand. At any time, therefore, there will be expanding industries and declining industries. A shift of demand from one commodity to another results in a fall in the demand for labour and other factors in one industry, and an increase in the demand for labour and other factors in another. If the labour could be easily transferred from the declining to the expanding industry no unemployment would occur. Labour, however, is not perfectly mobile, and even during the Great Depression there were expanding industries in some areas in which the level of unemployment was much lower than the average for the country as a whole. Such expanding industries were the motorcar industry in the Midlands and the new light industries that came to be established on the outer fringe of London. Where a declining industry is highly localised, a trade depression is exaggerated, and unemployment will be above the average, as in the distressed areas before 1939.

Unemployment due to a change in demand is called *structural unemployment* because it is caused by a change in the country's industrial structure, the switching of production from one kind of work to another. Such a change produces unemployment only because of the immobility of factors of production. It is possible, however, for structural unemployment to occur when an industry suffers a decline in the demand for its product without any compensating new demand arising. This is most likely to occur in the case of an industry manufacturing chiefly for export. It was largely because of the contraction of its export trade that the Lancashire cotton industry declined.

(b) *Technical progress.* Frictional unemployment, too, may result from the invention of a new machine or an innovation which may reduce the demand for labour in the industry concerned. The invention of the automatic loom, for example, reduced the demand for weavers in both the cotton and woollen industries. The introduction of office machinery—typewriters, computers, book-keeping machines, etc.—has resulted in the employment of fewer clerks, except, of course, where for other reasons the volume of work has increased. We have already seen that, even if in the short run machines have displaced some labour in the industries in which they have been introduced, in the long run a new or increased demand for labour has generally arisen elsewhere. Fewer people may be required in weaving, but more people perhaps will be wanted for the manufacture of looms. Fewer clerks may be needed, but instead there will be an increased demand for labour in industries making office machinery. Since, however, economic progress often causes people to lose their jobs, it has been thought only equitable to give them compensation in the form of "redundancy payments."

(iii) *Seasonal unemployment.* In some outdoor occupations, such as building and road making, bad weather often causes a suspension of work, so that temporary unemployment occurs. The weather, too, may prevent a fishing fleet putting out to sea. In some occupations there is a demand for labour only at certain periods of the year—hop-picking, potato-lifting, fruit-gathering, entertaining at holiday resorts, etc. Irregularity of employment at the docks led at one time to the amount of labour available often being greater than the amount required. Sometimes, however, it may be possible to combine seasonal occupations, such as the raising of sugar beet in summer with working in the sugar factory in winter.

(iv) *Residual unemployment.* This includes all those people who, on account of physical or mental disability, are of so low a standard of efficiency that few, if any, occupations are open to them. Payment of standard rates of wages, too, makes it more difficult for people so handicapped to find work. During both world wars the demand for labour exceeded the supply, but unemployment did not completely disappear. In addition, there are a few people who prefer to work no more than the minimum necessary for bare subsistence!

(14) FULL EMPLOYMENT AS A POLICY

There is not complete agreement as to what is meant by full employment. Lord Beveridge defined it as a situation where there are "more jobs than men" but other economists would consider this to be a state of "over-full" employment. A condition of full employment can be said to exist if the number of unfilled vacancies is equal to the number of people who are out of work. In such a case the reason why people are unemployed is to be found in the fact that labour is not perfectly mobile. The principal aim of a policy of full employment is to eradicate mass unemployment due to a general deficiency of demand. Other causes of unemployment are mainly frictional in character. As a result, full employment does not mean that there is work for everybody at all times. In such conditions, however, the volume of unemployment should be small, only comprising an ever-changing group of people transferring from one kind of work to another.

In spite of the prolonged depression of the 1930s, it was not until 1944 that the State accepted responsibility for full employment. The classical doctrine that supply creates its own demand remained unshaken, in spite of the efforts of the under-consumptionists, until Keynes put forward the view that deficiency of demand was due to the level of investment being too low. He, therefore, took the view that the Government itself should undertake investment when private investment was insufficient to provide full employment.

In 1944 the Government published a White Paper on *Employment Policy*, in which it declared itself "prepared to accept future responsibility for taking action at the earliest possible stage to arrest a threatened slump."[1] Lord Beveridge described this declaration as "epoch-marking,"[2] for previously the British Treasury had always clung to the view that the State was powerless to increase permanently the volume of employment. A few days after the White Paper came the publication of Lord Beveridge's *Full Employment in a Free Society*, giving a comprehensive survey of the unemployment problem, together with proposals for maintaining full employment. Unemployment between the two wars was not a problem of cyclical fluctuations, but was, Beveridge says, "a problem of general and persistent weakness

[1] Cmd. 6527 (H.M.S.O.). § 41.
[2] Lord Beveridge: *Full Employment in a Free Society*, Postscript.

of demand for labour," the root of the trouble being the existence of "a chronic deficiency of demand."

He laid down four conditions for the maintenance of full employment:

(*i*) There must be adequate expenditure, public and private, in order to create sufficient total income to prevent a deficiency of demand. In a trade slump it may be necessary for the Government deliberately to unbalance the Budget in order to stimulate demand.

(*ii*) The location of industry must be controlled. Where industries are highly localised, changes in demand may cause structural unemployment of so severe a character as to produce pockets of mass unemployment. This danger is lessened the greater the diversity of industry in an area.

(*iii*) There must also be organised mobility of labour, for, in a progressive economy, there will always be some industries which are declining while others are expanding. A policy of full employment does not mean, therefore, that labour can be guaranteed employment in a particular job in a particular place. When frictional unemployment occurs it will be necessary to retrain for work in other occupations those who are unemployed on this account.

(*iv*) If inflation is to be avoided the trade unions must adopt a responsible attitude to the situation.

Lord Beveridge did not aim merely at levelling out the ups and downs of the trade cycle. It was not enough for the Government to undertake public works in times of trade depression. What is required is a level of investment that will give full employment. Therefore if private investment proves to be insufficient to achieve this aim it must be supplemented by public investment. At the present day almost half the total investment in Great Britain comes from the public sector.

(15) PROBLEMS OF FULL EMPLOYMENT

Experience has shown that the maintenance of full employment produces problems of its own:

(i) *The danger of inflation is increased.* There are two reasons for this:

(*a*) Over-investment is likely to occur. It is impossible to calculate exactly how much public investment is required to yield full employment, neither more nor less. In its anxiety to ensure full employment, a Government may be inclined to undertake too much investment, and so a condition of inflation will be induced, with the demand for labour greater than the supply.

(*b*) *The wages policy of the trade unions.* Full employment puts the trade unions in a strong bargaining position. In the past, in times of depression, trade unions have had to submit to some reduction in money wages, and have had to wait for times of boom to secure wage increases for their members. If full employment is permanently maintained the situation becomes quite different—conditions are favourable to the trade unions all the time. If over-full employment exists, the problem will be intensified, for shortages of labour in many occupations will lead to proposals being put forward for raising wages in those occupations in order to attract more labour to them. Since in these conditions, however, labour can be drawn only from other occupations, wage increases will be demanded elsewhere as a means of retaining labour! Increased wages in one occupation lead to increased wages in others. In these conditions, costs can generally be passed on to consumers, and so rising wages are followed by rising prices, which in turn give rise to further demands for wage increases. In this way the inflationary spiral is kept in motion, and is difficult to arrest.

It was for this reason that the British Government in 1964–66 tried to persuade the trade unions to agree to an "incomes policy," under which increases in wages would be related to the rate of increase in productivity.

(ii) *A maldistribution of resources may occur.* Another serious danger is that economic resources will not easily move from one occupation to another. Changing conditions may reduce the demand for factors in one employment and increase the demand for factors in another. Instead of a transfer of factors taking place there will be demands for the declining industry to be subsidised—especially if it happens to be a nationalised industry, such as the railways—or protected by a tariff if foreign competition is severe. If economic forces are not allowed to determine the distribution of factors among different occupations the assortment of goods produced will not be that which the community as a whole prefers.

(iii) *The quality of labour may fall.* There are three reasons for this: (a) the high demand for labour makes it possible for the least efficient workers to secure employment; (b) the removal of the fear of losing one's job may, often subconsciously, cause many workers to put forward less effort, and some may deliberately slack; and (c) many workers frequently change their jobs. In spite of all this, however, the productivity of labour may rise, as it has in Great Britain during the past ten or fifteen years, as the result of the employment of more efficient capital.

In order to check inflation it has been necessary on several occasions since 1951 to damp down the expansion of credit. In most cases this policy was reversed immediately there was any increase in unemployment. A more determined effort to put an end to inflation occurred during 1957–58, with the result that for the first time since the State accepted responsibility for full employment, an expansionist policy had to be adopted in 1958–59 to restore the situation. The success of this policy in restoring full employment gives hope that a recession can be overcome if action is taken in time. It is clearly easier to prevent development of a serious slump than to overcome one if it should occur.

The long period of full employment since 1945 has tended to push the fear of unemployment somewhat into the background. At the present time when full employment appears to be the "normal" condition, the main concern has now become the rate at which production can be increased, that is, economic growth.

(16) INTERNATIONAL ASPECTS OF FULL EMPLOYMENT

The level of employment in a country such as Great Britain is to a large extent dependent on the prosperity of the export trade. In the past the trade cycle has been an international phenomenon, and fluctuations in business activity in this country have generally been accompanied by similar fluctuations in other parts of the world. The chief exception occurred in the late 1920s when Great Britain, after returning to the gold standard, ran into a slump three years ahead of the rest of the world. A decline in world trade is specially disadvantageous to Great Britain, for in addition to the loss of trade, there is also a decline in the income from the invisible items in the balance of payments. To be successful, therefore, a full employment policy needs to be international, and so all countries must strive towards this end. A balance of payments should balance, and surpluses should be lent or invested abroad. Multilateral trade must be encouraged.

The increased importance of the United States to the world economy, and the greater dependence of Western Europe on that country as a market for manufactured goods, may make it difficult to prevent a trade slump there from crossing the Atlantic. In a depression the United States can be expected to reduce its imports, and as a result the export industries of Great Britain and other countries will suffer.

Any sign of a recession of business activity in the United States is therefore closely watched by Great Britain. During the past fifteen years there have been four recessions in the United States, but only the first, that of 1948–49, had any serious consequences for Great Britain. The devaluation of sterling in 1949 was the result of a combination of circumstances, but the American recession was an important factor in the situation. The American recessions of 1953–54 and 1957–58 had surprisingly little effect on Great Britain, perhaps because of their mildness. What the effect, however, would be on Great Britain of a serious slump in the United States can only be conjectured, but it is well to remember that the American Government, like many others, is pledged to maintain full employment.

RECOMMENDATIONS FOR FURTHER READING

G. Crowther: *An Outline of Money*, Chapters 3 and 5.
G. Haberler: *Prosperity and Depression*, Part I, Chapters 1–8.
W. H. Beveridge: *Full Employment in a Free Society*.
R. F. Harrod: *The Trade Cycle*.
P. A. Samuelson: *Economics*, Chapters 12 and 13.

QUESTIONS

1. What is meant by the trade cycle? Describe critically any one explanation of the phenomenon. (Exp.)

2. "At one period the individual does better service to the community by saving all the money he can: at another by spending all he can afford." Discuss the soundness of this view and what conditions warrant additional saving and what conditions warrant extra spending. Do you regard it as the social duty of persons in England at the present time to save all they reasonably can or put their earnings into circulation so as to encourage extra production? (L.C. Com. Econ.)

3. What are the principal types of unemployment considered with reference to their major causes? (I.B.)

4. "Saving always equals investment." "It is because saving gets out of line with investment that variations in the level of national income occur." Discuss. (C.I.S. Inter.)

5. Explain the meaning of (*a*) saving, and (*b*) investment, in modern economic theory. What consequences can be expected if investment exceeds saving during (*a*) a period of less full employment; (*b*) during full employment? (A.I.A.)

6. Examine the meaning of full employment and the conditions for attaining it. (C.I.S. Final.)

7. "To secure at the same time a high average level of employment, rapidly expanding money rates (for work of given productivity) and a reasonable stability in the value of money passes the wit of man." (A. C. Pigou.)
Comment on this statement. (A.C.C.A. Final.)

8. What is meant by redundancy of labour? Suggest ways of reducing it. (I.B.)

9. "There may easily arise situations leading to unemployment, which the stabilisation of aggregate demand is unable itself to cure, although it may greatly ease whatever process of cure takes place."
Suggest some possible situations of this kind and some possible cures. (D.P.A.)

10. "By far the most important 'cause' of unemployment in a modern capitalist country is a deficiency in total expenditure." Discuss. (G.C.E. Adv.)

11. What do you understand by structural unemployment? Discuss possible remedies. (G.C.E. Adv.)

12. What factors influence the level of investment in an economy? (G.C.E. Adv.)

13. "Unemployment persists only because labour is immobile and trade unions refuse to accept cuts in money wages." Discuss. (G.C.E. Adv.)

14. "An increase in investment leads to an increase in employment *via* the multiplier." Explain carefully what is meant by this statement, making clear the assumptions necessary for it to be true. (G.C.E. Adv.)

15. Explain the meaning of the acceleration principle and discuss the conditions under which you would expect to find it operative. (Final Degree.)

16. "Experience suggests that of the three objectives—full employment, stable prices and free collective bargaining—it is possible to have any two, but not all three simultaneously." Comment. (Final Degree.)

17. Why have the severities of the pre-war trade cycle disappeared? (Final Degree.)

CHAPTER XXX

PUBLIC FINANCE

I. PURPOSES AND PRINCIPLES

(1) PURPOSES OF TAXATION

In early days Governments imposed taxes to raise revenue only to cover the cost of administration and defence, and in the case of despotic monarchs the personal expenditure of the ruler. Some services, such as the maintenance of law and order at home and defence against external enemies, it was recognised at quite an early date, could be provided more efficiently by the State than by individuals, and taxes raised to cover their cost could be regarded as payments for services provided by the State for the community as a whole.

During the past fifty years or so the British Government has vastly increased the range of services provided by the State, some indication of which can be obtained from a perusal of the items of Government expenditure listed in Table LXV on p. 538. It will be noticed that defence is still the principal purpose for which taxes are raised, though total expenditure on the social services falls only slightly short of it. Of the social services education and the health service are the most costly, but considerable sums too are expended on housing, pensions, national insurance, national assistance, family allowances and child care, most of these things requiring to be supplemented by further sums from local rates. Subsidies to agriculture, primarily for the purpose of reducing food prices, are another important object of expenditure. Quite a considerable sum too is required to pay the interest on the national debt.

As a result, the State has become the greatest spender of money in most countries today. At the present time taxation in Great Britain absorbs 25% of the national income. There is sometimes a tendency to regard money paid in taxes as lost, whereas in fact what happens is that the spending of the money is transferred to the State, most of it being returned to the community as a whole in the form of a great variety of services.

This huge volume of expenditure enables the State to exercise a great influence on the economy of the country. Nowadays, however, taxes are no longer imposed merely to cover unavoidable cost of

administration and the cost of services provided by the State, for
taxation has become an important instrument of economic policy.

TABLE LXV

Government Ordinary Expenditure

Items of Expenditure	1965–66	196–[1]
	£ million	£ million
Debt services	1,175	
Supply Services:		
1. Defence—		
Army	556 ⎫	
Navy	544 ⎪	
Air	562 ⎬ 2,120	
Ministry of Aviation (Defence) . .	255 ⎪	
Other Defence	203 ⎭	
2. Civil—		
I. Government and Exchequer . . .	109	
II. Commonwealth and Foreign . .	217	
III. Home and Justice	174	
IV. Industry, Trade and Transport . .	543	
V. Agriculture.	339	
VI. Local Government, Housing and Social Services	2,923	
VII. Education and Science	410	
VIII. Museums, Galleries and the Arts . .	10	
IX. Public Buildings and Common Government Services	189	
X. Smaller Public Departments . . .	8	
XI. Miscellaneous	92	
Total Ordinary Expenditure .	8,482	

[1] For the latest figures

(2) THE BUDGET AS AN INSTRUMENT OF ECONOMIC POLICY

The Budget is generally presented to Parliament by the Chancellor
of the Exchequer early in April. It is an estimate of revenue and
expenditure for the ensuing financial year. In times of financial crisis
revised interim budgets have had to be introduced in the autumn, as in
1931, 1947, 1955, 1961 and 1964.

In recent years two new practices have grown up in connection with
the Budget. Shortly before Budget day a number of White Papers are
published—the Economic Survey, National Income and Expenditure
and the Balance of Payments. These give details of the country's
balance of payments, the national income and summaries of production
of the basic industries—coal, iron and steel, textiles, agriculture—the
distribution of labour among different industries, investment in various
industries and personal expenditure on consumers' goods. For all

these items comparison is made with the previous year, and in the Economic Survey prospects for the current year are considered. These surveys of the nation's economic position give a fairly clear indication of the lines on which the Budget should be framed, and a Chancellor of the Exchequer cannot altogether ignore them. Though the actual Budget details of any rearrangement of taxation or expenditure are kept a close secret until they are announced in Parliament, the general framework of the Budget can often now be more clearly foreseen.

The second of the two recent changes in budgetary practice is the presentation of a full statement of all Government income and expenditure on both current account and capital account, some items of income and expenditure, mainly but not entirely of a capital nature, being shown "below-the-line." The modern British Budget therefore shows a true picture of Government income and expenditure. Before this practice was adopted, the Budget often showed a substantial surplus when actually there was a deficit if all items were taken into consideration. When the aim has been to use the Budget to check inflation a surplus of income has generally been required over all expenditure, both above and below the line. In general, it is doubtful whether all below-the-line expenditure should be covered by taxation, since the chief item comprises loans, which will eventually have to be repaid.

On p. 538 Government Ordinary Expenditure is shown. Consider now the following table giving "below-the-line" expenditure for the same year (Table LXVI).

It will be seen that most of the expenditure "below-the-line" consists mainly of capital items. Thus, the British Budget now shows what the Government intends to spend during the ensuing year on both current and capital account.

The following are some of the main ways in which the Budget can be used as an instrument of economic policy:

(i) *To stimulate recovery from a trade recession.* Except in time of war, it used to be a maxim of orthodox finance that the Budget should be balanced each year, that is, there should be neither a large surplus nor a large deficit. In the latter years of the Great Depression it was suggested that the Budget should be deliberately unbalanced (a policy known as "deficit financing") in order to promote recovery. Faced by a serious slump, this course might be necessary, but in the case of a recession it may be sufficient simply to reduce taxation. The Budget of 1958 was of this kind, and it was highly successful.

(ii) *To check inflation.* The aim of a disinflationary Budget is to reduce the amount of purchasing power in the hands of the community, and this is done by increasing the level of taxation so that a substantial

surplus is achieved. The first Budget of this type was the interim
Budget of November 1947, and since then this policy has been adopted
on a number of occasions. It is extremely doubtful whether by itself
this type of budget can be successful. If the increased taxation falls on
commodities it will raise their prices, thereby raising the cost of living
and leading trade unions to demand higher wages. As a result, the
inflationary spiral may be stimulated instead of checked.

TABLE LXVI

Government "Below-the-line" Expenditure

Items of Expenditure	1965–66	196–[1]
	£ million	£ million
Loans to Nationalised Industries	712	
Loans to Local Authorities	320	
Post-War Credits	17	
Loans for New Towns Developments . . .	52	
Loans for Overseas Assistance	81	
Loans to Private Industry	31	
Other items	57	
Total "below-the-line" Expenditure . .	1,270	

[1] For the latest figures.

(iii) *To reduce inequality of incomes.* In Great Britain inequality of
incomes has been greatly reduced by a steeply progressive income tax
and surtax, as a result of which one requires to have a gross income of
£10,000 a year in order to have £6,000 a year left after payment of
tax (see Table LXVII below). The accumulation of large fortunes has
been rendered difficult to achieve, partly because the ability to save has
been reduced, and partly because of a progressive scale of death duties,
rising to 80% of large estates, has greatly reduced the amount that can
be inherited. The number of people in Great Britain with incomes of
over £6,000 after payment of tax was 7,000 in 1938, only 200 in 1954,
but 14,000 by 1963. Between 1954 and 1963 the number of people with
incomes of less than £500 after tax declined by 6½ million, while the
number with incomes of over £1,000 after tax rose by 3½ million.
Inequality of income is still further reduced by the provision by the
State of social services which, though available to rich and poor alike, are
generally of most benefit to people in the lower-income groups.

(iv) *To assist the balance of payments.* Duties on particular imports may
be imposed or increased as in 1964–66 for the purpose of curtailing the
demand for these goods in order to reduce imports.

(3) PRINCIPLES OF TAXATION

Adam Smith enunciated four canons of taxation. In the first place, he said, the amounts people paid in taxes should be equal, by which in fact he meant proportional to their incomes. Secondly, he said that there should be certainty with regard to the amount to be paid, for it should not be a tax-gatherer's business to squeeze as much as possible from the taxpayer. Thirdly, there should be convenience of payment and collection. Fourthly, economy should be observed, so that taxes should not be imposed of a kind where the cost of collection was excessive. It has been estimated that in the case of some former taxes the expenses of collection absorbed as much as 85% of the yield. A serious objection to bringing small incomes within the orbit of income tax is the heavy cost of collection.

The proportional principle. Under this system, if a man with an annual income of £350 paid £35 in taxes, a man with an income of £5,000 would pay £500. Adam Smith supported the principle that taxation should be proportional to income, because he considered it to be the most equitable method of raising revenue open to the State. It was certainly more equitable than equality of payment—a fixed sum per head—as in the case of some poll taxes,[1] and as may occur with taxes on necessary foodstuffs. The Law of Diminishing Marginal Utility, however, shows that the marginal utility of £1 of income is much greater to the man with an income of £350 than to one with an income of £5,000. The revenue required by a modern Government is too large, however, to be raised merely by taxing the wealthy.

The progressive principle. Under a progressive system the amount of tax to be paid increases more than proportionately with income. Where great inequality of income exists this is generally regarded as being more equitable than the proportional system. Thus, on an income of £500 a year a tax of £50 might be paid (that is, 10%), and on £2,000 a year £300 (15%). The progressive principle would be easiest to carry out under a single tax system—that is, where each person was subject only to one tax based on his income. For reasons to be shown later, this method is impracticable, and in Great Britain revenue is raised partly by taxes on income and partly by taxes on commodities. As a result of taxation of commodities, the burden of taxation is more widely distributed, but some commodity taxes tend to be proportional to income, or sometimes even regressive. For example, a tax on necessary foodstuffs will result in a large family being more heavily taxed than a small one. The British income tax is

[1] By the Poll Taxes of 1378-80 each person was not, however equally taxed. A whole village was assessed at so much per head, but the rich paid more than the poor.

T

now steeply progressive. This is achieved by granting taxpayers certain allowances according to their circumstances, as for example, a personal allowance for a single person, a large one for a married man, allowances for children and dependent relatives, and also an allowance for earned income, as distinct from income from investments. After these allowances have been deducted from a person's income the remainder is subject to tax, the first portion at a low rate, the second at a higher rate and all above that at the full standard rate. On the highest incomes there is an additional levy, known as surtax. The following table shows the percentage of income taken in Great Britain in 1965–66 by income tax and surtax over a range of incomes for a married man with one child under eleven years of age, where the whole income is derived from salary or wages:

TABLE LXVII

A Progressive Income Tax

| Annual income | 1965–66 | | 19– | |
	Income tax and surtax	Tax as percentage of incomes	Income tax and surtax	Tax as percentage of incomes
£	£			
500	None			
600	2	⅓		
800	40	5		
1,000	89	9		
2,500	571	22		
5,000	1,418	28		
10,000	4,111	41		
50,000	39,824	79		
100,000	85,449	85		

Table LXVIII (page 543) shows the progressive character of death duties in this country today.

(4) DIRECT AND INDIRECT TAXATION

Taxes are of two main types—direct and indirect. Some taxes are placed on commodities or services, as for example, purchase taxes on furniture, electrical goods, jewellery, etc; duties on beer and spirits; and motor car road fund licences and driving licences. In all these cases the tax is paid indirectly as part of the payment for a commodity or for a permit to do something, and often the taxpayer does not realise what proportion of his expenditure on these things consists of tax. In the case of these taxes how much a person pays depends on the extent to which he uses the taxed commodities and services. Direct

TABLE LXVIII
A Progressive Scale of Death Duties

Value of Estate	Tax (Per Cent)
Under £5,000	Nil
£6,000	1
£7,000	2
£8,000	3
£10,000	4
£15,000	8
£20,000	12
£30,000	18
£50,000	31
£100,000	45
£500,000	65
Over £1,000,000	80

taxes comprise income tax, surtax, and profits taxes. Direct taxes are often paid directly by the taxpayer to the State, though many people have income tax deducted from their wages or salaries by their employers. Thus indirect taxes are outlay taxes, whereas direct taxes are taxes on income.

Consider now Table LXIX, which shows Government revenue:

TABLE LXIX
Government Ordinary Revenue

Item	1965–66	196– [1]
	£ million	£ million
Inland Revenue:		
Income tax	3,592	
Surtax	200	
Death duties	280	
Stamp duties	75	
Profits taxes	445	
	4,592	
Customs and Excise:		
Alcoholic drink	616	
Tobacco	1,054	
Oil	711	
Purchase tax	647	
Other	180	
	3,373	
Motor vehicle duties	234	
Total from taxes	8,199	
Broadcasting receiving licences	57	
Miscellaneous	269	
Total ordinary revenue	8,525	

[1] For the latest figures.

As with expenditure there are also 'Below-the-line' items of revenue, many of which are capital repayments. In the Financial Statement for 1965–66 the value of these items was not shown separately, the items in Table LXVI being given net.

It will be seen from Table LXIX that in 1965–66 the four principal direct taxes[1]—income tax, surtax, profits tax and death duties—accounted for £4,592 million out of a total revenue of £8,525 million, that is, approximately 55%. A hundred years ago more than two-thirds of the British Government's revenue was derived from indirect taxation. From the point of view of equity, however, direct taxation, because it can be directly related to the ability to pay, is to be preferred to indirect taxation. In consequence, as Government expenditure increased, there was at first a tendency to seek the additional revenue in direct taxes, with the result that by 1913 the yield from both groups of taxes was about the same. In the 1930s about 60% of the State's revenue came from direct taxes, but the peak was not reached until 1945, when over 65% of revenue came from taxes of this kind. Since that date the tendency again has been for the proportion of indirect taxation to increase, as direct taxation appears to have a greater disincentive effect than indirect taxation.

The effect of inflation, however, is to extend income tax to the lower-income groups, unless allowances are increased. The allowance of £340 for a married couple in 1965–66 was worth only half the allowance of £225 of the pre-1939 period, so that in effect income tax in 1966 was payable at a lower level of *real* income in that year than in 1939.

Upon what things should indirect taxes be imposed? Most people would agree that common necessaries of life should be excluded. Luxury goods therefore appear to be the things suitable for taxation, but it is often very difficult to draw a sharp line of demarcation between luxuries and other things, and if luxury goods are rigidly defined the total yield from taxes on them is not likely to be very great. The first principle of indirect taxation is to spread taxation over as wide a range of things as possible, so that people of all tastes are brought within the net. No one tax can then be singled out and criticised alone, but criticism, if any, must be levelled at the system as a whole. The smoker may ask why he has to pay more tax than the non-smoker; the beer-drinker wants to know why he pays more than the teetotaller; the motorist complains of the tax on petrol, different groups of consumers and shopkeepers complain of the various purchase taxes and so on. The wider the range of complaint, the more equitable probably is a system

[1] Since 1962 capital gains also have been taxed.

of indirect taxation! It is sometimes said that indirect taxes, unlike direct, can be avoided by forgoing the consumption of goods that are taxed, but this argument is baseless if the tax net is widely spread. Nevertheless, the taxation of commodities is likely to reduce their consumption. Goods in fairly inelastic demand, therefore, are those most suitable to be taxed (see para. 5).

II. EFFECTS OF TAXATION

(5) THE INCIDENCE OF TAXATION

The incidence of a tax is upon the person who pays it. This is not quite so obvious as it appears at first sight. In the case of income tax the incidence is always on the person receiving the income, for income tax cannot be shifted to someone else, a person's income always being reduced by the exact amount of the tax.

In the case of an indirect tax, however, one cannot be sure in advance whether the incidence of the tax will be on the buyer or on the seller of the commodity, or whether it will be divided between them. Suppose a specific tax of £2 is imposed on an electric radiator costing £6. If the price is immediately raised to £8 the incidence of the tax is clearly on the purchaser; for he has now to pay £2 more than previously for this commodity—that is, the old price plus the full amount of the tax. If the demand for electric radiators is perfectly inelastic the price will remain at £8 and the full incidence of the tax will then be on the purchaser. If, however, the demand for electric radiators is fairly elastic the quantity demanded will fall off as a result of the increase in price. In order to keep up sales, the price may have to be reduced to (say) £7. In such a case, buyer and seller each pay half of the tax, so that the incidence of the tax is partly on the buyer and partly on the seller. If the demand for the commodity is perfectly elastic the incidence of the tax will be entirely on the seller, since at any price above £6 sales will drop to zero (see Figs. 85, 86 and 87).

From this it follows that the commodities most suitable for taxation (from the point of view of maximising revenue) will be those the demand for which is inelastic. Unfortunately, however, many commodities in fairly inelastic demand are common necessaries of life, whereas the demand for some luxury goods is inclined to be more elastic. Semi-luxuries, such as tobacco and alcoholic drink, have to bear an increasing burden of taxation because experience has shown the demand for them to be fairly inelastic.

A similar argument can be applied to the National Insurance contributions of employer and employee. These payments are, in effect, taxes on the employment of labour. A perfectly inelastic demand for labour would result in an increase in wages sufficient to cover fully the cost of the employee's contribution; a perfectly elastic demand for labour would result in a fall in wages exactly equal to the employer's contribution.

(6) SOME ECONOMIC EFFECTS OF TAXATION

(i) *A deterrent to work.* Heavy direct taxation, especially when closely linked to current earnings, can act as a serious check to production by encouraging absenteeism, and making men disinclined to work overtime. The introduction of the system whereby deductions from wages for income tax are based on current earnings, the P.A.Y.E. system, emphasises the link between tax and earnings, and so influences production. The high level of tax, the method of collection and the fact that taxation is progressive and therefore falls most heavily on marginal income makes absenteeism from work appear less costly to a workman when it results in a reduction in his tax deduction as well as in his wages. The effect is to make overtime payments often appear less, instead of greater, than the standard hourly rate, for tax on marginal income is always at the highest rate that particular taxpayer is called upon to pay. For example, Table LXVII above shows that on £800 a year £40 has to be paid in tax, an average over the whole income of 1s. in the pound. On overtime, however, he would probably pay the standard rate (8s. 3d. in 1965–66), the difference in the rate of tax being very great when the overtime earnings raise income to a level where tax is imposed at a higher rate. When, therefore, as part of a disinflationary policy higher taxation has been required, the increase has tended to fall on indirect taxes, since to increase direct taxes might, it was thought, cause a fall in output. Direct taxation may often check the desire to work, but indirect taxation may actually increase the incentive to work, since more money is then required to satisfy some wants, the indirect taxes having made goods dearer than they were before.

(ii) *A deterrent to saving.* Taxation will clearly reduce people's ability to save, since it leaves them with less money at their disposal. Taxation may therefore act as a deterrent to saving. However, this will not always be the case, as it will depend on the purpose for which people are saving. Just as a fall in the rate of interest may make some people strive even harder to save, where they are saving for a particular purpose, so increased taxation may make such people redouble their efforts in order to be able to save as much as before. Much personal saving was formerly for purposes for which provision is now made by social insurance—sickness, old age, etc.—covered by a compulsory deduction from income similar to a tax. More than half of total saving, however, is now provided by institutions—insurance companies, building societies, etc.—and by the undistributed profits of limited companies. Both distributed and undistributed profits are subject to Corporation Tax in Great Britain at the present day. Heavy taxation of profits makes it more difficult for businesses to build up reserves to cover replacement of obsolete or worn-out capital.

(iii) *A deterrent to enterprise.* Those economists who regard profit as a reward earned by the more successful entrepreneurs condemn taxes on profits because they consider such taxes to be checks on enterprise. It is argued that entrepreneurs will embark upon risky undertakings

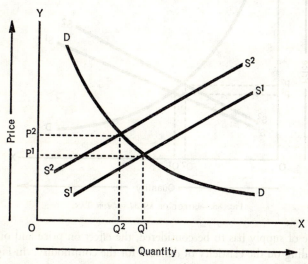

FIG. 85.—EFFECT OF SPECIFIC TAX.

only when there is a possibility of earning large profits if they are successful. Heavy taxation of profits, it is said, robs them of their possible reward without providing any compensation in the case of failure. As a result, production is checked and economic progress hindered. It may be, too, that full employment provides conditions in which many of even the less efficient firms make profits, and so there may be greater justification for taxation of profits in such conditions.

(iv) *Taxation may encourage inflation.* We have already seen that one of the methods used to fight inflation is to budget for a large surplus, the object being to reduce by increased taxation the amount of purchasing power in the hands of consumers. With full employment, however, increased indirect taxation will lead to demands for higher wages, thereby encouraging inflation. A general increase in purchase taxes pushes up the Index of Retail Prices, and so brings in its train demands for wage increases.

(v) *Diversion of economic resources.* Only if there are no hindrances to the free play of economic forces will resources be distributed among occupations in such a way as to yield that assortment of goods and services desired by consumers. Taxation of commodities is similar in effect to an increase in their cost of production. Thus, the influence of a

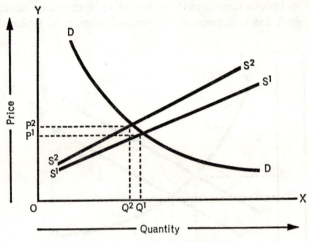

FIG. 86.—EFFECT OF AN *ad valorem* TAX.

change of supply has to be considered, the effect on price and output depending on the elasticity of demand for the commodity. In Fig. 85 the effect of a specific tax is shown. * IN PROPORTION TO VALUE.

Fig. 86 shows the effect of an *ad valorem* tax. In both cases the effect is to reduce output and raise price. How much price rises will depend on the elasticity of demand for the commodity. Only if demand is perfectly elastic will there be no increase in price (Fig. 87). Only if supply is perfectly inelastic will there be no reduction in output.

Differences in taxation may cause resources to move from the heavily taxed to more lightly taxed forms of production. This result may, of course, be desired on non-economic grounds. Where local rates are high, the establishment of new industry is discouraged, and new firms will seek sites where rates are lower. In the international sphere taxes on imports will divert production from "low-cost" to "high-cost" areas, with the result that the total world output of goods will be less than it might have been.

(7) TAXABLE CAPACITY

Over the past hundred years the level of taxation has increased enormously in all countries, and time and time again there have been protests that the limit of taxable capacity has been reached. It is extremely difficult, however, to determine what is the taxable capacity of a people, but this is not unconnected with the purposes to which the proceeds of taxation are put. The limit must be the point beyond which the additional taxation would produce economically harmful results that outweigh the gain to the community from the use of the money raised by taxation.

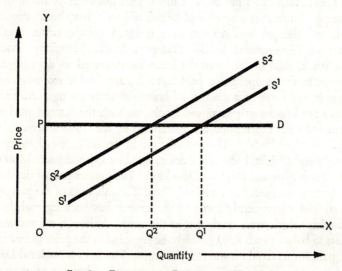

FIG. 87.—ELASTICITY OF DEMAND AND TAXATION.

It has been suggested on a number of occasions that in Great Britain the limit of taxable capacity had been reached. Everything, however, depends on what the State does with the revenue it raises. At the present day a great deal of it is returned to the people in the form of social services. The more the State does for its people, the greater the amount of taxation they are able to bear. Nevertheless, it must not be forgotten that taxation can be a deterrent both to work and to saving.

The extent of the increase in taxation in Great Britain can be seen from the fact that in 1913 taxation was equal to 10 per cent. of the national income; a quarter of a century later it reached 20 per cent.; and by 1965 it had risen to over 25 per cent. Taxation in the United States is equal to 22 per cent., and in Sweden to 19 per cent. of the national income.

III. THE NATIONAL DEBT

(8) PUBLIC DEBTS

Public debts are of two main types, depending on the purpose for which the money was borrowed:

(i) *Reproductive debt.* When a loan has been obtained to enable the State or Local Authority to purchase a real asset, the debt is said to be "reproductive." In Great Britain many Local Authorities formerly owned gas, electricity and tramway undertakings, the money for their acquisition or construction being borrowed. Most borrowing by Local Authorities has been of this type, most recently mainly for housing. Since 1945 a number of British industries have been nationalised, and the previous owners have received compensation in the form of Government Stock—Transport Stock, Electricity Stock, Gas Stock, etc. In this way the State has increased its debt by the amount of the compensation paid, but it has acquired in exchange real assets in the form of a number of industrial undertakings. All these stocks are known as guaranteed stocks, as both the interest paid on them and their redemption are guaranteed by the Government.

(ii) *Deadweight debt.* The second type of public debt is known as "deadweight" debt, because it is not covered by any real asset. Most of the British National Debt is of this kind. The greater part of the debt has been accumulated in financing Great Britain's wars of the past 250 years, and consequently most of the money has been expended on materials which were dissipated at the time. Although no real asset exists to balance such debt, it might be regarded as the price the nation has paid for its freedom and independence. The British National Debt had its origin in 1694 in William III's necessity to borrow in order to prosecute war against France. Each succeeding war in which Great Britain has been engaged has seen a large increase in the debt while, in the interval between wars, it has been only slightly reduced, although, in the half-century preceding the outbreak of war in South Africa in 1899 it had been reduced by one-quarter. During the First World War the debt increased by eleven times, to £7,800 million; at the end of the Second World War it had reached the colossal sum of £25,000 million. In Victorian days there were reasonable hopes that the debt would be completely paid off in the near future, but two costly world wars have put an end to such plans. Indeed, the debt has considerably increased—by nearly £5,000 million—since the last war. In addition there is the external debt, mostly owing to the United States (under the Washington Loan Agreement of 1945) and to Canada. Repayment of this external debt in annual instalments began in 1952 and will continue to the year 2001. A further £900 million was borrowed in 1965 from foreign central banks, repayable by 1970, to cover a large deficit in the balance of payments.

Floating and Funded Debt. Most of the National Debt is funded, that is, it exists in the form of long-term Government Stocks, such as Consols, War Loans, Saving Bonds, etc., which are dealt in on the Stock Exchange. The Floating Debt is short-term borrowing. It originated in the need of the Government to incur expenditure in anticipation of revenue, most of which comes in during the last quarter of the financial year. This floating debt now consists of Treasury bills, and Ways and Means Advances. In 1910 Treasury bills amounted to only £36 million, but in 1965 totalled over £5,500 million. Before 1914 the Floating Debt comprised only a small fraction of the total National Debt; in 1965 $12\frac{1}{2}\%$. The orthodox financiers of the pre-1914 period would have severely condemned such an expansion of the floating debt, which they considered should be kept to a minimum, since they thought that all long-term borrowing should be funded. The chief objection to this method of borrowing is that it makes borrowing too easy.

(9) THE BURDEN OF THE NATIONAL DEBT

The extent of the burden on a nation of a public debt depends in the first place on whether it is an external or an internal debt. If one country obtains a loan from another it means that it can import from abroad goods and services to the value of the loan without at the time having to export anything in exchange. When interest on the loan has to be paid and the principal repaid these payments can be made only by exporting goods and services, without receiving any imports in exchange—"unrequited" exports as they are sometimes called. Thus the burden of the debt is thrown on to the balance of payments, which in consequence becomes more difficult to balance. If, however, the foreign loan is used for the economic development of the country, as were the nineteenth-century loans to the United States and present-day loans to the developing nations, the ultimate effect may be to increase productive capacity to such an extent that the loan can be quite easily repaid. Similarly, the Washington loan of 1945 enabled Great Britain to make a more rapid recovery from the effects of the war.

In the case of internal debts, the debt is owed by the State chiefly to its own citizens, or to institutions such as banks and insurance companies or even to Government departments. Interest payments are raised from the taxation of the community, but are paid back to members of the same community. Such payments are said to be merely *transfer payments*, for the total wealth of the community as a whole is not affected, however great the total debt may be, except for the cost of its management. People as a whole pay taxes to the State to enable the State to pay them interest, but the two groups—taxpayers and interest receivers—are not exactly the same, although those who pay most in taxes are likely to include those who receive most in interest. The size of the debt, however, will have an important effect on the amount of taxation to be levied. Whereas, in 1939 interest on the British National Debt required taxation of about £234 million per year, in 1965–66 it required taxation amounting to about £1175 million, without in either case making any repayment of debt. The main drawback of heavy taxation is that it may hinder production. An increase in the value of money following a deflationary policy will increase the burden of the National Debt, just as inflation will decrease it.

In comparing the burden of the National Debt at two different periods a comparison of the amounts paid in interest does not form a very reliable guide owing to changes in the value of money. Account must be taken of other factors. The interest payable on the debt can be calculated per head of the population or as a percentage of either the national income or total Government revenue. In 1938 interest on the debt required 22% of Government revenue, but in 1965 less than 12%, but this exaggerates the fall in the burden of the debt, for the range of the Government's expenditure widened enormously during the intervening years. If the interest on the debt is calculated in proportion to the population we find that in 1815 it came to an average of £4, in 1914 to only 9s., in 1938 to £5 and in 1965 to £12 per head. If, however, we allow for the fall in the value of money due to inflation we see that the burden of the debt in 1914 was less than a tenth of what it had been in 1815, and in spite of two world wars less of a burden today than it was in 1815. Probably the best method, however, is to relate the burden of the debt to the national income. In 1938 the interest on the British National Debt was equal to 5% of the national income, but by 1965 it had fallen to a little over 4%. Comparison on this basis with earlier years, however, is not possible, because national income statistics are not available for years before 1941.

(10) THE NATIONAL DEBT AND MONETARY POLICY

The huge increase in the floating debt and the fact that the National Debt now shows a tendency to expand even in time of peace has made the management of the debt an important factor in monetary policy. Indeed, according to the Radcliffe Report (1959), the National Debt "has come to be an integral part, even an indispensable part" of the

British financial system, since the management of the debt provides the monetary authorities with an opportunity of influencing the economic system. Management of the National Debt covers (i) the issue of new stocks and redemption of old stocks; (ii) operations in the markets for "gild-edged" securities by the Government broker; and (iii) the provision of capital when required for nationalised industries and local authorities.

Excluding bank-notes, the total debt of the public sector in 1965 was as follows:

TABLE LXX

The Debt of the Public Sector

				£ million
Foreign debt .	.	.	.	2,900
Funded debt .	.	.	.	18,000
Savings Certificates, etc. .	.	.	.	3,000
Floating debt.	.	.	.	6,100
The National Debt.	.	.	.	30,000
Debt of Local Authorities	.	.	.	8,100
Debt of Public Corporations .	.	.	.	7,000
Total .	.	.	.	45,100

Holders of the debt are Government departments, including the Issue Department of the Bank of England, insurance companies, pension funds, commercial banks, trustee savings banks, merchant bankers, discount houses, building societies, overseas and foreign banks.

The intervention of the Government broker in the securities market has resulted in the prices of Government stocks being largely determined by the Government itself. The aim is to influence the prevailing rate of interest in order to restrict the demand for real resources of both the public and private sectors of the economy to the available supply of these resources. Only a small part of new issues of Government stock is taken up by investors, the remainder being held back and gradually released to the market through the Government broker, who also buys up a little at a time those stocks that are nearing their date of redemption.

IV. LOCAL TAXATION

(11) LOCAL RATES

The Central Government levies taxes; the Local Authorities levy rates. Since 1925 there has been a single rating authority in each area, but previous to that date different Local Authorities, often with overlapping boundaries, levied rates for different purposes.

Nowadays only 25% of the revenue from rates is used entirely for local purposes, the remainder being employed on the administration of many services on behalf of the Central Government, which supplements the local rates by a grant from the national exchequer. Some of the cost of the health service, police, education and the maintenance of roads are provided for in this way. Some services are of a more definitely local kind, such as the provision of public parks, libraries and museums.

Rates are assessed on property, each house, shop, workshop, factory, etc., being given a rateable value, assessed according to its size, situation, etc. The owner or occupier of the property pays rates in proportion to its rateable value. For example, if a local authority imposes a rate of 21s. in the pound the rates to be paid for a house of rateable value of £30 would be 30 × 21s.—*i.e.* £31 10s.

Serious objections have been raised to the basing of the assessment of rates on property. In the first place, a rate of (say) 15s. in the pound will not produce the same sum in every local authority's area. Where most of the property consists of industrial premises and small dwelling-houses, as in some manufacturing towns, the yield per head will be much smaller than in an area where there is a high proportion of good residential property, as at many seaside and inland resorts. Differences in the burden of rates between one area and another were one of the causes influencing the location of industry between the two wars.

The calculation of rateable values is now undertaken by the Inland Revenue authorities, and so assessments have been standardised throughout the country. Government grants, too, have been modified in favour of the poorer authorities. In spite of these reforms, however, the main objection still remains: ownership or occupation of property does not form a good basis for taxation, for it does not closely relate the amount to be paid to ability to pay. Under the present rating system an old couple living on retirement pensions may pay the same amount in rates as their next-door neighbours with perhaps four or five times their income. As a result, local taxation often tends to be regressive. The Allen Report (1965) found that rates were in fact a regressive form of taxation. In 1966 it was proposed to reduce the rates of people with low incomes or large families, the cost to be borne mainly by the Exchequer.

The increasing cost of Government services that have to be provided locally has drawn attention to the increasingly heavy burden of local rates. Reform of the method of assessment to bring it more into line with ability to pay—the basis of income tax—has so far found little favour. It has been suggested, however, that one way to alleviate the burden would be to transfer some local expenditure from Local Authorities to the Central Government. For example, to relieve Local Authorities of the cost of teachers' salaries would take from them their heaviest item of expenditure, which at present absorbs more than one-third of their total revenue. It seems likely that more expenditure will be transferred from Local Authorities to the Exchequer in the future.

RECOMMENDATIONS FOR FURTHER READING

H. Dalton: *Public Finance.*
U. K. Hicks: *Public Finance.*
A. R. Prest: *Public Finance.*

QUESTIONS

1. Consider the effects of different forms of taxation on the incentives to work and to save. (R.S.A. Adv.)

2. Why should a good system of taxation include a variety of taxes? (A.I.A.)

3. What is meant by the incidence of a tax? Trace the incidence of an indirect tax, like the tobacco tax. (B.S. Inter.)

4. "The old theory of taxation has been killed by the double need to maintain incentive in the industrial system and to control private spending." Discuss this statement. (I.B.)

5. What are the characteristics of a good tax system? Explain what is meant by the incidence of taxation. (C.C.S. Inter.)

6. Discuss the merits and demerits of indirect taxation. (Exp.)

7. What is meant by progressive taxation? On what grounds can it be justified? (C.C.S. Final.)

8. It has often been claimed that indirect taxation is inequitable and that to the maximum possible extent taxation should be direct. Do you agree with this view? Illustrate your answer by reference to any current developments with which you are familiar. (C.I.S. Final.)

9. In what circumstances might the instrument of taxation be used other than for raising revenue? (I.H.A.)

10. Explain how it is possible for the reduction of a duty on a particular commodity to lead to an increase in the total revenue yielded by the duty. Give examples. (B.S. Final.)

11. (a) Name Adam Smith's Canons of Taxation.

(b) Indicate, if you can, what modifications they require to adapt them to modern conditions. (A.C.C.A. Final.)

12. Distinguish between direct and indirect taxation. What determines the relative amounts raised by each method? (C.C.S. Final.)

13. Explain the statement: "Budgetary policy cannot now exist independently of monetary policy but must be integrated with it." (I.M.T.A.)

14. What are the characteristics of a good system of taxation? Explain what is meant by (*a*) progressive taxation, (*b*) the incidence of taxation. (C.C.S. Final.)

15. Discuss the advantages and disadvantages of high graduated death duties as a means of increasing revenue. (D.P.A.)

16. Distinguish between direct and indirect taxation and discuss the relative merits of each type. (G.C.E. Adv.)

17. Describe the main categories of government expenditure in the United Kingdom. What forces have determined the size of each category? (G.C.E. Adv.)

18. Discuss the arguments that have been put forward in support of the view that the size of the public debt is unimportant. (Final Degree.)

19. "Since all taxation results in a transfer of income to the State, it matters little whether the transfer is effected directly by a tax on incomes, or indirectly by taxes on particular goods and services." Discuss. (Final Degree.)

20. Since a government can borrow only what people have saved why is a budget deficit financed by public borrowing inflationary? (Final Degree.)

ADDITIONAL EXAMINATION QUESTIONS

1. Examine the advantages and disadvantages of the institution of private property. (R.S.A. Adv.)

2. There has been much talk about incentives to increase production. Which incentives would you place first, and why? (I.T.)

3. "We never find monopoly undiluted by competition and very rarely find competition undiluted by monopoly." Explain and illustrate this statement. (L.C. Com. Econ.)

4. Outline a policy which could be expected to raise the standard of living of an under-developed country. Illustrate your answer by reference to a particular country. (I.B.)

5. What considerations influence a young person in his choice of occupation? (C.C.S. Final.)

6. Write brief notes on three of the following:
   (1) Malthus;
   (2) indirect taxation;
   (3) The World Bank;
   (4) fixed costs and variable costs. (I.B.)

7. "Great Britain can only support her present population if at least half the people live in great cities." (Hicks.) Discuss this statement in its bearing upon the problem of agricultural development in Great Britain. (I.B.)

8. "Capital goods are unquestionably productive—and nobody likes to part with his money. These two facts are sufficient to explain, and justify, the payment of interest on capital." Do you agree? Explain the point at issue. (L.G.B.)

9. Compare the advantages and disadvantages which consumers may derive from production by a monopolist. How far would your arguments be modified if the monopolist were a public board? (I.M.T.A.)

10. Write a short essay on what you think should be the aims of economic policy. (I.B.)

11. What is meant by economic growth? How can it be fostered in Britain? (I.B.)

12. Explain the difficulties to be overcome in making an estimate of whether, over a period, the real income of a community has risen or fallen. (C.I.S. Final.)

13. Write notes on two of the following:
   (a) Price discrimination;
   (b) Backward sloping demand curves;
   (c) The acceleration principle;
   (d) Complementary goods. (C.I.S. Final.)

14. Should workers' contributions to social insurance be regarded as a tax, or as the purchase of insurance? (C.I.S. Final.)

15. It has been said that the difference between the clearing banks and the

merchant banks is that the former live on their deposits and the latter on their wits. Comment on this statement. (I.B.)

16. "In spite of the fundamental resemblance between international trade and domestic trade, there are also points of difference." Explain this statement. (C.C.S. Final.)

17. Explain the terms: (a) quasi-rent; (b) consumer's surplus; (c) invisible exports; (d) devaluation. (C.C.S. Final.)

18. Should manufacturers be allowed to fix the retail prices of their products? (C.C.S. Final.)

19. Explain the difference between a worsening of the terms of trade, and an adverse movement in the balance of payments of a country. Which, in your opinion, is likely to be economically more disadvantageous for Great Britain? (C.I.S. Final.)

20. Is resale price maintenance less of an evil than simple monopoly? (C.I.S. Final.)

21. Consider the case for and against increasing diversification of a firm's products. (C.C.S. Final.)

22. What sort of legislation, if any, is economically desirable to influence the price of land? (C.C.S. Final.)

23. What is the International Monetary Fund? Describe carefully how it is able to extend short-term credits for member nations. (G.C.E. Adv.)

24. Describe what you consider to be the chief objectives of government policy affecting the economy as a whole. To what extent do these conflict with one another? (G.C.E. Adv.)

25. What would be the effects on the demand for motor cars (both new and old) and the extent of their use of:

    (a) a decrease in national income;

    (b) an increase in the annual vehicle licence fee;

    (c) an increase in the tax on petrol? (G.C.E. Adv.)

26. Compare income distribution before tax in the United Kingdom in 1938 and the present day. What have been the principal causes of the change between the two periods? (G.C.E. Adv.)

27. "Nationalisation of industries is unimportant; the real issues concern public control rather than public ownership." Discuss. (G.C.E. Adv.)

28. What have been the causes of the rapid increase in the British output of agricultural products during the last twenty years? (G.C.E. Adv.)

29. How can the Government influence the distribution of income? Refer in your answer to the actual conditions in the United Kingdom. (G.C.E. Adv.)

30. Why do primary product prices tend to fluctuate between wider limits than the prices of industrial products? (G.C.E. Adv.)

31. Discuss the arguments for and against the levying of local rates upon industrial premises. (Final Degree.)

32. Examine the case for and against short-time working as a means of dealing with redundant employees. (Final Degree.)

33. What are the main problems that would arise in the United Kingdom if the pace of automation were rapidly increased? (Final Degree.)

34. What would be the effect on the price of advertising space in newspapers of:

    (a) an increase in the demand for newspapers;

    (b) the introduction of a new B.B.C. television channel;

    (c) the introduction of a new commercial television channel?

35. How can the theory of consumer behaviour help in appraising the relative merits of distributing goods by rationing as against distributing by the price system?

36. Distinguish between the economic consequences of (a) an exceptionally cold winter following upon an exceptionally mild winter, and (b) a long-run decline in average winter temperatures.

INDEX